Anke Niederau

The Big Book of Nail Diseases

Cause • Podiatry diagnosis • Therapy • Prophylaxis

Verlag Neuer Merkur GmbH

Deutsche Bibliothek Cataloguing in Publication Data
A catalogue record for this book is available from the Deutsche Bibliothek's website: http://dnb.ddb.de.

P.O. box 1253, 82141 Planegg
Germany

Anke Niederau
The Big Book of Nail Diseases
ISBN 978-3-95409-049-5
Based on the third revised and extended German edition 2016

Translated from German by Martina Tollgreve, Montreal/Canada
Layout/Design: Martina Stolzmann
Cover photo: © Fotolia/Amboss
Print: Neografia, a. s., Martin-Priekopa, Slowakei

This book is a reference guide for all colleagues already working in practice and for those who routinely deal with podiatry issues. I hope to deliver a better understanding of existing nail diseases and, at the same time, to illustrate therapeutic treatment options for use by podiatrists and pedicurists. Please note that not all nail diseases and their therapeutic treatments are mentioned. I, therefore, invite you to contact me to discuss or exchange different therapeutic treatment options, experiences and recommendations.

Interdisciplinary teamwork with other medical practitioners, such as physicians, homeopaths, orthopedic shoe specialists, physiotherapists and caregivers, provides development potential and creates career opportunities.

We, therefore, play an indispensable role in the interdisciplinary treatment network where the goal is to develop shorter treatment periods and achieve faster therapy success.

I would like to mention that I could not have written this book alone. My special thanks go to Karl Ziebolz who was an inspiration during my educational training to become a medical podiatrist. I would also like to thank my husband Bruno and my children who greatly contributed to the success of this book with their feedback and constructive criticism.

Valuable advice and recommendations from colleagues were very much appreciated during the writing of this reference book. My special thanks go to Elke Pätzold, Brigitte Rathenow, Heidi Gerstner, Jeanette Ziebertz-Kracke, Beate Teubner, Liesel Sayferth, Peter Kovar, Wolfgang Knörzer, Ira Bruchardt and Thomas Seibt.

I am also grateful to Dr. Albert Strasser of Vienna (Austria), surgeon and specialist for wound healing (www.wundmed.com) for extensive information and images on "diabetic-neuropathic onychopathy (dno)".

Ocean Pharma, Bernd Stolz, Remmele's Propolis, Hellmut Ruck, Eduard Gerlach, 3TO, Greppmayr, VHO, Erkodent, Brigitte Rathenow and Süda kindly provided images and texts published in this book. Thank you to Regine Richard and Susanne Bender for assisting me with the drawings.

Anke Niederau

1 Introduction

Why is a basic knowledge of causes, diagnosis and treatment options of nail diseases so important?

For every podiatrist, pedicurist and any healthcare practitioner, it is crucial to identify nail abnormalities and nail growth disorders and, after a thorough anamnesis and diagnosis, to develop and execute an adequate treatment plan, working together with a physician or homeopathic practitioner.

For a proper diagnosis, the following issues must be taken into account:

Anamnesis
- age
- previous illnesses (e.g.: circulatory disorder, diabetes mellitus)
- dietary habits
- congenital or acquired foot and toe deformities
- growth rate
- mechanical stress on the nail
- socks and shoes (fit accuracy is important since otherwise first deformities can develop)

Diagnosis
- static of the foot
- careful inspection of the nails (ensuring good lighting conditions is important)
- infections on one or multiple nails
- asymmetrical infection (local)
- symmetrical infection (might be an indication for general disorder)
- examination of nails should be performed with a magnifier
- examining nails under an examination light helps detect subungual clavus or small nail tips in the sulcus
- microscopic examination by a physician
- nail mycosis (bacteria) requires a bacterial culture

The following aspects are also important for the proper examination of nail mycosis:
- When and where did it start?
- What are the symptoms?
- Comparing the infected nail to a healthy nail. What are the differences?

Causes for nail abnormalities and nail growth disorders:
- hereditary cause (congenital foot and toe deformities)
- trauma or disease-related causes (circulatory disorder)
- harmful substances (chemicals, medication, toxins)
- infection of the nail (onychomycosis)

Additional causes for nail abnormalities and their descriptions are mentioned in chapter 9 and 10.

Special attention must be paid to the characteristic shine of a healthy nail, the shape, colour and thickness of the eponychium and the nail wall, where an excavator (double instrument or another blunt probe) is the most suitable instrument for a thorough examination. It enables the detection of clavus or ingrown nails. More often, this examination reveals multiple nail abnormalities which must be documented with a photograph or a drawing. The PodoCam camera (former Becker company now Anton Gerl, Cologne) enables an accurate evaluation of abnormalities on nails and skin. It is a valuable tool that ensures high-quality care for the patient.

The PodoCam is a user-friendly camera for all clinics with an EDP-system. It has an intuitively designed interface and delivers high-resolution images. The camera automatically assigns the images to each patient and facilitates the transfer of multimedia images.

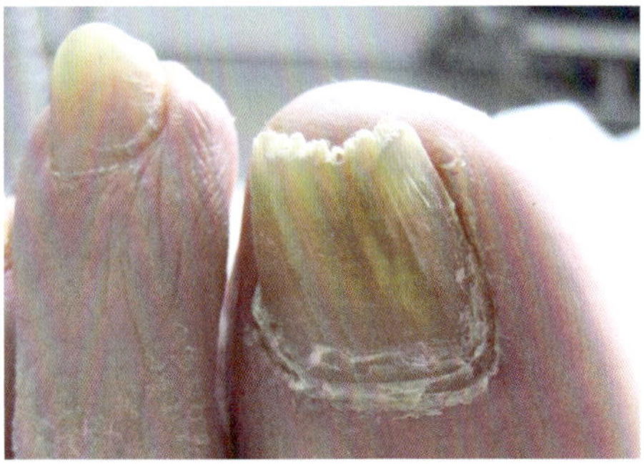

Image 1.1 A nail with multiple disorders: possible onychomycosis, onychauxis, onychorrhexis, onset of pterygium

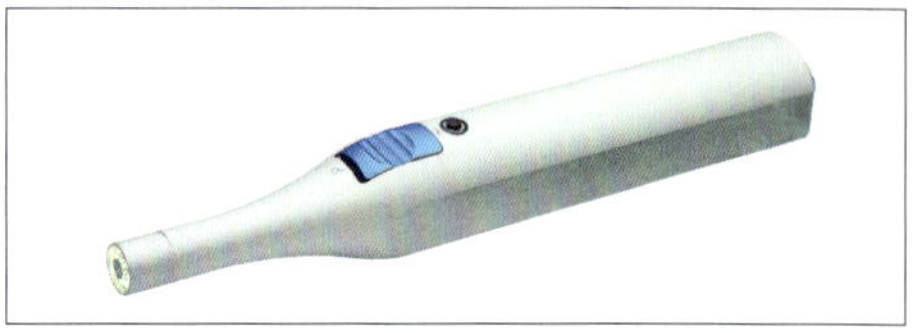

Image 1.2 PodoCam

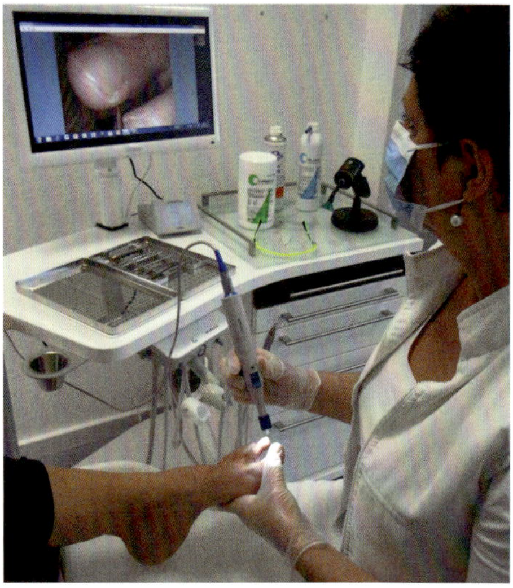

Image 1.3 The PodoCam in the clinic (images 1.2 and 1.3 curtesy of the former Becker company)

Image documentation and interdisciplinary communication are easily retrieved by the podiatrist at any time. The slim design and integrated LED light source allow the examination of hard-to-reach places. The camera reveals even the smallest details and delivers crisp clear images. For wound treatment, it is positioned at a distance of 1 centimeter from the wound margin or nail wall. The camera can be cleaned easily and sterilized between patients. The simple USB plug-and-play installation works on any computer or laptop and the image enlargement feature (up to 200 X) works on any iPad, monitor or smartphone. Virtual image transfer is an excellent communication tool that allows improved communication and understanding, especially for patients with neuropathic disorders. Thanks to this combination of visualisation and understanding, treatments, such as brace therapy, are easily presented to the patient and discussed. For interdisciplinary referrals, images can be sent along with a short text ensuring legitimate traceability and verification.

For any busy podiatrist, the PodoCam is a revolutionary multifunctional instrument used to obtain accurate diagnoses and precise documentation. It is also an excellent communication tool that no professional should be without.

Proper documentation ensures optimal interdisciplinary treatment consultation options between physicians, podiatrists and other professionals.

This book is intended to offer diagnosis and treatment assistance for nail abnormalities and disorders in practice, as well as in the field of prophylaxis, since many nail abnormalities could be prevented with proper, patient-oriented preventive treatments.

2

The structure of nails

The **nail (Lat.: unguis, Greek: onyx)** is a skin appendage that consists of 100 to 150 horn cell layers which can be between 0.05 millimeters (nail of an infant) and 0.75 millimetres thick.

Nail formation (onychisation) is a cornification process that starts behind the nail fold. The horn cells consist of hard keratin with a high percentage of sulphur double-bond compound and a homogeneous arrangement of keratin filaments (essential component of keratin). Horn substance is primarily composed of chains of protein molecules, the polypeptide chains. The nail grows continuously: fingernails approximately 1 millimetre per week and toenails approximately 1 millimetre per month (see chart 2.1).

Nail formation (onychisation)

Nail formation is a cornification process that foregoes the forming of keratohyalin. Keratohyalin is a protein structure found in granules in the stratum granulosum. These small dense granules are collected in the cells. During further cornification, keratohyalin is first transformed to eleidin (a fat- and protein-rich acidophilic substance) and then keratin. The keratin is transported into the stratum lucidum. This layer has the appearance of a thin line preventing dehydration.

Nail plate (corpus unguis)

The nail plate is formed in the germinal matrix (nail matrix). One third of the horn substance is created by the stratum granulosum (granular layer) of the nail bed and the remaining part of the nail plate is formed by the lunula. The nail is composed of three layers: the dorsal layer (dorsal nail), consisting of hard keratin; the intermediate layer (intermediate nail) made up of keratin with cell structures and cell nucleus residues; and the palmar layer (ventral nail), a soft keratin layer that is connected to the nail bed with longitudinal strings. The nail plate pushes from the germinal matrix on the nail bed towards distal direction. The nail bed exhibits groove-like structures connecting the nail plate to the nail bed.

The nail plate curves in two directions (longitudinal and transverse direction) increasing the nail's stability.

Various factors determine the colour of a nail:

- the capillaries of the nail bed (surface with tiny blood vessels underneath the nail)
- keratin (horn substance) which exhibits a yellowish to greyish colour
- pigment-forming cells (melanocytes) found in matrix and the nail bed area

The thickness of the nail plate increases towards the distal end and is thinner in the germinal matrix area.

Nail matrix (radix unguis)

The matrix (germinal matrix) produces cells that become the nail plate. The lunula (lat.: small moon) is the visible part of the matrix, the whitish crescent-shaped base of the visible nail.

Nail bed (hyponychium, solum unguis)

The nail bed exhibits tiny longitudinal grooves, similar to a corrugated sheet, connecting the nail bed to the nail plate.

Nail wall (perionychium)

The nail wall is the cutaneous fold overlapping the sides and proximal end of the nail.

The crescent-shaped proximal part of the nail with the underlying matrix is covered by the perionychium and the epithelial cuticula (cuticle).

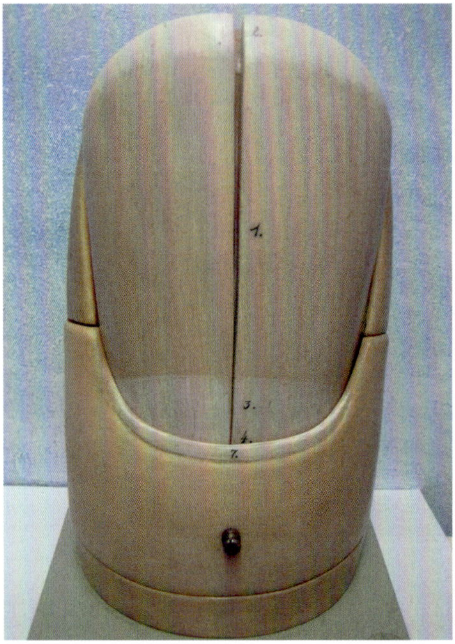

Image 2.1

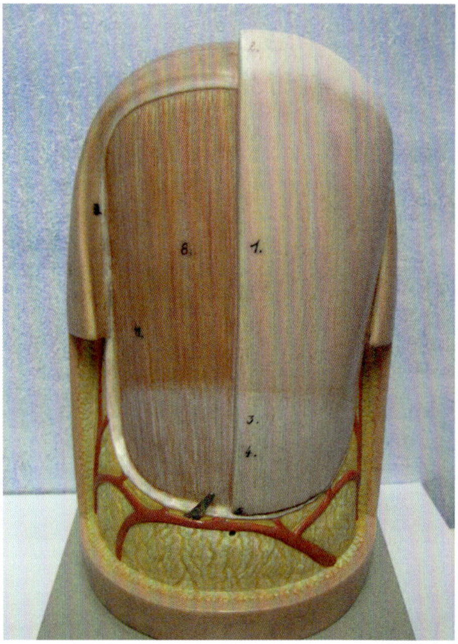

Image 2.2

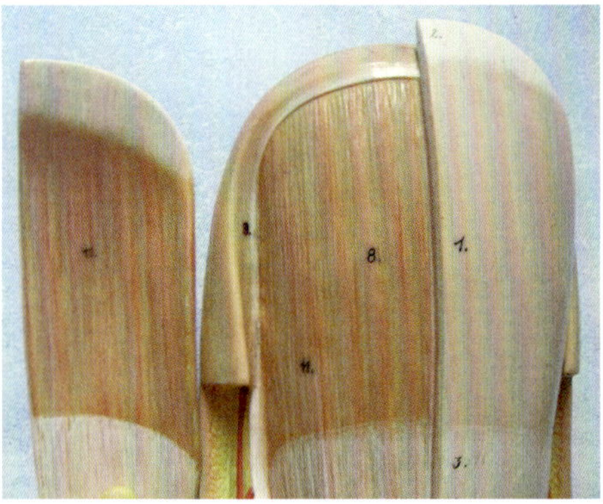

Image 2.3

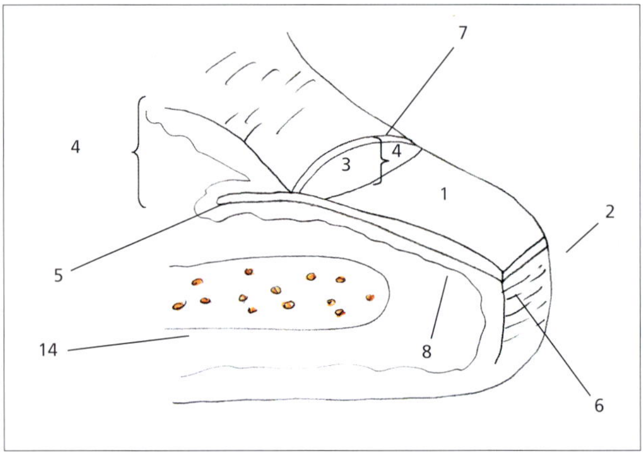

Image 2.4

Images 2.1 to 2.4 inscription

1 Nail plate (corpus unguis)
2 Margo liber, free margin
3 Lunula, whitish crescent-shaped-base
4 Radix unguis, nail root
5 Matrix, germinal matrix
6 Lateral Margo liber, lateral free margin
7 Cuticula, cuticle
8 Hyponychium – solum unguis, nail bed
9 Sulcus unguis, nail fold
10 Intermediate nail with papilla grooves
11 Hyponychium – solum unguis, nail bed with papilla grooves
12 Perionychium – Vallum unguis, nail wall
13 Sole horn
14 Bone, phalanx

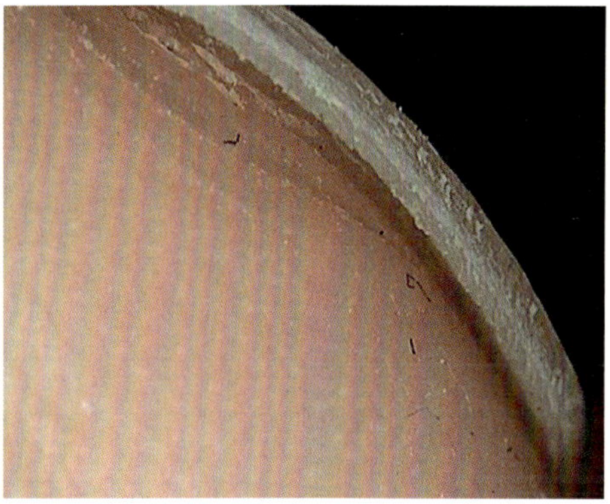

Image 2.5 The three horn layers of a nail

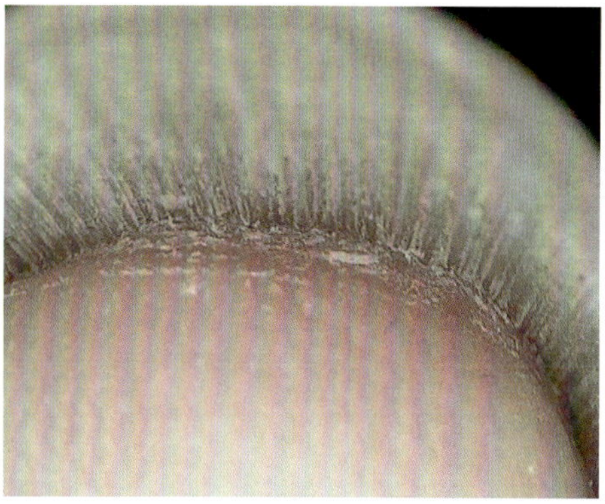

Image 2.6 Distal view of the ventral nail at the transition to the sole horn (PodoCam).

Nail fold (sulcus unguis)

The sulcus unguis is the transition between the nail plate and the nail wall.

Cuticle (cuticula)

The cuticle is located on the proximal perionychium (nail wall). It is located on the back of the nail like a dense, thin fold and acts as a protective seal for the nail sinus. Damaging the cuticle can cause severe nail growth disorders due to bacterial or fungal infections.

Sole horn

The sole horn is located under the distal free margin. It is a horny structure that prevents the detachment of the nail from the nail bed and forms a protective barrier for the nail plate against germs and foreign particles.

Function

The nail has mainly a protective function. It protects the distal phalanx, the fingertip and the surrounding soft tissues from injuries. It also serves to enhance precise delicate movements and functions as a tool, enabling, for instance, a so-called "extended precision grip (e.g. pulling out a splinter) and certain cutting or scraping actions.

Nails grow continuously. Fingernails grow approximately 1 millimetre per week and require, on average, six months to regrow completely. Toenails are thicker and grow at a slower rate. They require about twelve months to regrow completely.

Development of the nail matrix begins towards the end of the third embryonic week when a slightly curved primary nail area forms exhibiting an arc-shaped margin. Granular cells slowly form the nail which grows from distal to proximal direction. At the end of the fifth month, the eponychium and the hyponychium form the matrix. After the sixth month, the nail grows from proximal to distal direction.

Nail growth disorders

Various external and internal factors affect nail development and can cause delayed growth. Some of the causes for nail growth disorders are listed below:

Accelerated growth	Delayed growth
Summer	Winter
Daytime	Nighttime
Pregnancy	
Minor injuries	
Nail biting	
Nail cutting	
Nails on the right hand	Nails on the left hand
Adolescence	Old age
Men	Women
Finger	Toes
Middle finger	Thumb and small finger
Ring finger	
Index finger	

Chart 2.1 Nail growth

Nail growth disorders caused by:

- Exogenous (external) factors (image 2.7)
  Exogenous nail growth disorders are physical traumas caused by injuries, chemical toxins, medication and foot and toe deformities.
- Endogenous factors (image 2.8)
  Endogenous factors generally affect not only the growth of one nail, but of all nails. Skin diseases and various underlying diseases are the cause. Mineral and vitamin deficiencies are also to blame.
- Genetic factors
  Mediana canaliformis nail dystrophy is a nail disorder characterised by a paramedian canal or split in the nail plate of one or more nails. Sandpaper nails are also caused by genetic factors.

Podiatrists and foot care professionals should be able to recognize the causes and appearance of nail diseases to initiate proper treatment.

Properly fitting shoes and socks also play an important role in the prevention of nail deformities. I advise my patients to consider not only the length of a shoe, but also the width plus the flexibility and height of the outer material.

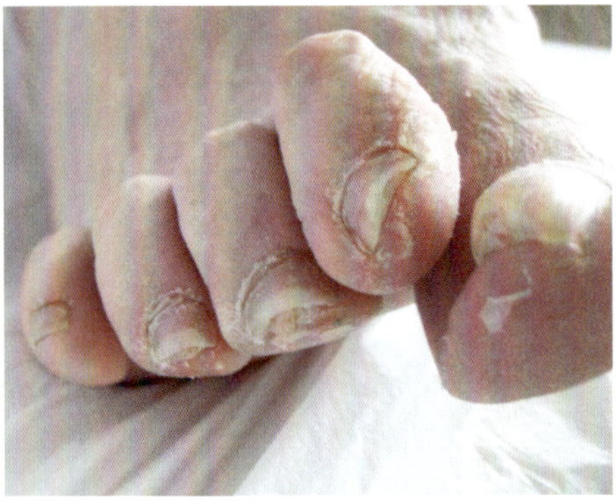

Image 2.7 Toe deformities (hallux rigidus, claw toe D2 to D4, digitus superductus D2)

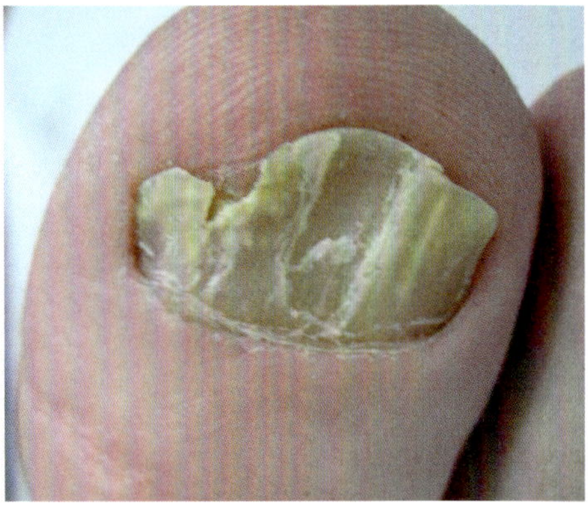

Image 2.8 Psoriatic nail

I demonstrate the importance of buying the correct shoe and sock size with the help of a caliper (images 2.9 to 2.14). Shoes that are too tight on top often lead to an uncomfortable, incorrectly fitting shoe. Purchasing properly fitting socks is equally important. I place the sock, without pulling on it, on the inner side of the foot and explain to the patient what must be considered when purchasing socks.

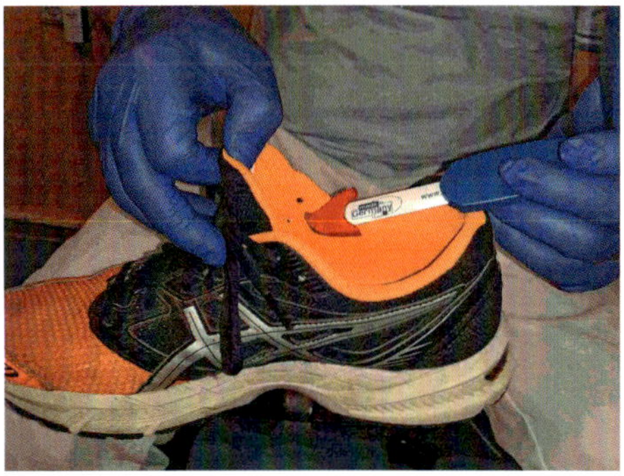

Image 2.9 Inside measurement

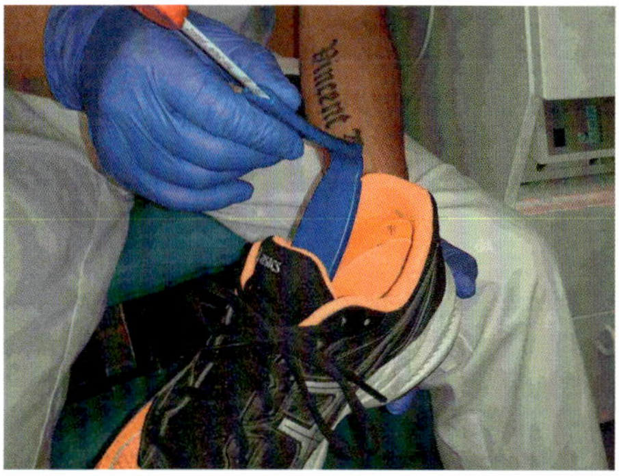

Image 2.10 Inside measurement

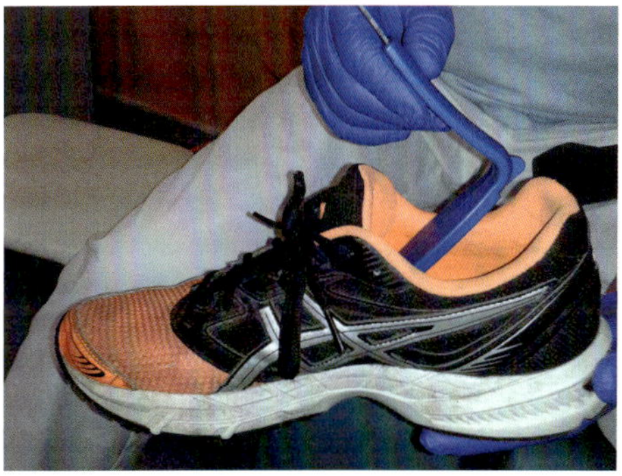

Image 2.11 Carefully remove the measuring device without changing the measuring scale

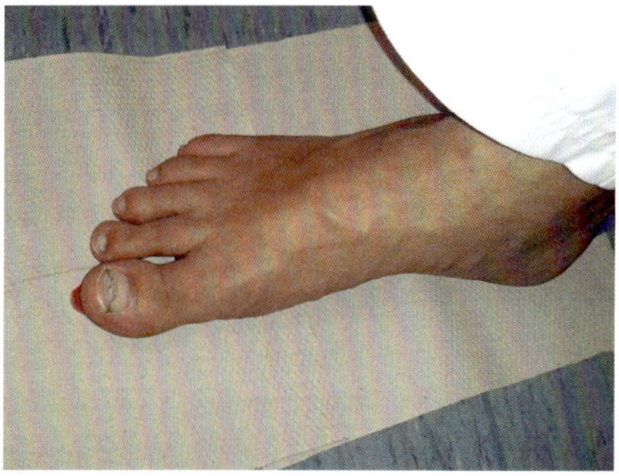

Image 2.12 The patient places one foot on the index. Conclusion: The shoe is too short.

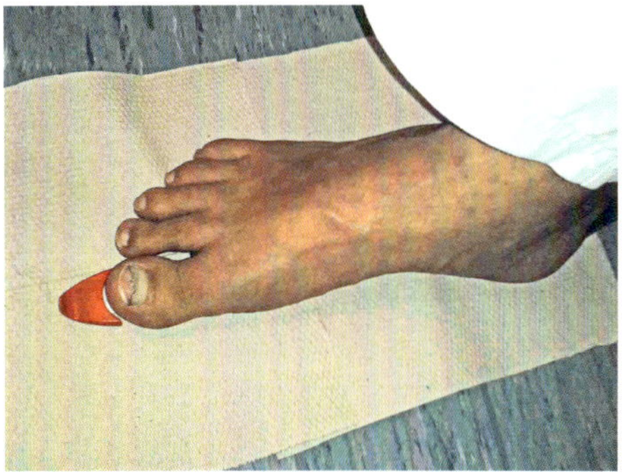

Image 2.13 Correctly fitting shoe

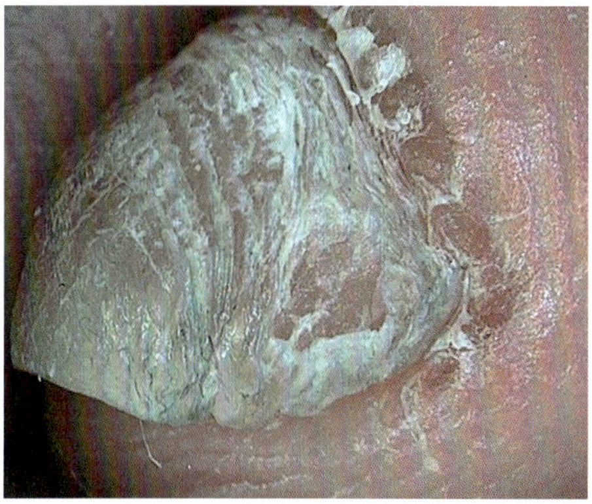

Image 2.14 Compressed nail caused by shoes that are too small

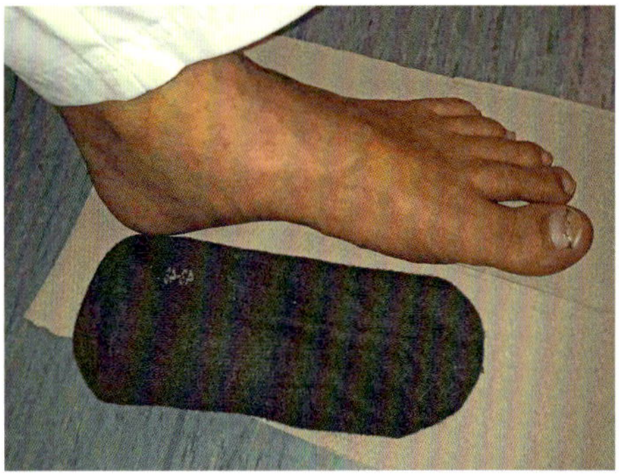

Image 2.15 Place the sock next to the foot

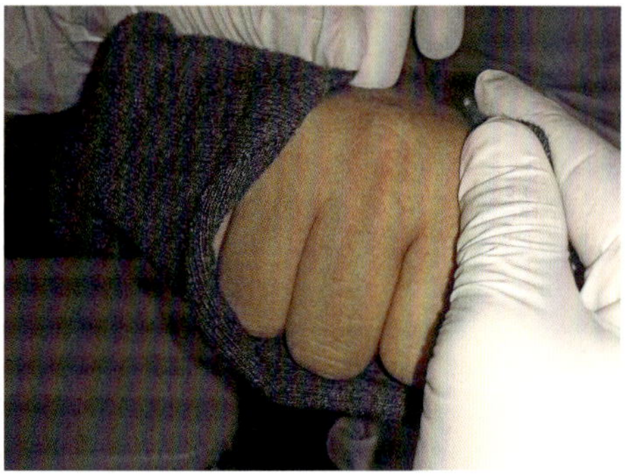

Image 2.16 Sock measurement on the hand with a relaxed fist

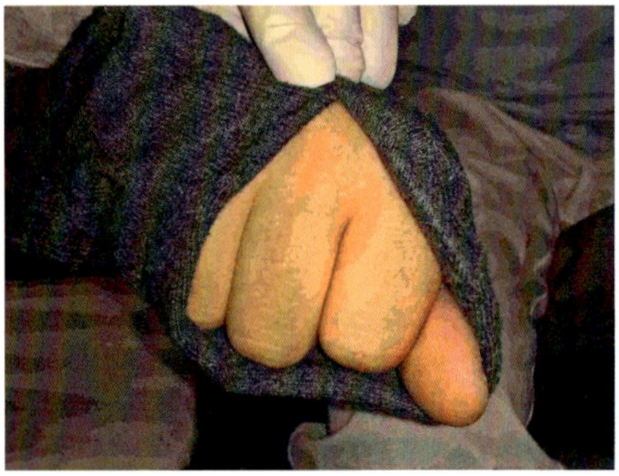

Image 2.17 Sock measurement: one finger's width above the knuckles of the metacarpus

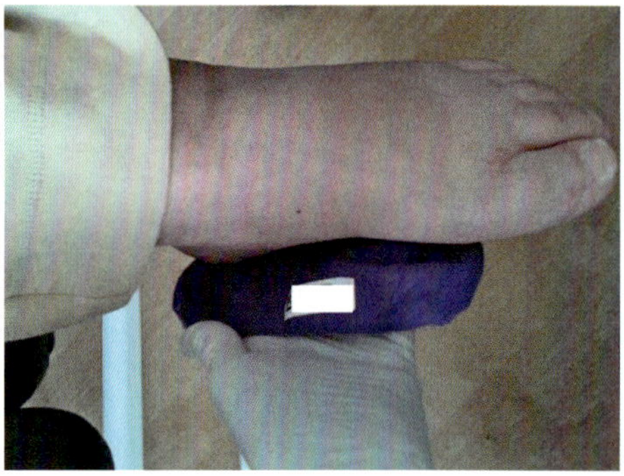

Image 2.18 These socks are too small

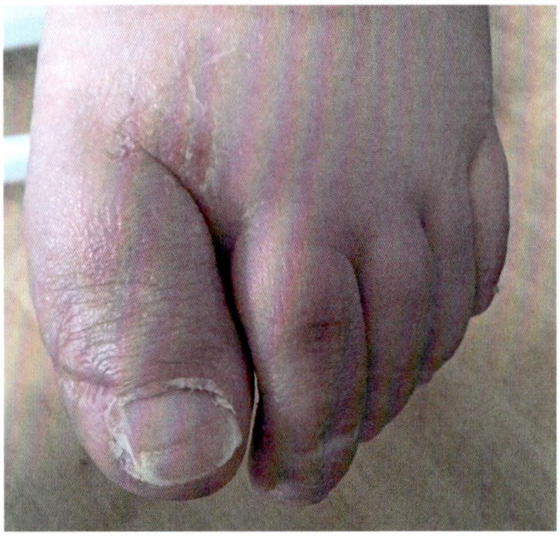

Image 2.19 Toe and nail deformities caused by incorrectly fitting socks

To determine the proper fit of a sock, you place the length of the sock around the patient's relaxed fist without pulling on it. If it overlaps by one finger's width, then the sock fits properly (images 2.15 to 2.19).

The same technique can be used for compression socks (images 2.20 to 2.22).

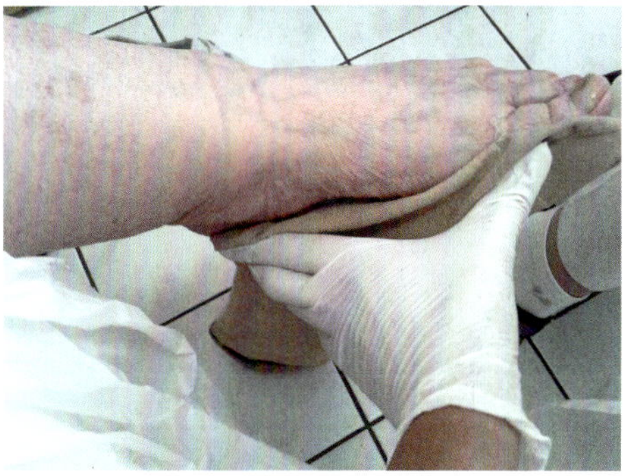

Image 2.20 Fitting of a compression sock

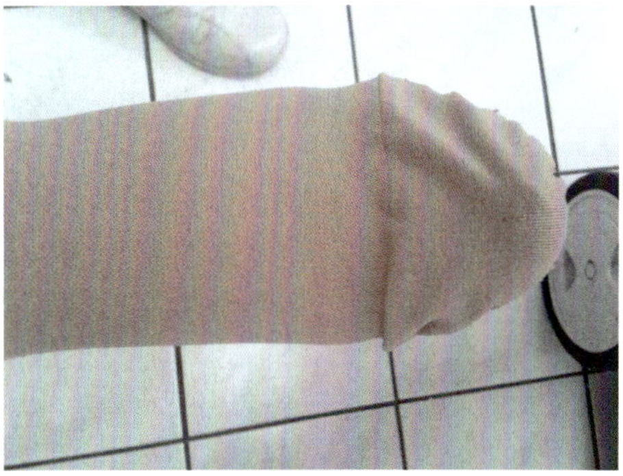

Image 2.21 Compression sock with soft tip

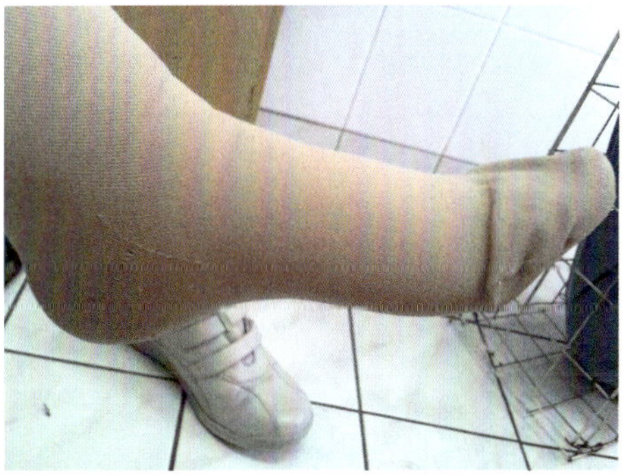

Image 2.22 Properly fitting compression sock

3

Nail diseases

3.1 Diabetic Neuropathic Onychopathy (DNO)

(As per Dr. Adalbert Strasser, Specialist Surgeon, WundMED, Vienna, Austria)

Definition
Pathological change of the toenails due to diabetic foot syndrome with peripheral polyneuropathy.

Causes
In diabetic foot syndrome, the neuropathic component pathogenetically damages the nerves of the nail matrix causing nail growth dysfunction.

Appearance
The result is uncontrolled growth of the nail whereby the nail plate becomes unusually thick. Horizontal and longitudinal grooves develop on the nail and necrotic tissue deposits form between the underside of the nail and the cuticle.

This disorder is often diagnosed as onychomycosis and, if treated incorrectly, it can have a devastating impact for the patient since, in the worst case, amputation of the end phalanges is the only option.

Patients not only dislike the appearance of their nails, but also experience pain. Often convoluted nail growth is accompanied by pressure pain, cuticle irritation, and inflammation-triggering osseous tissue irritation of the end phalanges. In addition, the thickened nail plate can cause severe pain and foot static dysfunction, thereby changing the patient's movement pattern.

The unphysiological movement pattern caused by the neuropathic foot combined with toe deformity creates atypical pressure points, thereby overstressing the foot and increasing uncontrolled nail growth. Socks that are too small or improper footwear promote the pathological gait pattern. The metatarsal advancement in diabetic foot syndrome also contributes to neuropathic onychopathy.

Complications
Wound healing complications deriving from DNO pose a high risk for diabetics, especially injuries in the nail area.

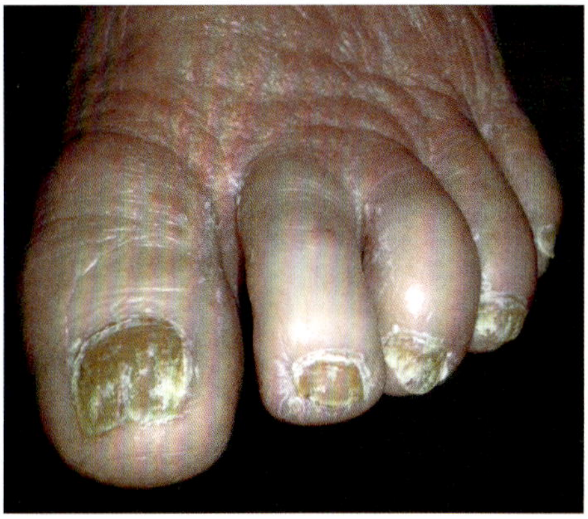

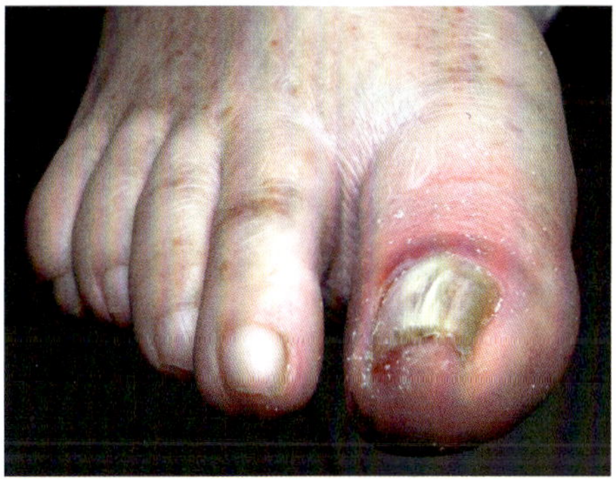

Images 3.1 and 3.2
Diabetic neuropathic onychopathy

Incorrectly performed foot care damages the sensitive cuticle and can lead to the development of whitlow, non-healing ulcerations, subungual abscesses, fistula formation and osteomyelitis of the end phalanges.

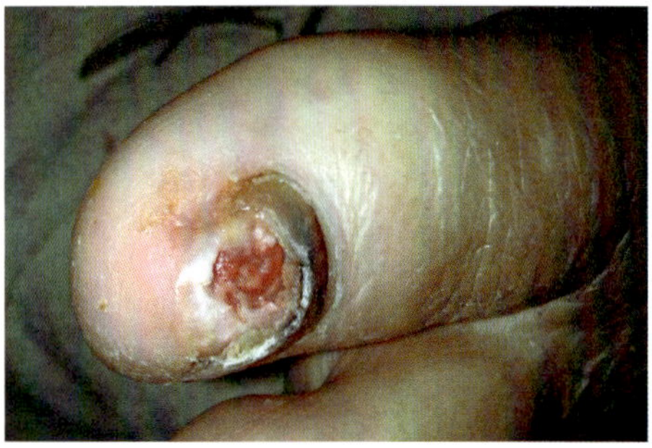

Image 3.3 DNO with subungual ulcer

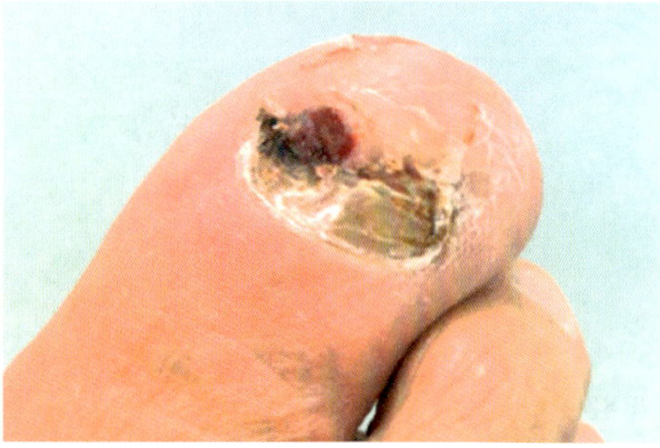

Image 3.4 DNO with subungual abscess

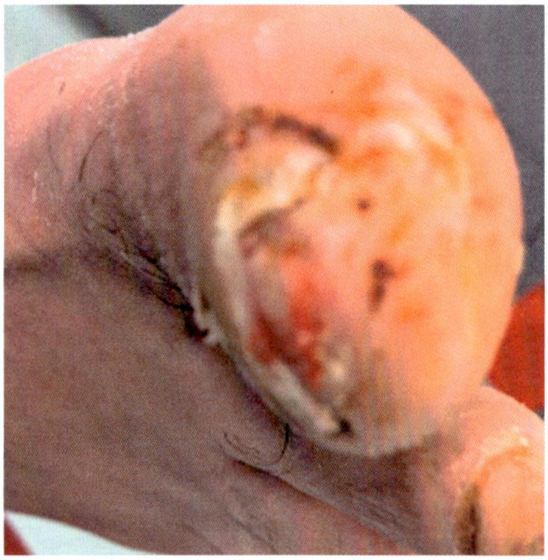

Image 3.5 DNO with subungual abscess-forming ulcer

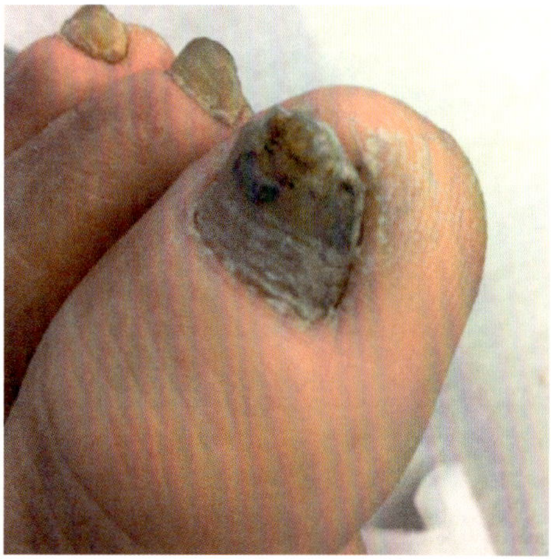

Image 3.6 DNO with subungual pressure hematoma

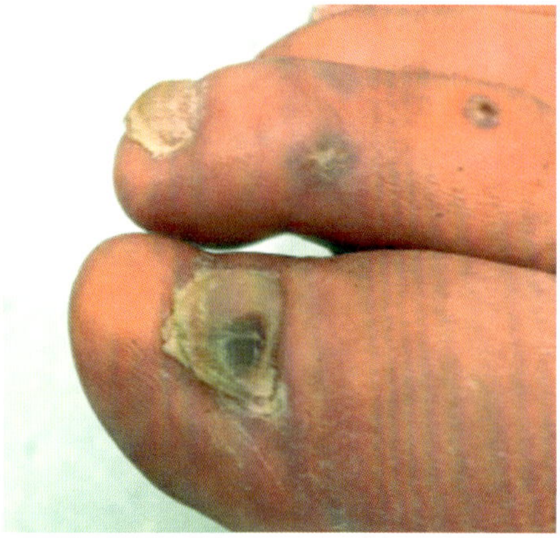

Image 3.7 DNO with subungual pressure hematoma

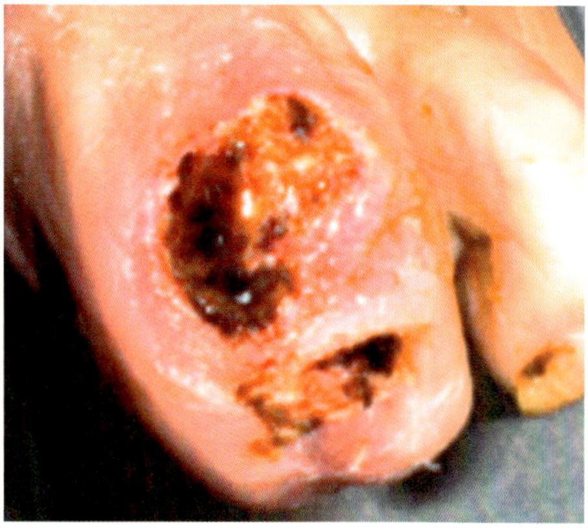

Image 3.8 DNO with fistula-forming osteomyelitis preceded by a pressure ulcer

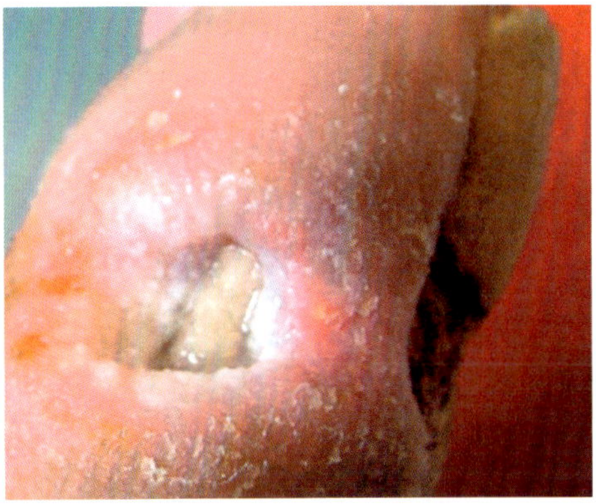

Image 3.9 DNO with osteomyelitis and abscess- and fistula-forming ulcer

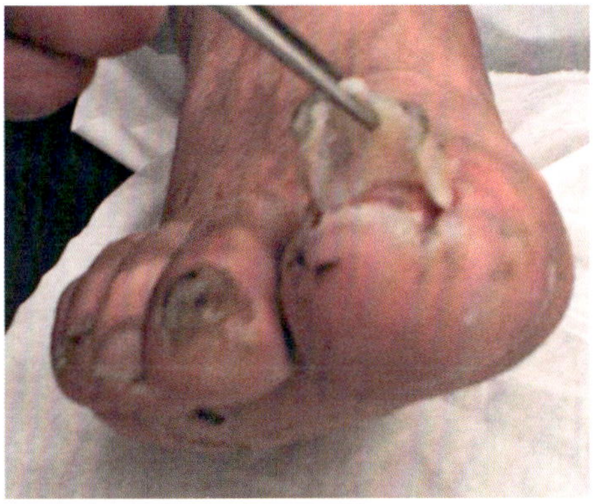

Image 3.10 DNO with detached nail plate

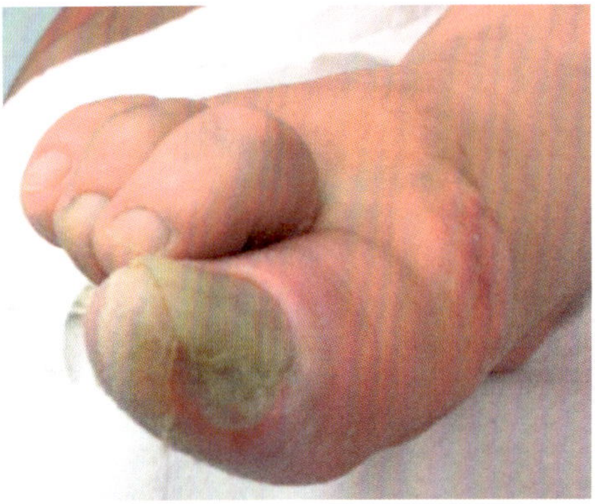

Image 3.11 DNO with abscess-forming and beginning fistula-forming paronychia

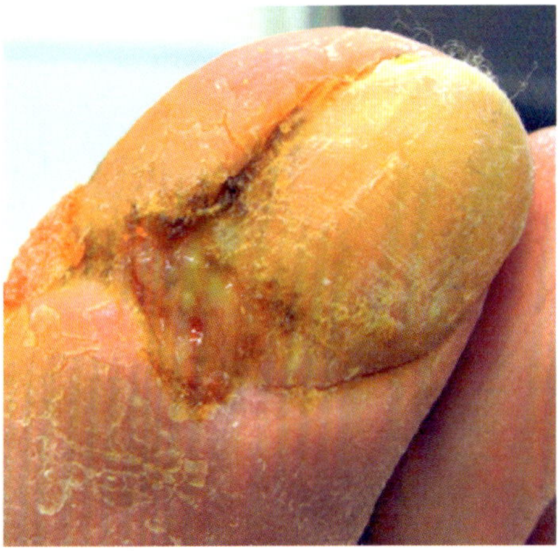

Image 3.12 DNO with abscess- and fistula-forming paronychia

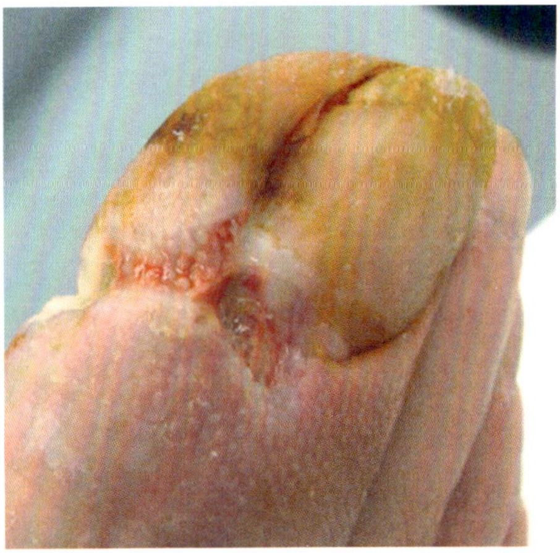

Image 3.13 DNO with abscess- and fistula-forming ulcer

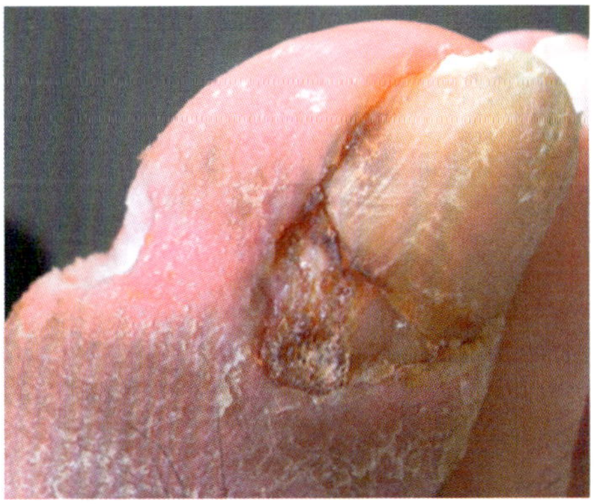

Image 3.14 DNO with osteomyelitis of the left big toe's end phalanx showing an abscess- and fistula-forming ulcer

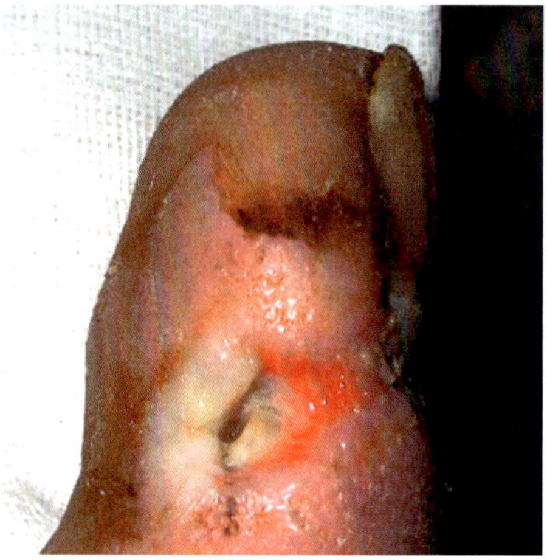

Image 3.15 Paronychia with abscess- and fistula-forming ulcer with osteomyelitis

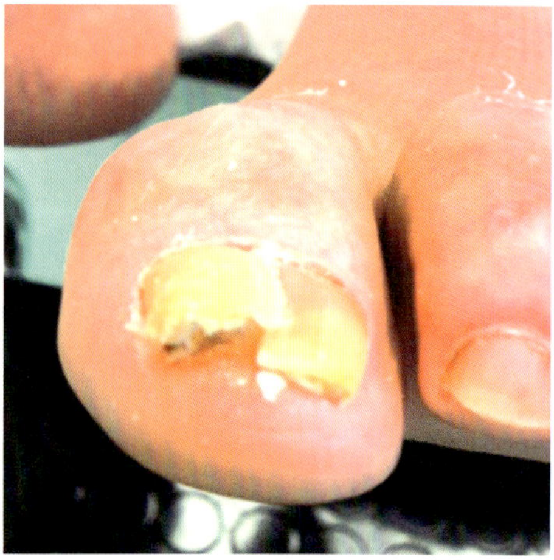

Image 3.16 DNO with split nail plate

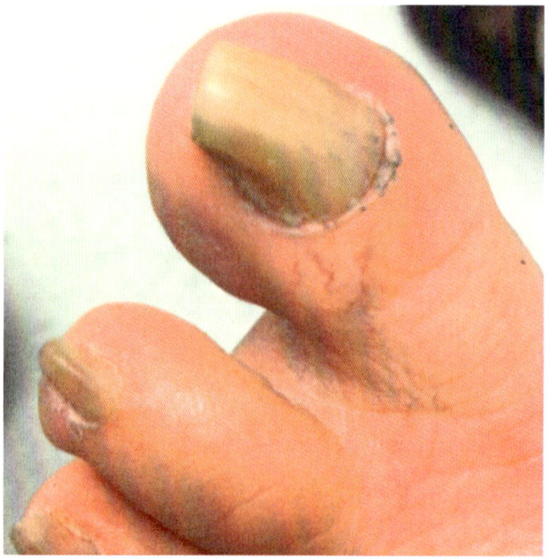

Image 3.17 Unguis convolutus

Treatment

To decrease pressure and pain, the thickness of the nail must be gradually reduced over a period of several months. The painful convoluted nails can be corrected with an adhesive non-wire brace using minimal activation force to avoid sulcus irritation. Applying tamponades aggravates the situation and can lead to the loss of the end phalanx. To rule out mycoses infestation, the affected nails should undergo a DNA analysis. If onychomycosis is present, treatment with Spirularin® is recommended. The active ingredient derives from the spirulina algae which fight bacteria, viruses and fungi. It is a gentle, natural and harmless substance yet very effective, which is proven by the results of many studies and practical experiences worldwide.

The above-mentioned treatment approach has helped me to improve the appearance of nails and to eliminate pain and discomfort for the patient.

The big toe is especially susceptible to pain and inflammation since it must absorb most of the pressure during movement. Close cooperation between diabetologist, orthopedic shoe maker and podiatrist is of the utmost importance.

In the acute phase a forefoot-relief shoe provides comfort for the patient but subsequently, wearing fitting orthopedic shoes is advisable since an arterial microcirculatory disorder aggravates the entire pathology.

Improper treatment can lead to limb loss.

If subungual abscesses with osteomyelitis of the nail plate are present, it is advisable to perform a sequestrectomy.

In addition to following sterile guidelines, frequent examinations, rinsing and strain relief are crucial.

The use of tamponades is discouraged since they host proteus and pseudomona organisms, according to Dr. Strasser's analysis of antibiograms. In case tamponade insertion is indispensable, it should never stay inserted longer than 24 hours and only sterile Ligasano® white tamponade should be applied.

Summary by Dr. Strasser
Due to the serious complications that are involved with nail disorders, diabetic neuropathic onychopathy is associated with diabetic foot syndrome. If fungi infestation is detected, it can be attributed to DNO syndrome.

DNO onychauxis with onychomycosis
With a beginning hallux rigidus and hammer toes, the nail thickness must be gently reduced over a longer period. An antimycotic treatment with spirulina algae extract and toe tape (if the toes are still flexible enough) provides relief.

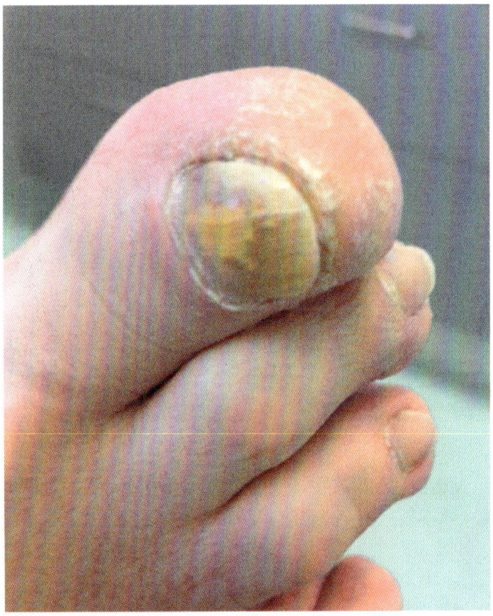

Image 3.18 Close-up of DNO

3.2 Unguis incarnatus (Greek: onychocryptosis)

The Latin name unguis incarnatus is more frequently used for an ingrown toenail (images 3.20 to 3.26).

Definition

Deeply embedded in the nail bed (image 3.21) with inward curved lateral nail edges (image 3.23) that are covered by the lateral nail wall. The front corners of the nail plate start to grow into the nail wall tissue (image 3.22) causing severe pain and inflammation if left untreated (image 3.23).

Causes

- excessive cutting of the nail corners
- pronounced transverse curvature of the nail plate caused by various factors
- changes of the nail plate's thickness and texture
- a reaction to a long-term inflammation in the nail fold, such as paronychia (tissue folds surrounding the nail), whereby the serous fluid dissolves part of the nail substance generating an uneven, partly jagged nail edge; this uneven edge prevents proper healing
- malpositioning of the foot or the toes, such as with hallux valgus, increase the damage
- wearing improper footwear
- diabetes mellitus, hormonal changes such as puberty or menopause, genetically determined sensitive skin

Various stages

- **Inflamed non-purulent:** Pressure applied by the deep lateral nail margin in the nail fold triggers inflammation displaying the classic signs, such as inflammatory reddening, swelling, pain, overheating and functional impairment in the nail fold and nail wall area.

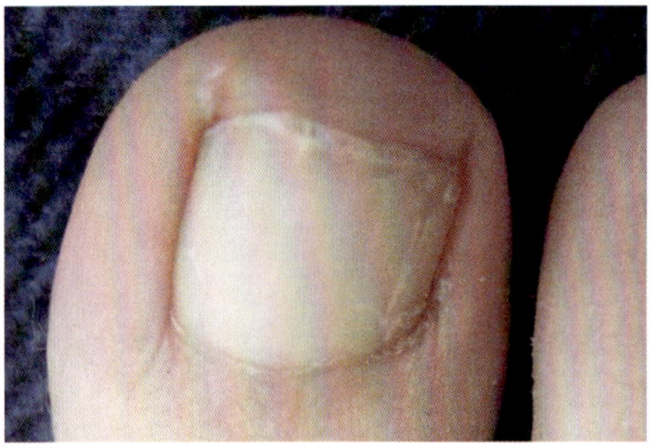

Image 3.20 Unguis incarnatus with slightly lateral pressure pain

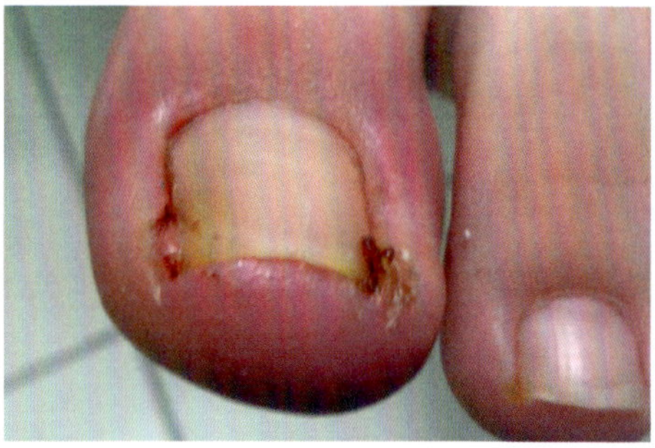

Image 3.22 Unguis incarnatus with painful inflammation

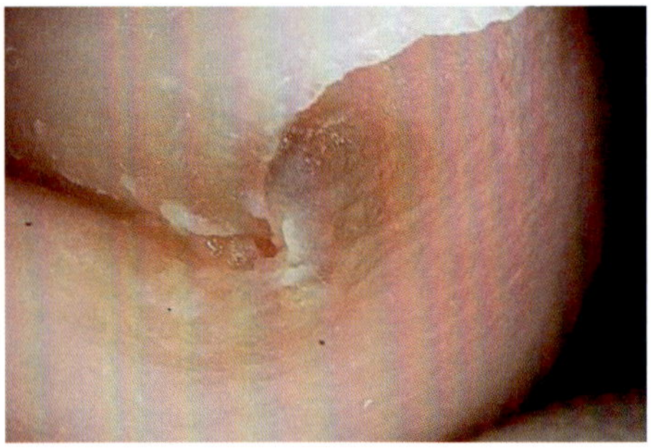

Image 3.21 Unguis incarnatus with slightly lateral and medial pressure pain

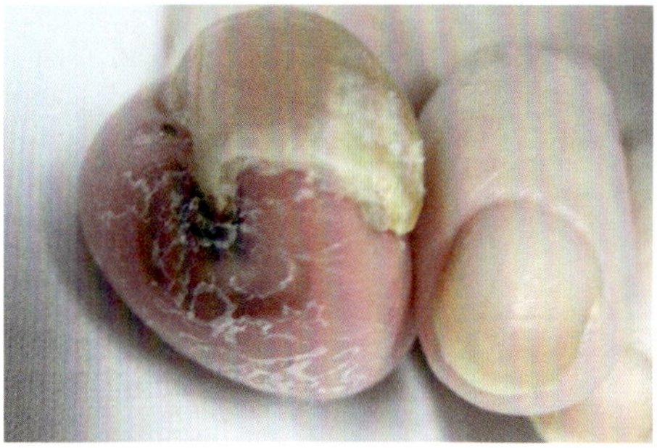

Image 3.23 Unguis incarnatus with granulation tissue and suppuration

- **Inflamed purulent:** The progressing inflammation promotes bacteria invasion through the widened nail fold causing acute paronychia (suppuration in the nail fold and under the nail plate). The purulent secretion often drains spontaneously or through applied pressure from the nail fold. The podiatrist can perform the initial treatment but must refer the patient to a physician for further treatment.

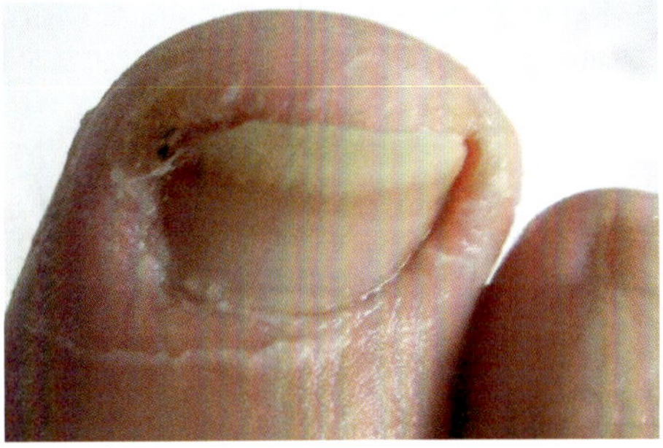

Image 3.24 Unguis incarnatus with slight lateral and medial pressure pain and minor inflammatory reaction

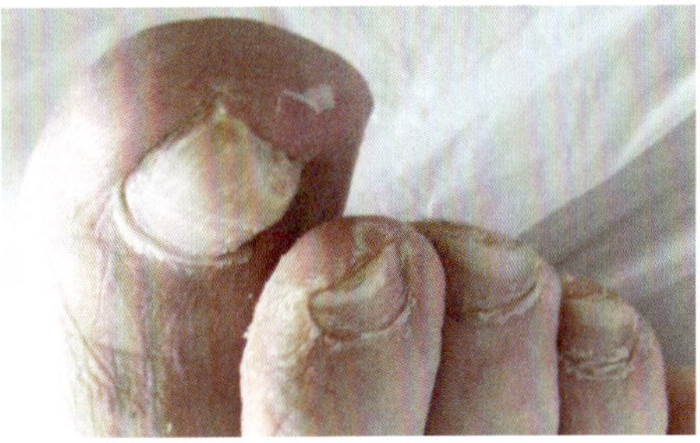

Image 3.25 Unguis incarnatus with slight lateral and medial pressure pain

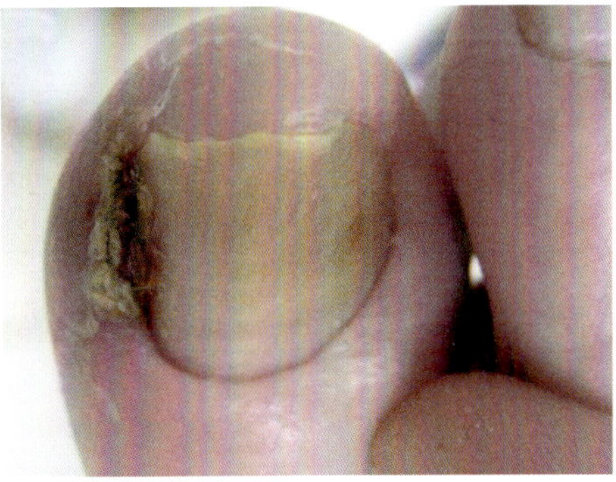

Image 3.26 Unguis incarnatus with granulation tissue and medial suppuration

- **Inflamed purulent with granulation tissue:** In the progressed stage of the unguis incarnatus, granulation tissue develops. During the chronic inflammatory process, granulation tissue with its own blood circulation forms, so-called proud flesh. This granulation tissue has the tendency to grow exuberantly over the nail plate. Here too the podiatrist only performs the initial treatment and refers to the patient to a physician for further treatment.

Complications

Lymphatic vessel inflammation (lymphangitis often incorrectly identified as sepsis) can lead to necrosis of the toe if the inflammation is left untreated. The irritation of a sharp nail corner increases cell division and aggressive granulation tissue develops. For patients who suffer from diabetes mellitus or circulatory disorders, prolonged paronychia can lead to toe amputation.

Wound documentation

Every wound care treatment must be documented (image 3.27 see following page) in writing, a photo can be added to complete proper documentation (images 3.28 to 3.30).

Treatment

- Working with sterile instruments is of utmost importance.

> Cooperation with a physician is crucial.

- After thorough disinfection (e.g., with octenisept or Prontoman), check the nail margin for irregularities, hyperkeratosis and clavi with a probe, a double-end instrument or a blunt nail knife.
- Smooth out minor irregularities with a nail splitter, gauge, corner file or diamond-fissure grinding instrument.
- Cut the skin-penetrating nail tip in a V-shape and remove with a corner nipper, gouge, nail splitter or diamond-fissure grinding instrument making sure

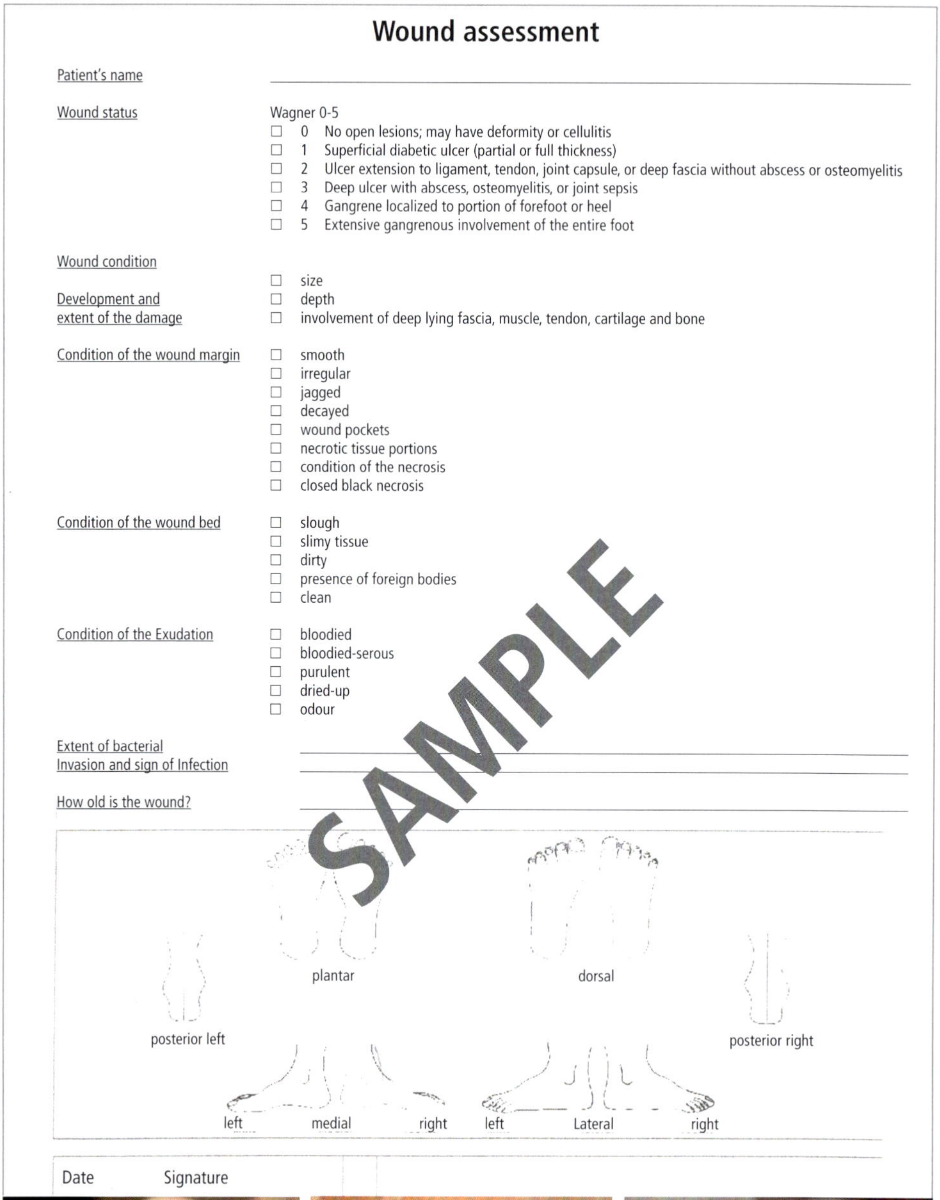

Wound assessment

Patient's name ______________________________

Wound status

Wagner 0-5

- ☐ 0 No open lesions; may have deformity or cellulitis
- ☐ 1 Superficial diabetic ulcer (partial or full thickness)
- ☐ 2 Ulcer extension to ligament, tendon, joint capsule, or deep fascia without abscess or osteomyelitis
- ☐ 3 Deep ulcer with abscess, osteomyelitis, or joint sepsis
- ☐ 4 Gangrene localized to portion of forefoot or heel
- ☐ 5 Extensive gangrenous involvement of the entire foot

Wound condition

Development and extent of the damage

- ☐ size
- ☐ depth
- ☐ involvement of deep lying fascia, muscle, tendon, cartilage and bone

Condition of the wound margin

- ☐ smooth
- ☐ irregular
- ☐ jagged
- ☐ decayed
- ☐ wound pockets
- ☐ necrotic tissue portions
- ☐ condition of the necrosis
- ☐ closed black necrosis

Condition of the wound bed

- ☐ slough
- ☐ slimy tissue
- ☐ dirty
- ☐ presence of foreign bodies
- ☐ clean

Condition of the Exudation

- ☐ bloodied
- ☐ bloodied-serous
- ☐ purulent
- ☐ dried-up
- ☐ odour

Extent of bacterial Invasion and sign of Infection ______________________________

How old is the wound? ______________________________

Date Signature

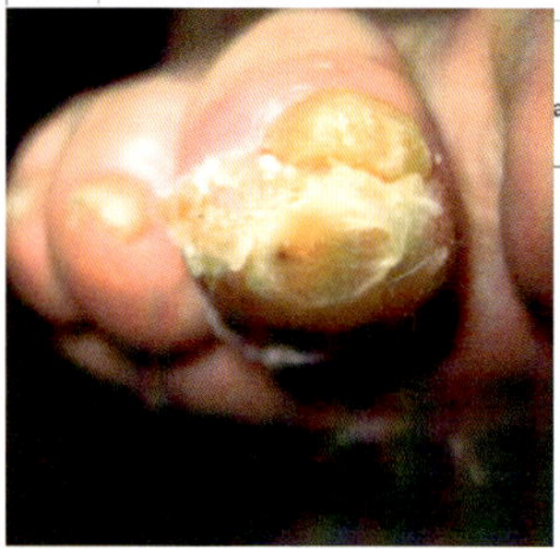

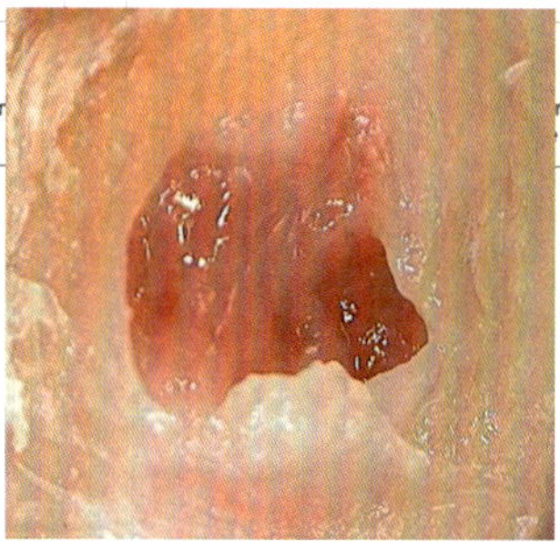

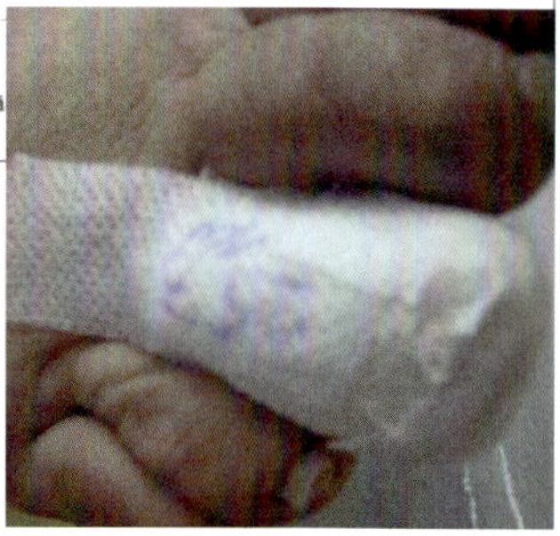

Image 3.27 Written wound documentation

Images 3.28 to 3.30 Wound documentation examples

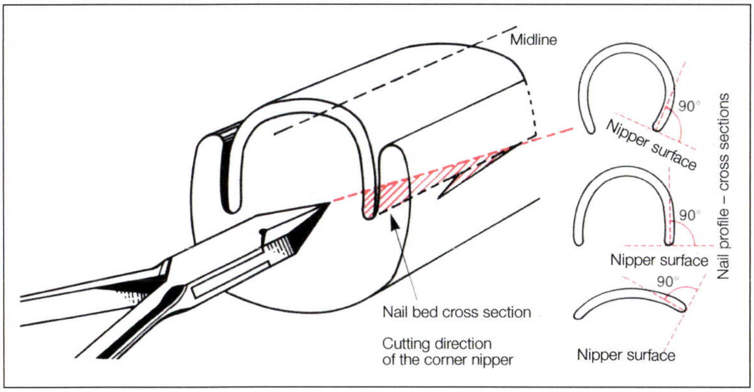

Image 3.31
Corner nipper cutting direction

Source:
Klaus Grünewald, Theorie der medizinischen Fußbehandlung, tome 1, 4th ed. 2012, Verlag Neuer Merkur

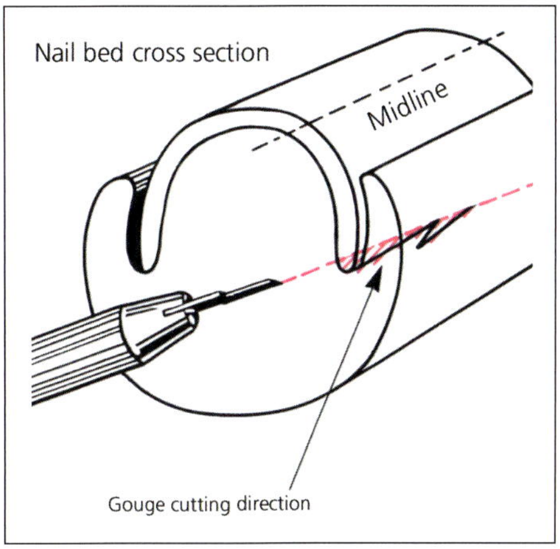

Image 3.32 Gouge cutting direction

Source: Klaus Grünewald, Theorie der medizinischen Fußbehandlung, tome 1, 4th ed. 2012,, Verlag Neuer Merkur

not to remove too much and not to leave sharp nail edges behind (images 3.31 to 3.34).

- Remove hyperkeratosis carefully from the sulcus with Prontoman spray (allow the spray to take effect for two minutes and, if needed, insert a thin spray-impregnated tamponade in the nail fold).
- For wound treatment in the sulcus area, use the following disinfectants: Pronto-Man gel, octenisept, Dolerma antiseptic nail fold oil, isopropyl 70 %, Calendula or colloidal silver.
- To stop potential bleeding, insert Clauden gauze or a gauze impregnated with a Policresulen concentrate solution, Copoline, fleece or cellulose strip into the fold and remove after three minutes. Nasal drops can also be used and are especially suitable for diabetic patients.
- After straightening the nail margin and removing sharp edges, insert Copoline or Ligasano tamponade in the nail fold.
- Apply nail correction braces, such as adhesive braces (BS brace, Gold brace (Goldstadt brace), Onychoclip brace, Erki brace) or spring-wire braces (Ross Fraser, 3TO, VHO, ORa). For how to properly attach the individual braces, see chapter 5.
- Apply a sterile dressing on the tip of the toe and ensure that there is no pressure applied to the toe.
- See the patient every day until the infection has subsided; following sterile guidelines is crucial.
- To promote faster healing, the patient can apply Spirularin nail serum on the nail and take frequent footbaths with sage, camomile, bran, thyme, horsetail or sea salt (one tablespoon in five liters of water at 37° to 38° C).

Prophylaxis

- correct cutting of the nail
- wearing properly fitting footwear
- careful cleaning of the sulcus with hyperkeratosis and clavus removal

Hygiene

- All infections are vulnerable to the invasion of the MRSA bacterium (methicillin-resistant Staphylococcus aureus). According to the Robert Koch Institute (German federal government agency and research institute responsible for disease control and prevention), the Staphylococcus bacterium has multiplied substantially. In 20% of the population, it is constantly detectable and in 50% of the population it is temporarily detectable. MRSA poses a high risk for patients with wound infections and a weakened immune system.

The German Federal Ministry of Health reports: "In Germany alone 400,000 to 600,000 people acquire nosocomial infections. These commonly called hospital-acquired infections are acquired during in-house or out-patient treatments claiming the lives of 7,500 to 15,000 people annually while traffic accidents are responsible for 3,475 deaths."

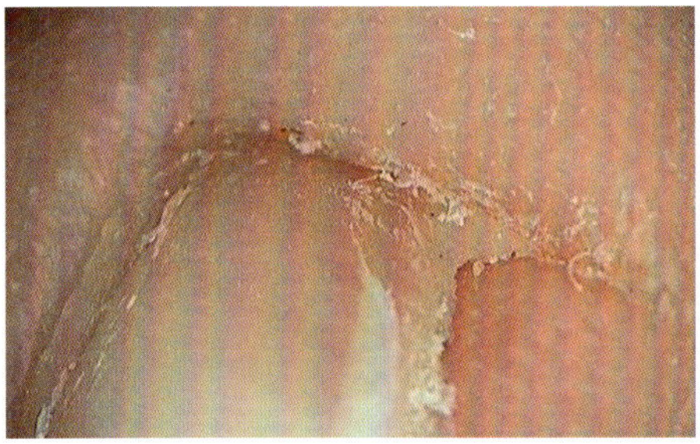

Image 3.33 Unguis incarnatus with painful inflammatory response (medial)

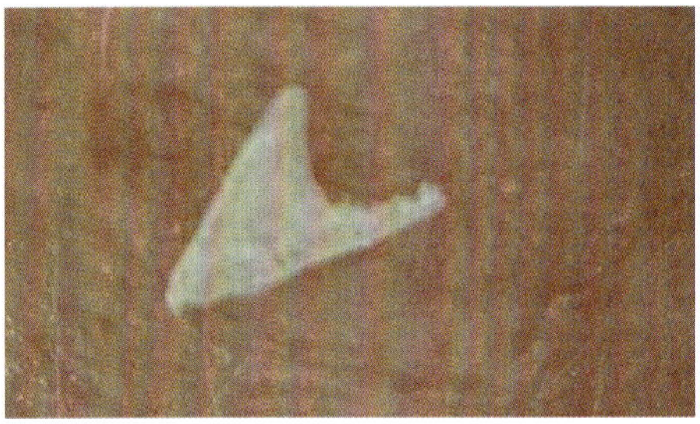

Image 3.34 After removal of the ingrown nail corner

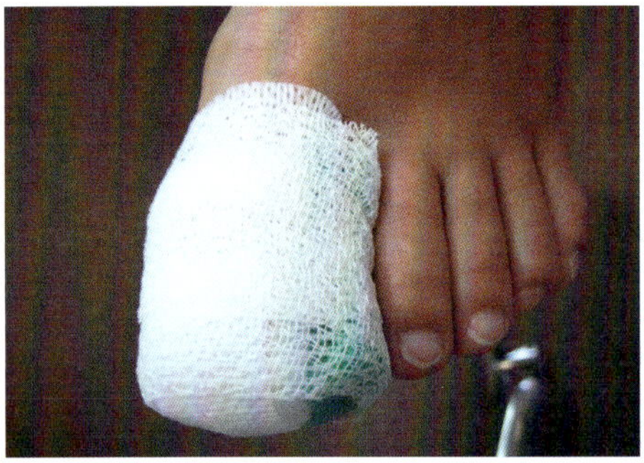

Image 3.35 Pressure relief

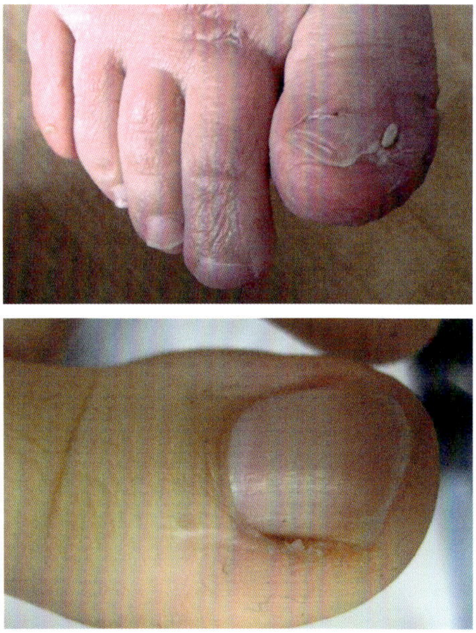

Images 3.36 and 3.37 Improperly performed Emmert's procedure

Risk factors for the practice

1. latent risk to the podiatrist's own health and the health of other patients due to infection and bacteria transfer
2. the detection of MRSA within a practice can lead to its temporary closing; infected staff members must take sick leave and are not allowed to be in the practice environment
3. following the hygiene guidelines for patients infected with MRSA is crucial

The above risk factors demand the following special treatment and hygiene standards:

- full anamnesis
- MRSA hygiene plan and implementation of hygiene measures in the practice environment
- offering and recommending care and medical products (e.g., Spirularin foot gel, mousse and cleaning lotions, skinicer® sedative shampoo) to patients and staff members since these products protect against Staphylococcus aureus and, in particular, MRSA.
- Proper preventative measures, such as frequent hand disinfection and following standard infection control guidelines, help prevent the spread of MRSA infections (image 3.38).

The guideline "At home follow-up care recommendation for patients with unguis incarnatus" can be found on the following page.

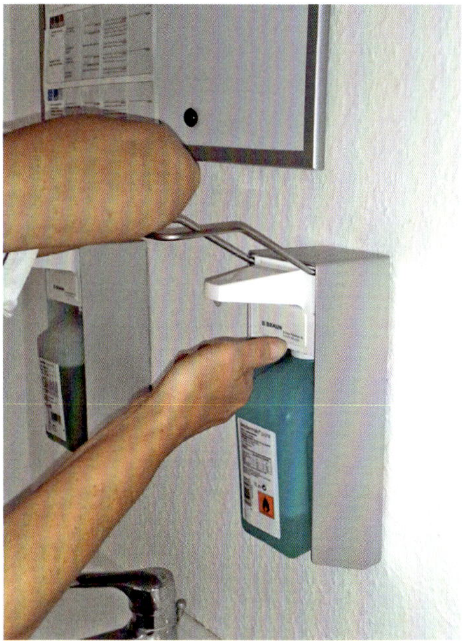

Image 3.38 Hand disinfection

At home follow-up care recommendations for patients with ingrown toenails

Dear Patient,

I am committed to perform your planned nail correction treatment with the utmost care and in accordance with the newest state of science and technology.

After care at home is important and will not only promote proper healing but also keep treatment costs low. I, therefore, have listed a few guidelines for you to follow at home.

General guidelines

Restrictive footwear (length, width, height) must be avoided!!!

Cut toe nails straight across (square shape) and not too short.

Wear socks made of cotton, wool, silk or bamboo.

Always dry toes and the area between the toes thoroughly after showering or bathing.

Allow the water to evaporate after showering or bathing.

Effective wound care

After the antiseptic foot bath, allow the water to evaporate before drying with a clean cloth.

Schedule daily visits with your podiatrist or physician to change wound dressing and tamponade.

Wear open-toed shoes such as sandals whenever possible.

Choose shoes that are not too tight or small if wearing closed shoes is inevitable.

Closed shoes must be of natural materials such as leather.

A moist environment in the foot area must be avoided!

Cooperation with the treatment specialist

You have chosen the gentle corrective procedure with nail correction braces.

The nail changes when it grows so the brace may loosen causing minor pressure discomfort.

If this happens, see your podiatrist who will remove callous skin on the nail fold, apply a fresh tamponade and refit, reposition or replace the brace.

Based on experience, approximately three braces are needed during a nail correction procedure.

Visits to the podiatrist's office can be minimized by applying special wound and healing ointment or cream to the nail fold while wearing the corrective brace and by rigorously implementing the above-mentioned guidelines.

Do not miss any follow-up appointments!

3.3 Paronychia/ Panaritium
(whitlow)

Definition
Painful acute inflammation of the nail wall area causing severe inflammation of the entire area around the nail (images 3.39 to 3.43).

Causes
- ingrown toenail (unguis incarnatus)
- tight footwear
- incorrect cuticle removal
- blow, pressure and injuries
- intolerance to certain medication, such as anti-rheumatic medication
- moist environment
- microorganisms, especially Staphylococcus (MRSA-risk), Streptococcus, Pseudomonas and fungi (Candida albicans); viruses such as Herpes simplex are rarely involved

Complications
- progressive stage: forming of granulation tissue and bone involvement
- lymph vessel inflammation (lymphangitis) and tissue destruction (necrosis)
- nail loss

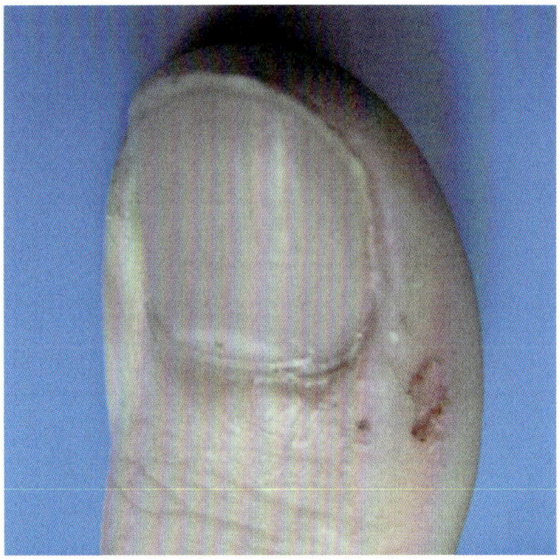

Image 3.39 Caused by working with chemicals

Treatment
Working with sterile instruments is of utmost importance!

Cooperation with a physician is crucial!

After thorough disinfection with octenisept (keep in fridge and apply cold reducing pain sensitivity) and ensuring that an ingrown toe nail is causing the inflammation, follow the treatment procedure for ingrown toe nails and carefully insert a sterile tamponade (e.g., Ligasano) impregnated with antiseptic ointment, Spirularin nail serum, Propolis solvent, octenisept gel, Prontoman gel, colloidal silver or

Image 3.40 Caused by toe crowding in a diabetic patient

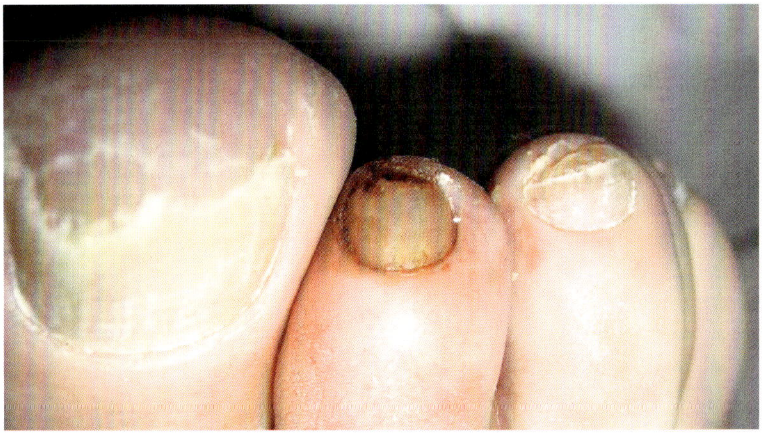

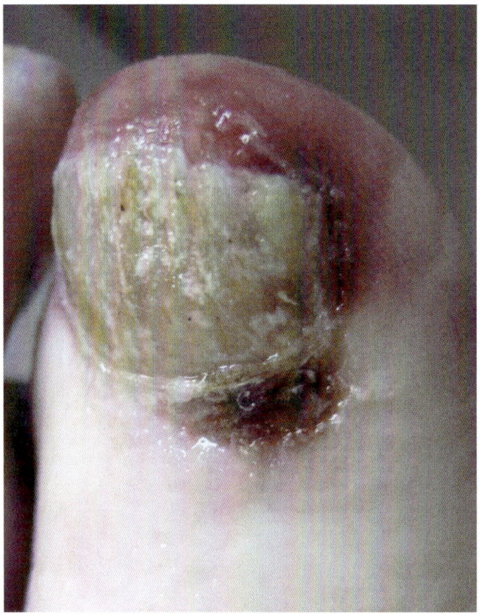

Image 3.41 Paronychia with suppuration and onychomycosis

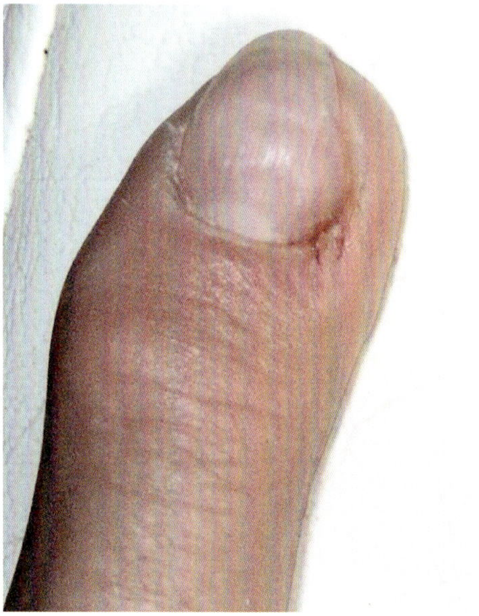

Image 3.42 Paronychia as a result of an incorrectly performed manicure

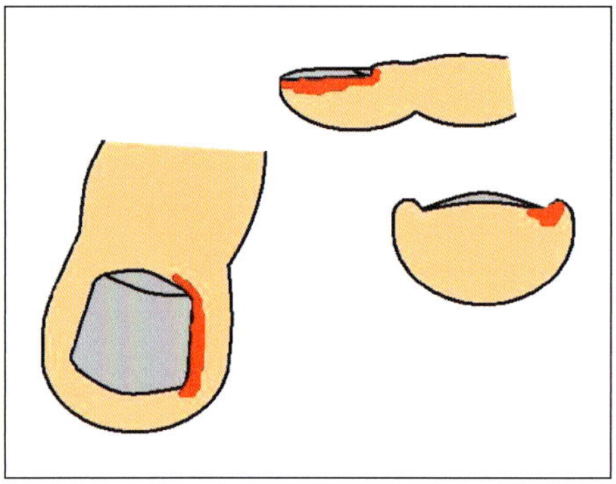

Image 3.43

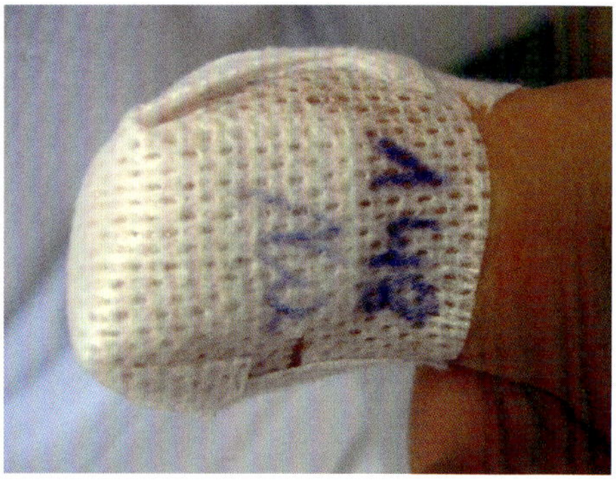

Image 3.44 Toe dressing

tea tree oil (careful as this might cause an allergic reaction) with a thin excavator into the nail fold. If necessary, apply a correction brace, preferably an adhesive brace, to relieve pressure.

An ozone steam application promotes healing. In addition, accurately performed wound care with sterile wound compresses and a proper toe dressing (image 3.44) as well as ensuring pressure relief are also important.

Prophylaxis

- pressure trauma prevention
- properly fitting foot wear
- adequate foot hygiene

3.4 Unguis convolutus
(pincer nail, rolled nail)

Definition
Unguis convolutus (pincer nail or rolled nail) is a nail deformity characterized by the transverse overcurvature of the nail plate, in which the lateral edges of the nail pinch the soft tissue (images 3.45 to 3.50).

Causes/symptoms/appearance
Unguis convolutus is the leading cause of unguis incarnatus (ingrown toe nail). The curved lateral nail edges promote hornification in the nail fold causing pain and discomfort.

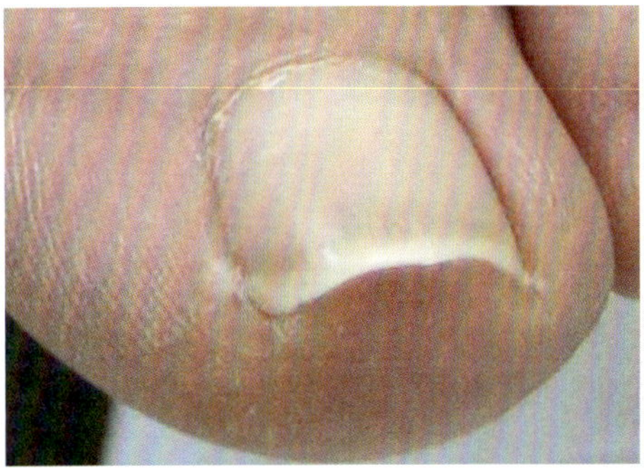

Image 3.45

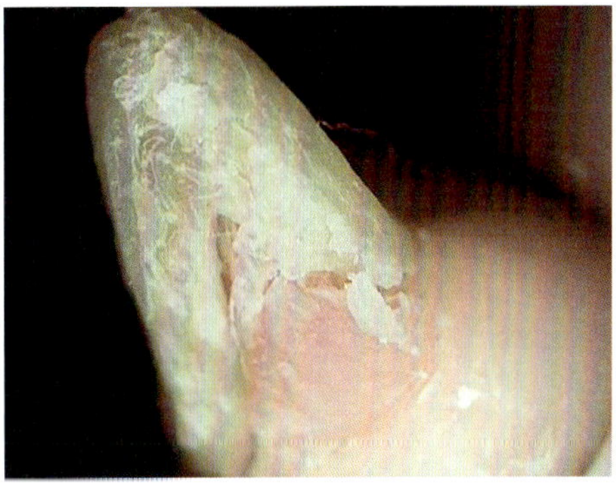

Image 3.46

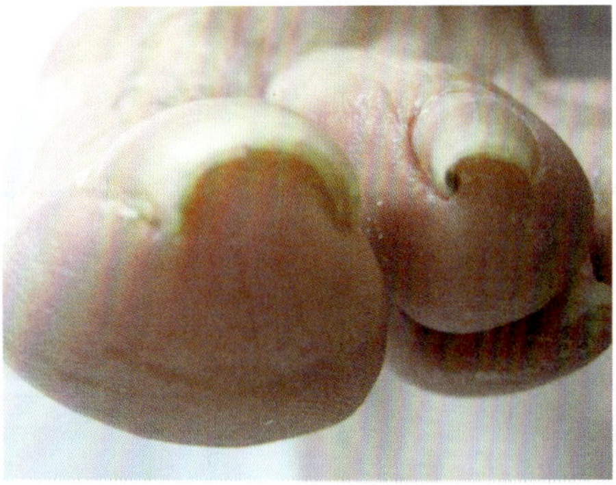

Image 3.47

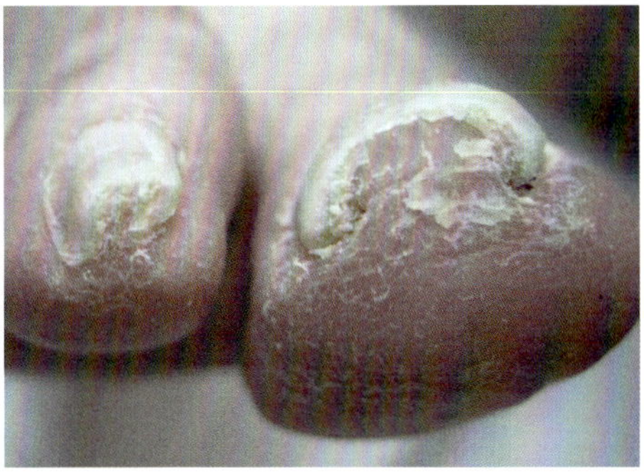

Image 3.48

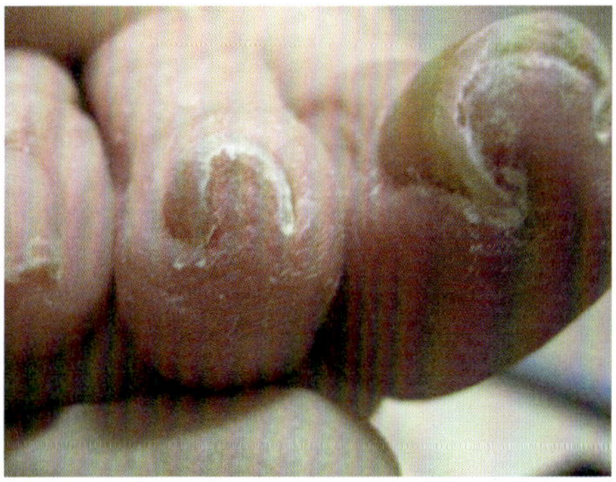

Image 3.49

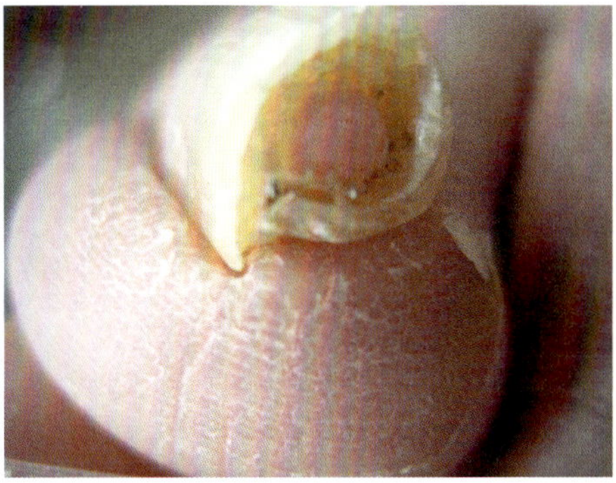

Image 3.50

Unguis convolutus presents itself in various shapes (morphology):

- omega shape (images 3.51 and 3.52)
- tile shape (images 3.53 and 3.54)
- plicated type (images 3.55 and 3.56)

Improper fitting footwear is the leading cause for nail plate deformities. However, metabolic disorders can also cause severe curving of the nail plate even within a period of a few weeks (images 3.57 to 3.59).

Furthermore, foot and toe deformities and hyperkeratosis in the sulcus account for unguis convolutus (image 3.60).

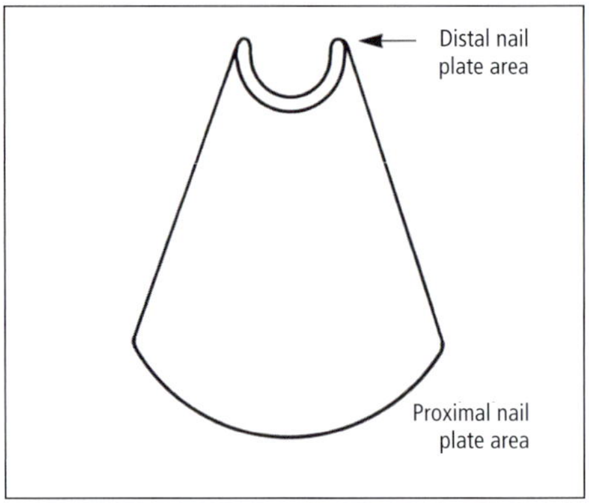

Image 3.51 Unguis convolutus (omega shape)

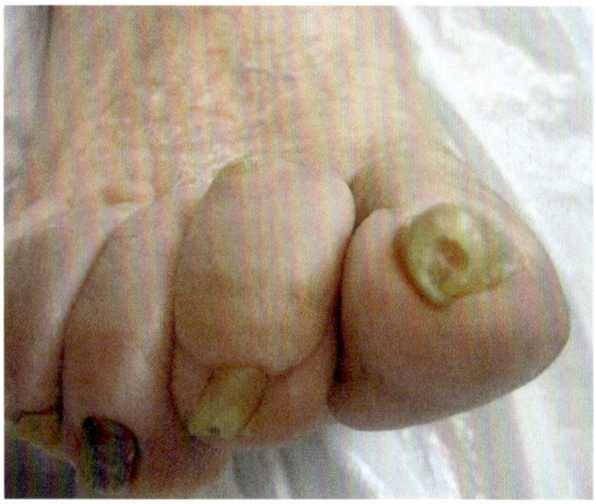

Image 3.52

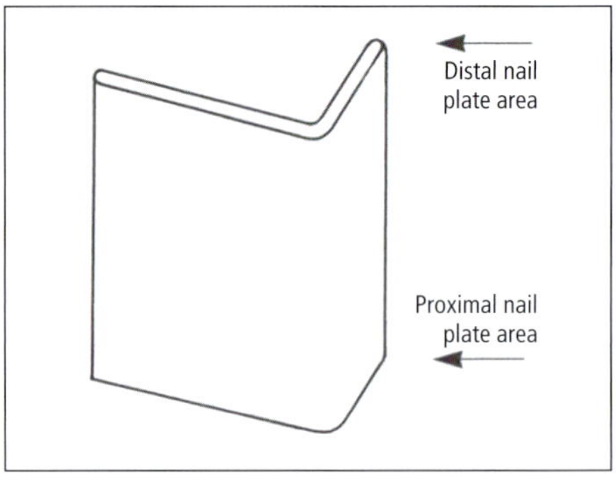

Image 3.53 Unguis convolutus (tile shape)

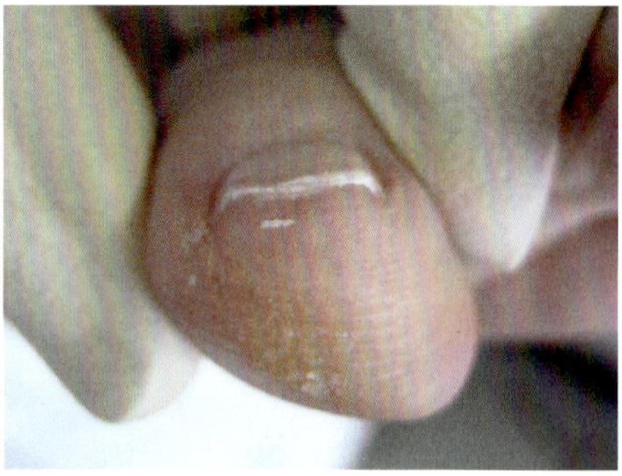

Image 3.54

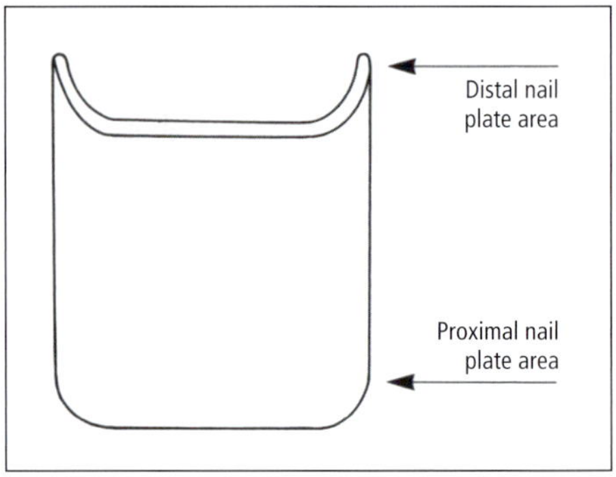

Image 3.55 Unguis convolutus (plicated type)

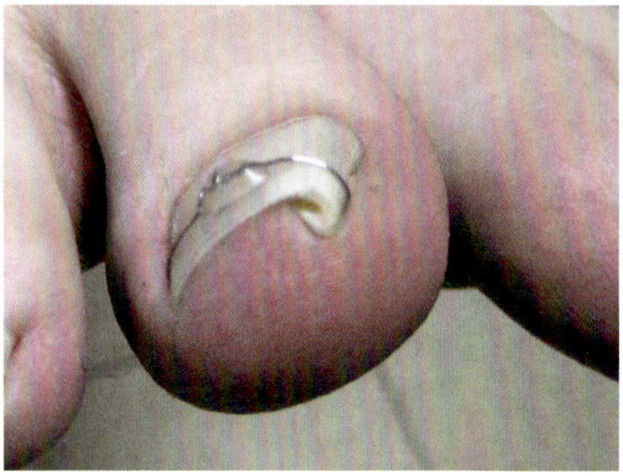

Image 3.56 Source: Brigitte Rathenow

Complications
- unguis incarnatus
- onychomycosis

Treatment
Cut the unguis convolutus in small stages with the tip of a nail nipper to prevent tearing (image 3.61). Remove excessive hornification in the nail fold with either a scalpel, medi-blade, cuticle nipper or a probe. If there are no signs of irritation cotton impregnated with urea solution (40%) or salicylic acid can be inserted in the nail fold to inhibit hornification.

Simply cutting away or grinding off the medial and lateral nail edge in the nail fold can inflict pain and is, therefore, not recommended. It creates a gap in the nail fold causing narrowing of the nail bed (chart 3.1).

The growing nail presses against the narrowed nail bed and deforms, causing pain and discomfort for the patient. Here the use of a nail correction brace is highly recommended.

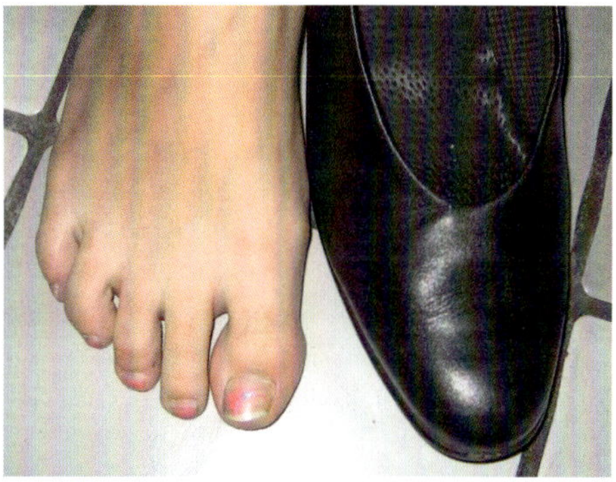
Image 3.57

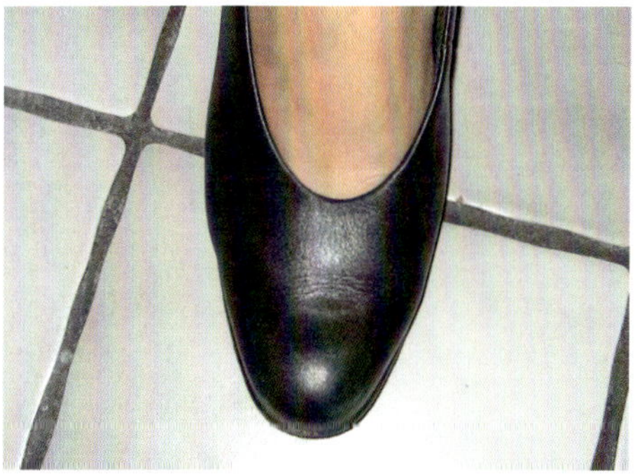
Image 3.58

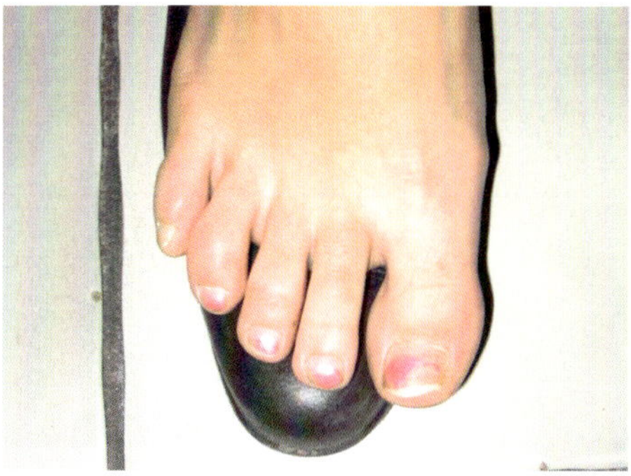
Image 3.59

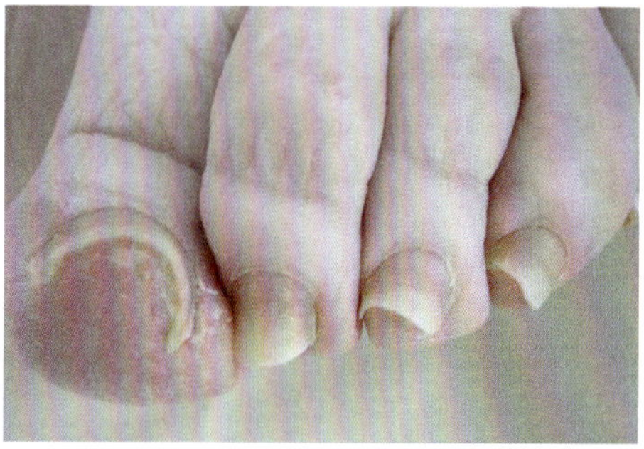
Image 3.60 Foot and toe deformities and hyperkeratosis in the sulcus

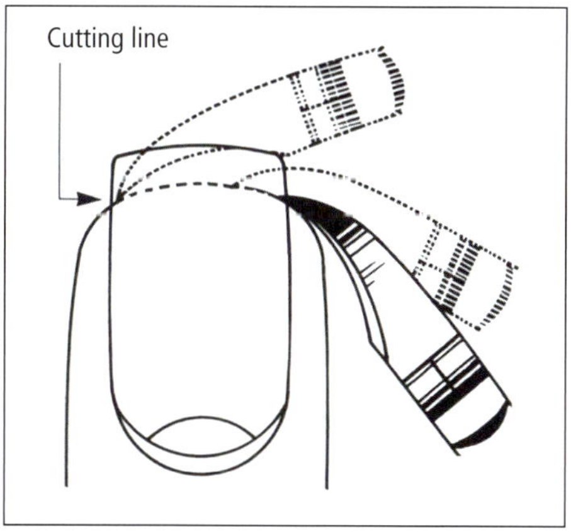

Image 3.61 Correct positioning of the nail nipper on the cutting line

Images 3.51, 3.53, 3.55, 3.61 and chart 3.1
Source: Klaus Grünewald, Theorie der medizinischen Fußbehandlung, tome 1, 4th ed. 2012,, Verlag Neuer Merkur

Nail and nail fold complications	Potential implications due to incorrect grinding	Potential implications due to incorrect cutting
tearing of the distal free nail margin under pressure	yes	no
overcurvature of the nail plate (unguis convolutus)	yes	yes
ingrown nail (unguis incarnatus)	no	yes
clavus formation in the nail fold	yes	yes
callus formation in the nail fold	yes	yes
nail bed deformity	yes	yes
hypersensitivity of the nail bed and distal free nail margin	yes	yes

Chart 3.1 Potential nail bed complications due to incorrect cutting or grinding of the nail plate

Taking contraindications into consideration, restoration of the original nail shape with the following orthonyxia braces has been proven to be an effective non-surgical treatment option: Ora brace (chapter 5.5), 3TO brace (chapter 5.3), Fraser brace (chapter 5.2), BS brace (chapter 5.9), Podofix brace (chapter 5.12), Goldstadt brace (chapter 5.8), Onyclip brace (chapter 5.11), Erki brace (chapter 5.13).

In less severe cases, permanent tamponades, such as gutta-percha wedges (chapter 7.5), sulci splints (chapter 7.7) or Smig (chapter 7.4) provide adequate results.

However, the patient must understand the importance of wearing proper footwear to achieve long-term success.

Prophylaxis

- Advise and inform parents:
  I visit playgroups and show the parents proper nail cutting techniques and what they must consider when they purchase footwear for their children. I do the same information sessions in kindergardens and schools and motivate the children in a playful setting to do foot exercises (additional suggestions upon request).
- Educate parents about the importance of properly fitting footwear.
- Cutting the nail correctly.
- Doing foot exercises to prevent foot deformity.

3.5 Onychomycosis
(Greek: mykos = fungus)

Definition
Fungal infection of the toenails or fingernails commonly caused by filamentous fungi (dermatophytes) that invade the nail bed (image 3.62).

Causes
A weakened immune system, microlesions, systemic diseases, a moist environment in footwear or poor hygiene promote pathogenic fungi colonization on or in the human organism. An infection is always preceded by cellular damage caused by trauma, circulatory disorder, diabetes or metabolic disorder (e.g., angiopathy).

DYM-system
D = Dermatophytes, 80% of infections, primarily found on skin and nails.
Y = Yeast fungi (atypical Candida infections), 15% of infections, affect the mucous membrane.
M = Mould fungi, 5% of infections. Affect the lungs.

Dermatomycosis: fungal infection of the skin (image 3.63)
Tinea pedis: dermatophytosis
Onychomycosis: fungal infection of the nail (images 3.64 and 3.65)
Trichomycosis: fungal hair infection
Thrush: fungal infection of the mucous membrane

By analysing DNA, scientists from the University of Mainz identified several hundred different types of fungi. Each cubic meter of air contains between 1,000 and 10,000 fungal spores. It is estimated that there are more than 1.5 million different types of fungal spores. A human being breathes in between 10,000 and 20,000 liters of air daily and every breath contains one to ten fungal spores.

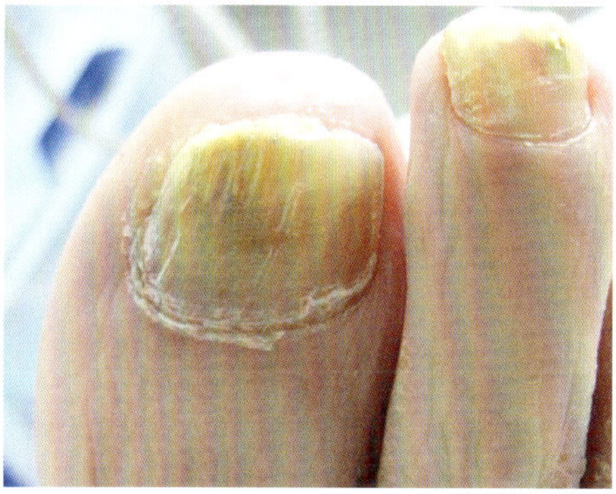
Image 3.62 Onychomycosis

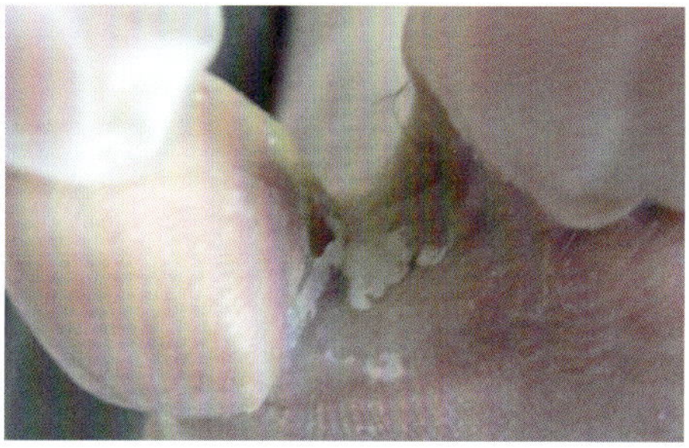
Image 3.63 Interdigital mycosis

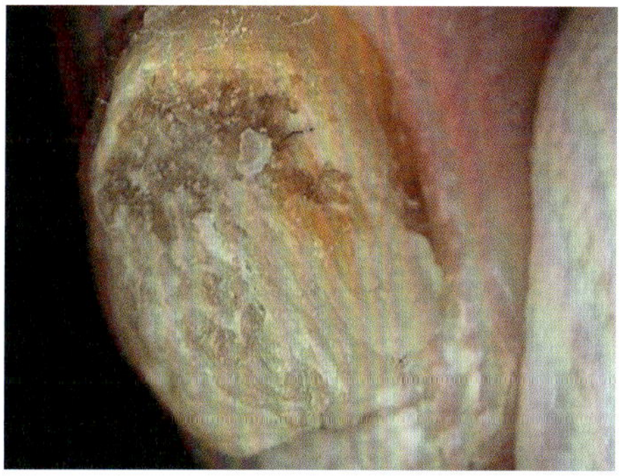
Image 3.64

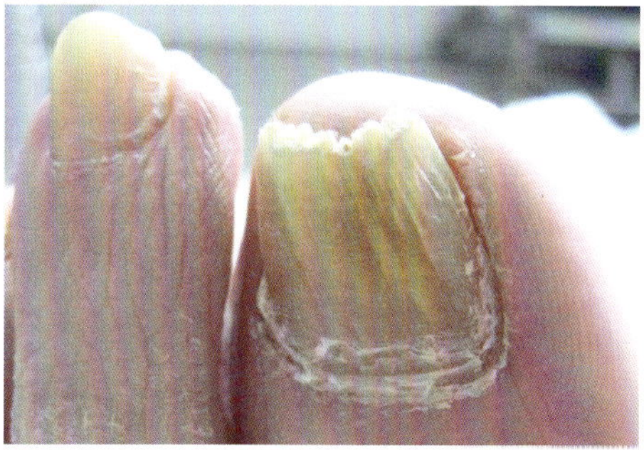
Image 3.65

Appearance and colonization

Onychomycosis starts 90 per cent of the time in the distal area of the nail plate, rarely in the centre or proximal area of the nail. An infestation of the matrix and nail bed epithelium is rather rare, if it does occur though, it prolongs the treatment significantly. Nails affected by a fungal infection are often dry and brittle and it is, therefore, important to not only treat the mycosis, but also to apply conditioning products such as Spirularin nail serum or nurturing nail oils by Gehwol, Sixtus, Peclavus, Allpresan etc.

There are six different types of mycosis:

1. DSO (distal subungual onychomycosis, images 3.66 to 3.68) is the distal subungual and lateral onychomycosis.

DSO is the most often occurring type of infestation. Pathogens first colonize the hyponychium and the distal parts of the lateral nail bed grooves and spread towards proximal direction in the nail epithelium and nail bed. Soft keratin formation and the development of small gaps in the distal nail plate promote a secondary microorganism infestation whereby the subungual tissue reacts with subacute dermatitis and hyperkeratosis. The nail plate becomes unusually thick, has a yellowish to brownish colour and the nail is no longer transparent. It can lead to onycholysis as the infection progresses. Onycholysis is the separation of the nail plate from the nail bed and from the distal or lateral nail margin towards proximal direction.

DSO is mostly detected in Trichophyton rubrum and other dermatophyte infections. However, mould fungi and other atypical Candida infections also belong to this type. These are often accompanied

From a therapeutic point of view, it is important to identify the degree of infestation of the nail plate.

- Stage 1: 30% of the nail plate
- Stage 2: 30 to 60% of the nail plate
- Stage 3: more than 60% of the nail plate

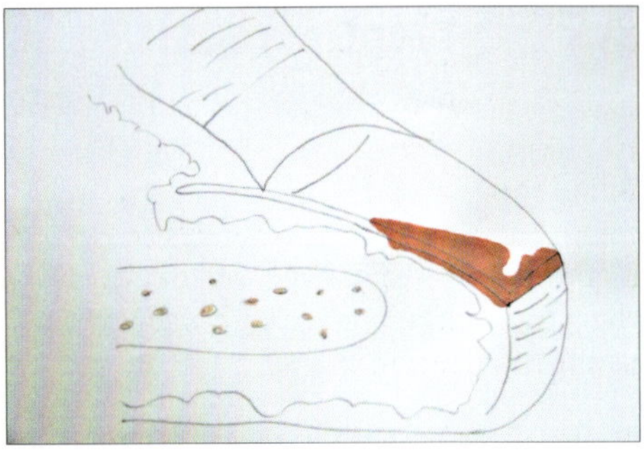

Image 3.66

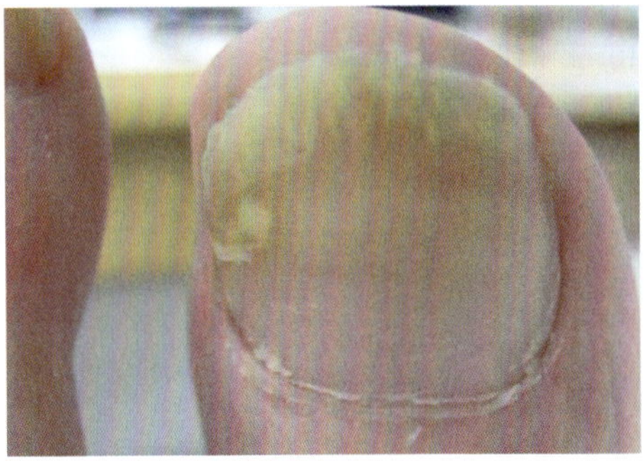

Image 3.67

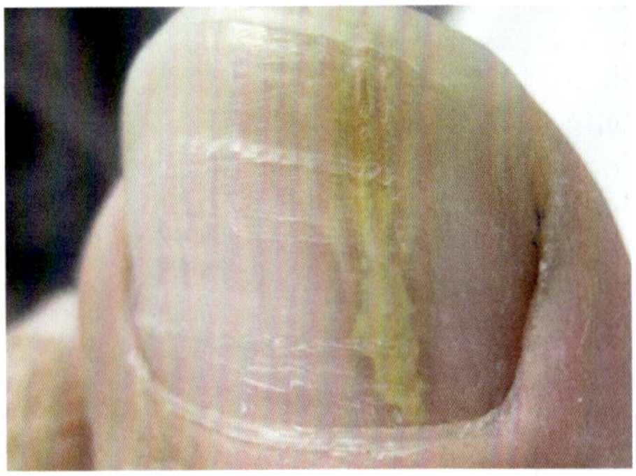

Image 3.68

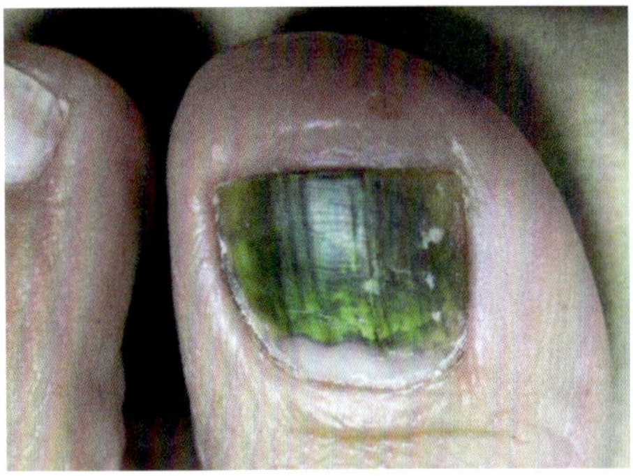

Image 3.69 Mould fungus

Mould fungi (image 3.69) always start from the distal and spread towards proximal direction and are triggered by Fusarium, Scopulariopsis brevicaulis and Aspergillus spp. With Fusarium and Scopulariopsis nail infection, the nail plate displays a white-yellowish to amber colour, while the Aspergillus types cause black or greenish discolouration.

2. PSO (proximal subungual onychomycosis, images 3.70 and 3.71)

PSO is a rare type of infestation. The fungi colonize the cuticle area. Injuries to the cuticle facilitate penetration and the fungi spread from the eponychium to the nail matrix where they penetrate the nail plate. Once the pathogens spread in the matrix further towards the distal direction, the entire nail plate has been infested.

The chronic irritation promotes subungual hyperkeratosis causing the proximal nail wall to become unusually thick. First a small white spot appears in the lunula area, then the nail wall thickens, damaging the cuticle. The nail displays a white or yellowish discolouration and looses its transparency. Trichophyton rubrum plays a key role in this type of infestation.

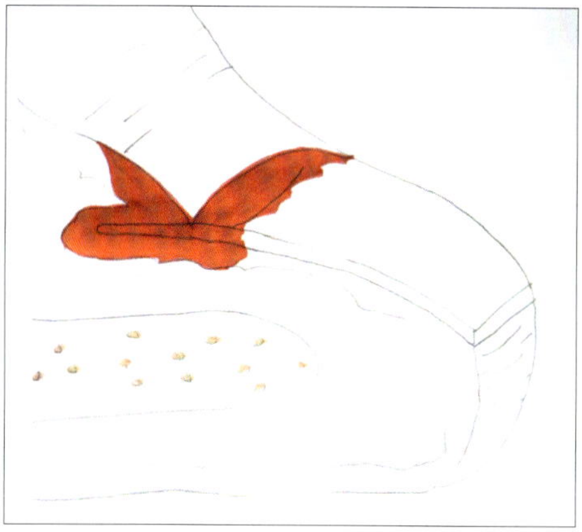

Image 3.70

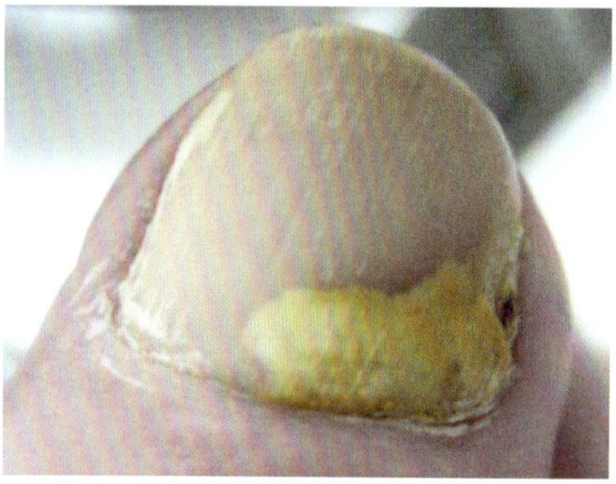

Image 3.71 Proximal subungual onychomycosis

3. TDO (total dystrophic onychomycosis, images 3.72 to 3.76)

TDO is divided in a primary and a secondary type. Both cause the complete infestation of the nail apparatus plus total dystrophy and onycholysis.

The primary type refers to chronic mucocutaneous candidiasis, a congenital immune defect that can trigger a life-long infestation of mucous membranes, skin and nails with candida albicans.

The proximal nail wall becomes extremely thick and is no longer distinguishable. An inflammatory reaction in the matrix and the nail bed impairs the development of regular nail structures.

The secondary type is the final stage of the previously mentioned infestation forms where the infestation has spread to the entire nail organ causing total dystrophy.

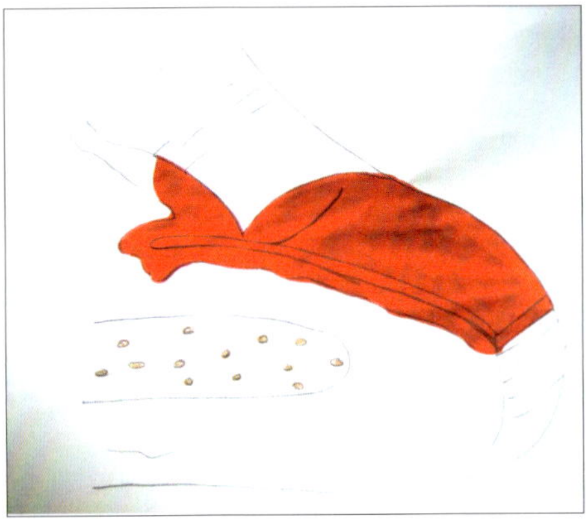

Image 3.72

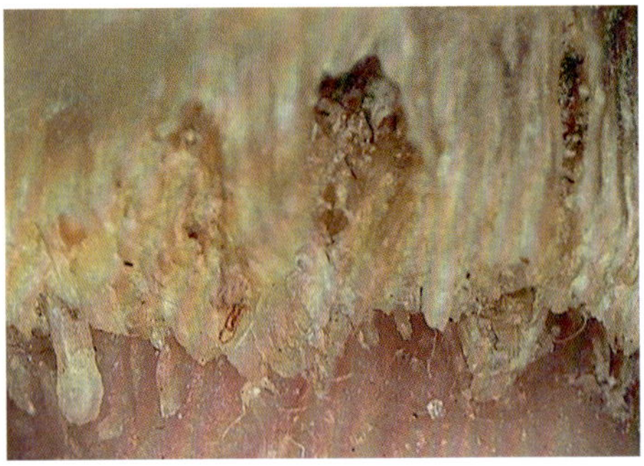

Image 3.73

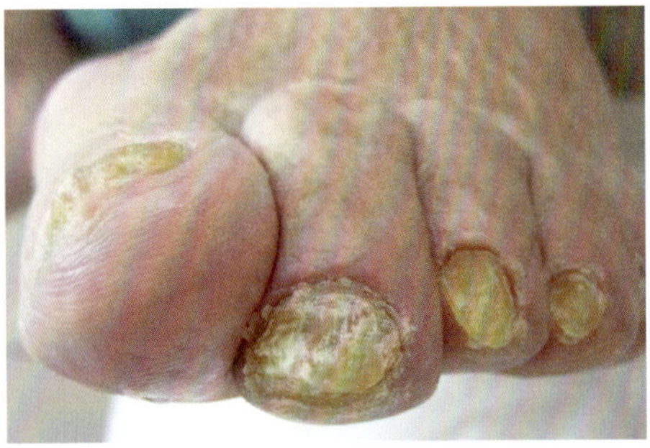

Image 3.74

Image 3.75

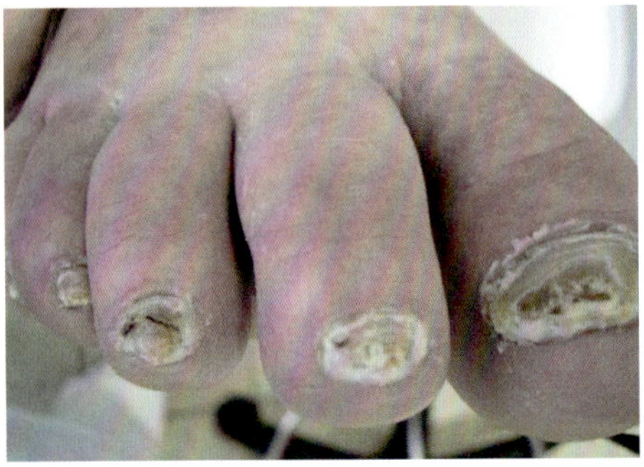

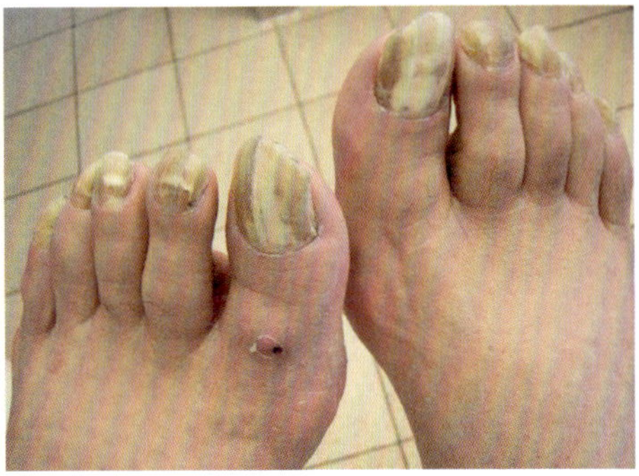

Image 3.76

4. WSO (white superficial onychomycosis) (images 3.77 to 3.79)

WSO is characterized by massive fungi penetration in the dorsal part of the nail plate whereby only the upper layers are affected (image 3.78). It is often accompanied by dermatomycosis. Often crowding and overlapping of toes are the cause. First, individual white spots develop which grow together over time covering large parts of the nail. The affected nail part appears white or yellowish; the nail surface becomes rough, soft and brittle.

In most cases, the thick white appearance on the nail is caused by the pathogen Trichophyton mentagrophytes, however several mould fungi, such as Acremonium spp., Aspergillus spp. and Fusarium spp., also have this appearance.

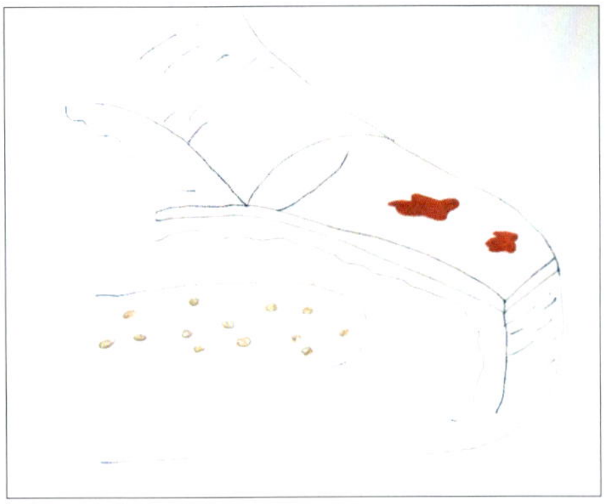

Image 3.77

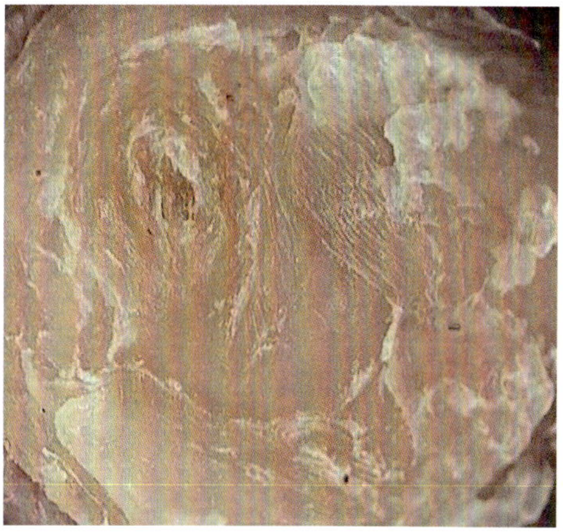

Image 3.78 Before treatment …

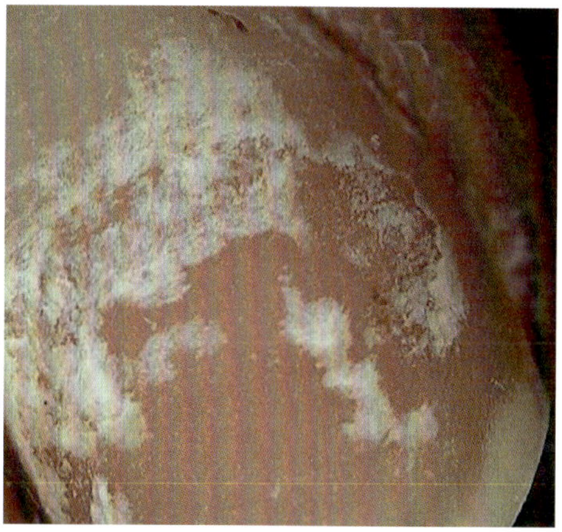

Image 3.79 … after grinding off the thick white layer (WSO)

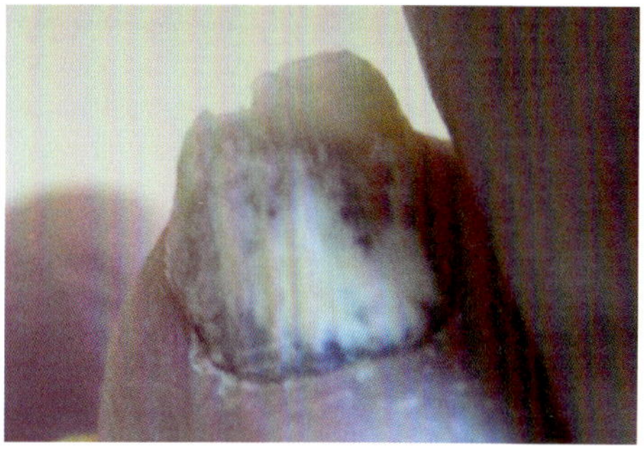

Image 3.80 Before treatment …

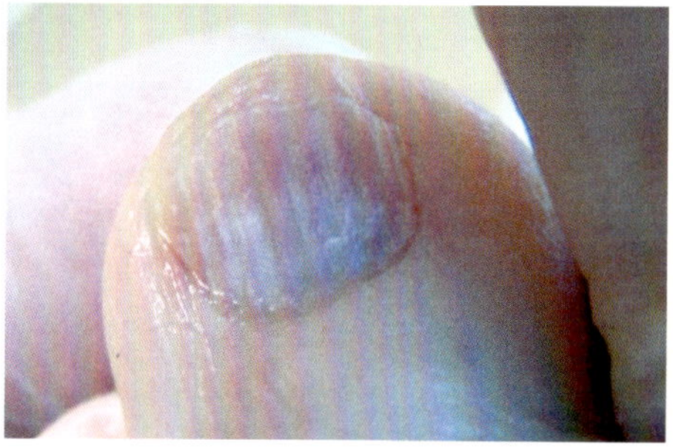

Image 3.81 … after grinding off the thick white layer (WSO)

5. CO (candida onychomycosis, candida paronychia with accompanied nail deformities, images 3.82 and 3.83)

Candida paronychia is often preceded by paronychia. It is characterized as a secondary pathogen penetration of the nail plate.

Fungal infestation can affect the distal-subungual, distal-lateral and proximal-subungual areas of the nail. Infestation to the proximal-subungual area is caused by an injured cuticle when yellowish-brown stripes appear parallel to the

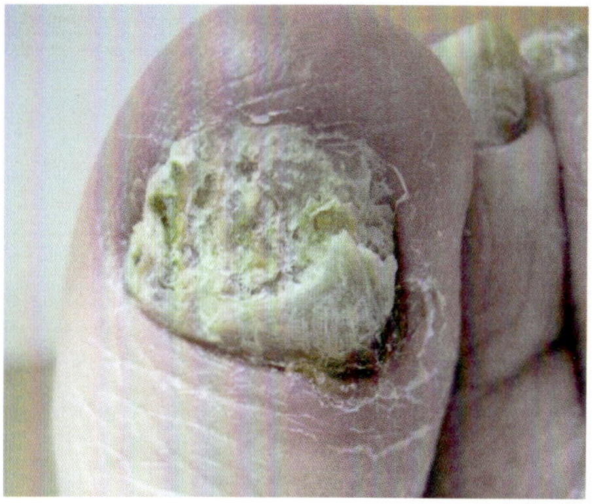

Image 3.82

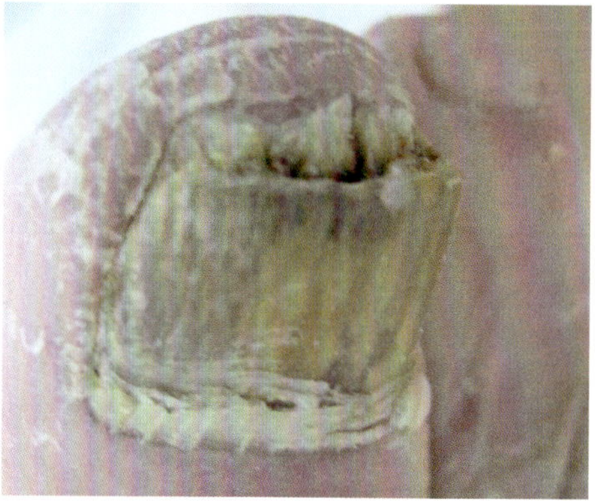

Image 3.83

lateral nail wall. The common pathogen is Candida albicans.

Candida onychomycosis develops with chronic mucocutaneous candidiasis or chronic recurrent paronychia. Patients with a severely impaired immune system (e.g., HIV patients) are especially vulnerable.

6. EO (endonyx onichomycosis) (image 3.84)

With endonyx onichomycosis the surface of the nail plate is infected similar to WSO. However, the pathogens can penetrate deep into the nail, damaging the keratin layers. Typical pathogens are Trichophyton soudanense and Trichophyton violaceum.

Pathogenesis

Person-to-person (spores) and animal-to-human transmission.

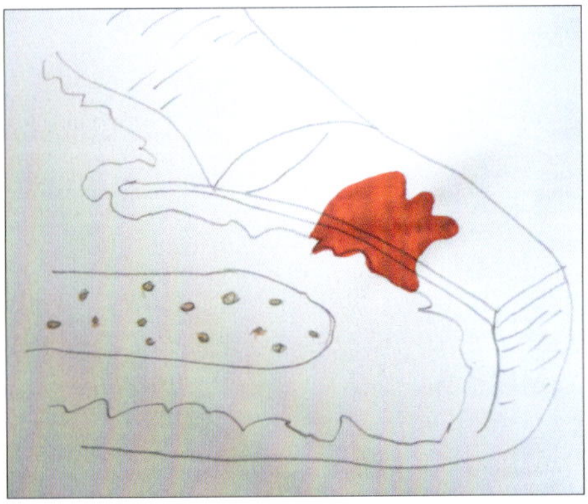

Image 3.84

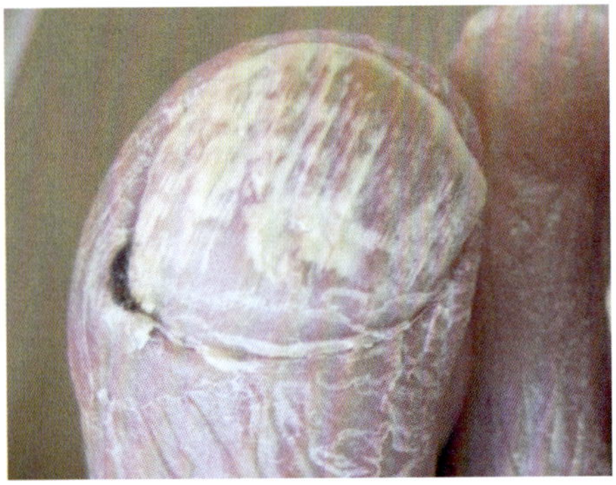

Image 3.85

Fungal hyphae and mycelium parts spread passively (e.g., soil movement, by being inhaled or eaten, propagation on or in plant seeds and on jam). Mycelium reacts sensitive to dryness, lack of an energy source, heat and cold (stress inducing) limiting their spreading potential.

Spores increase the spreading potential of fungi significantly by reproducing sexual spores (meiospores) and asexual spores (mitospores, conidiospores). Furthermore, they are dispersed by wind and can survive stress periods.

Spores are often equipped with reserves, exhibit a thick cell wall, are coloured, sticky and dry (biologically inactive). A 1989 research study revealed that by preserving the dermatophytes in paraffin oil Trichophyton rubrum can survive 142 months and Trichophyton mentagrophyte 74 months. The mould fungus Scopulariopsis brevicaulis can even be cultured after 137 months.

Potential contamination causes

Saunas, public pools and showers are known breeding grounds for fungi and walking barefoot, poor foot hygiene, hyperhidrosis, being overweight, orthopedic misalignment and incorrect footwear also play an important role. Improper footwear and certain sock materials are the main reason for heat accumulation, excessive skin moisture and for promoting harmful microflora in the foot area. Diabetic patients with circulatory disorders and patients with PAOD suffer from an impaired immune system making them vulnerable for infections.

Studies focusing on the effect of sock or stocking fabric on the growth behaviour of human-pathogenic fungi reveal that sock fibres can either promote or slow down the growth of fungi. Polyamide sock fibres with a high elastane share and silk fabric significantly promote the growth of Trichophyton rubrum, Trichophyton mentagrophytes and Candida albicans.

What are the different stages of onychomycosis?
- nail surface appears dull and lacks shine (images 3.86 and 3.87)
- discolouration of the nail bed (images 3.88 to 3.90)
- gradual callus formation under the nail causing the nail to detach from the nail bed (images 3.91 to 3.93)
- nail becomes brittle and displays small cracks (image 3.94)
- complete destruction of the nail (image 3.95)

Differential diagnosis

Mycosis is often confused with the following nail disorders. A medical clarification by a physician is therefore imperative:
- psoriasis
- onychogryposis
- medication-induced nail dystrophy
- eczema nail (neurodermatitis)
- paronychia

Complications
- nail loss (onychomadesis)
- permanent damage of the nail bed and the penetration of foreign bodies and microorganisms
- bacteria are generally unable to penetrate healthy skin layers, a fungi infestation, however, enables them to break into the skin causing additional infections and deterioration
- key bacteria (humid bacteria), such as Pseudomonas aeruginosa or Proteus mirabilis, cause gram-negative infections.

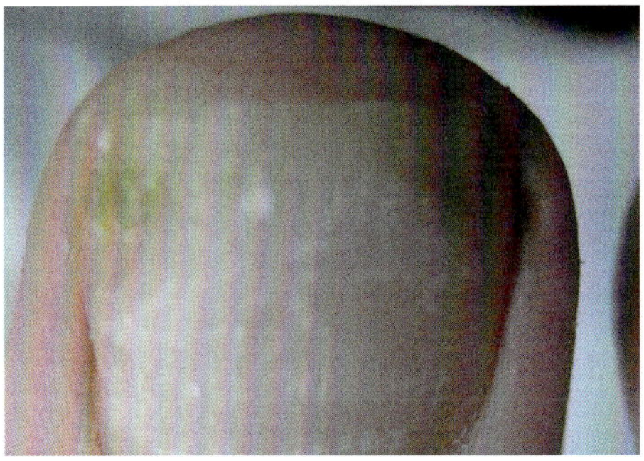
Image 3.86 Onset of onychomycosis

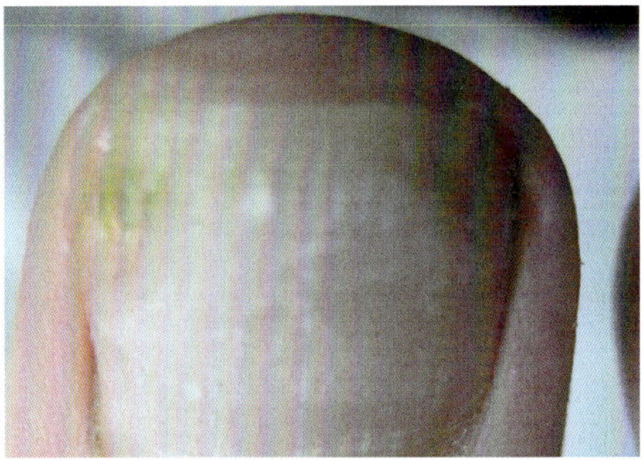
Image 3.87 Onset of onychomycosis

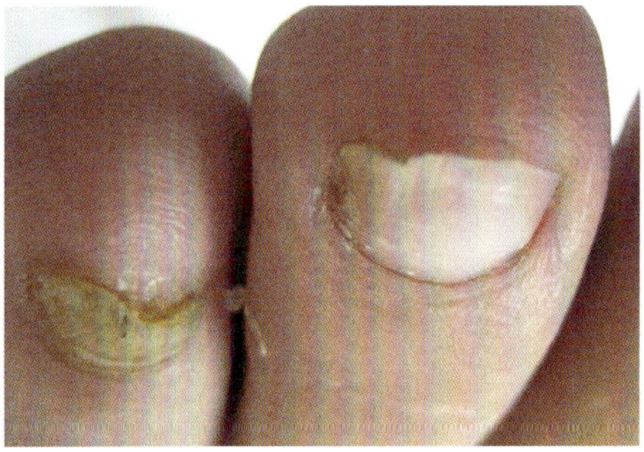
Image 3.88 Onychomycosis displaying yellowish discolouration

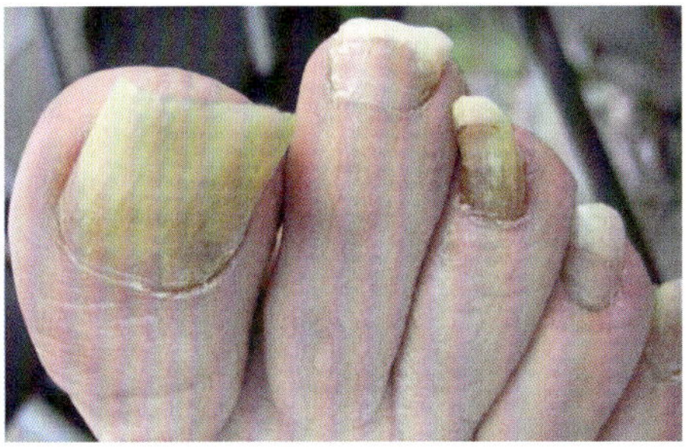
mage 3.89 Yellowish discolouration of the nail caused by onychomycosis with onycholysis

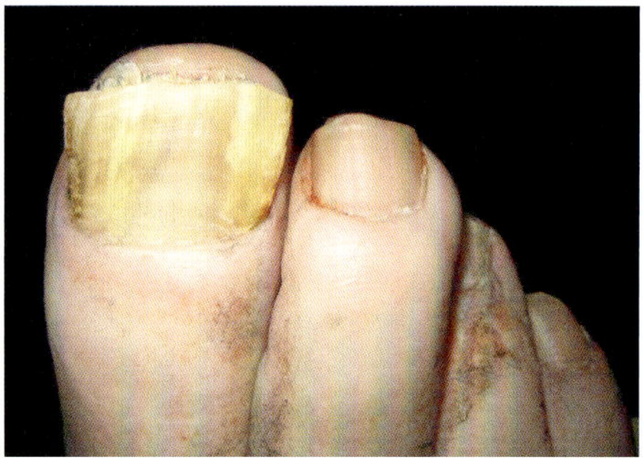

Image 3.90 Yellowish discolouration of the nail

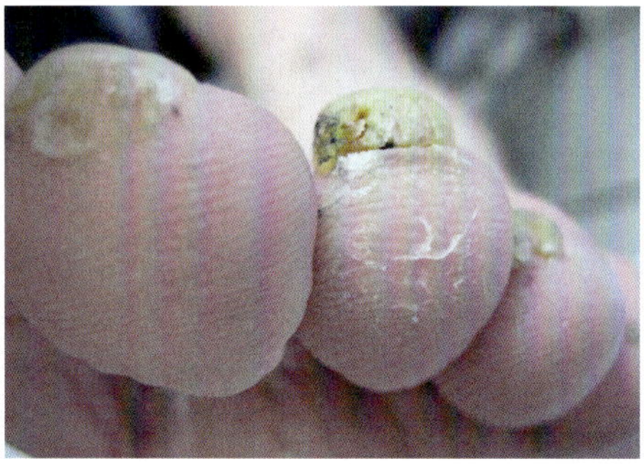

Images 3.91–3.93 Callus formation under the nail plate, caused by mycosis. This results in onycholysis.

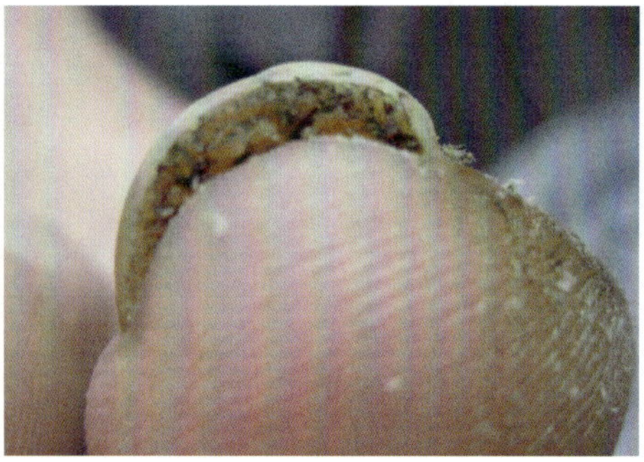

Image 3.92

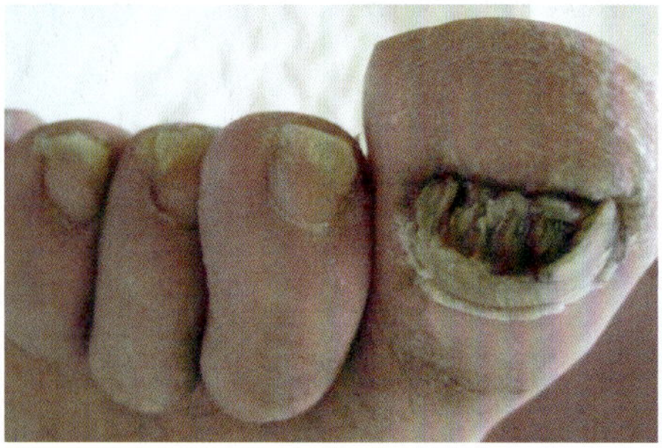

Image 3.93

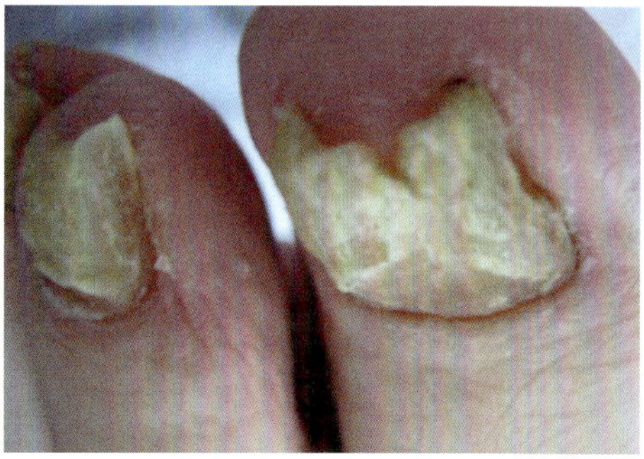

Image 3.94 The nail becomes brittle and displays cracks

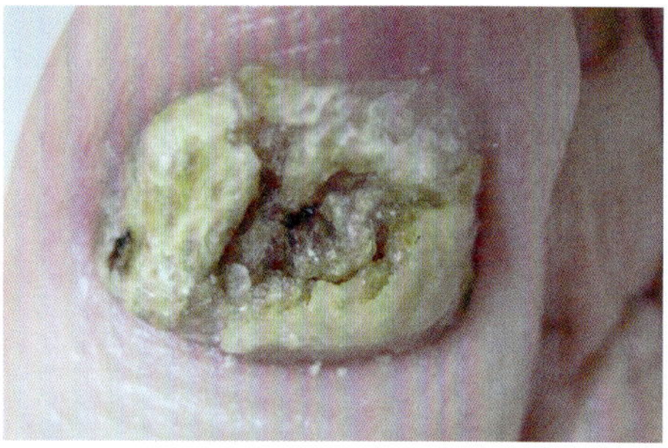

Image 3.95 Complete destruction of the nail plate

Treatment

Cooperation with a physician is crucial!

The objective is to break the mycosis infestation cycle permanently.

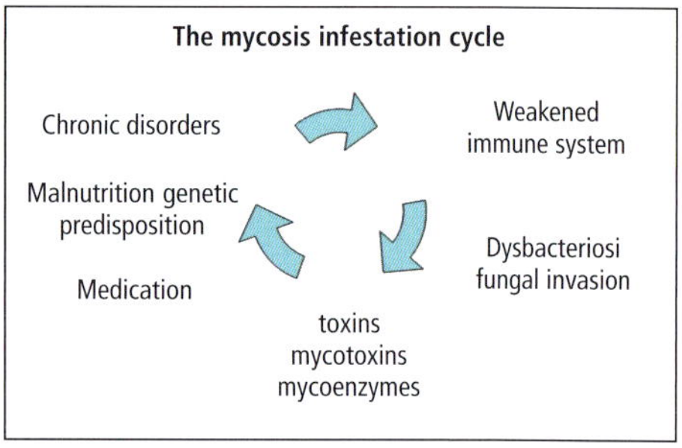

Image 3.96 The mycosis infestation cycle

12 imperatives for podiatrists for the proper diagnosis and treatment of nail and foot mycosis
by Dr. med. Pierre Foss, dermatologist and specialist for cytological mycosis diagnostics

1. No nail fungi without foot fungi.
2. Therefore: The antimycotic treatment must include the entire foot, not just the nails.
3. Nail and foot mycoses easily spread to other skin surfaces as often seen with a pedocrural infectious unit in a previously infected lower leg mycosis).
4. Therefore: In case of severe mycotic infections of nail and foot, protect the lower legs preventatively with broadband antimycotic ointments.
5. It must be explained to the patient that nail and foot mycoses can easily spread to other skin areas such as the groin area, the axils, the scalp, the thighs, etc., especially if he/she has a weakened immune system.
6. Nail fungi are especially problematic for diabetic patients since they are at high risk to develop diabetic foot syndrome.
7. Properly treating severe nail mycosis generally takes a whole year.
8. Systematically grinding off the infected nail areas while protecting the nail fold and perforation therapies for stable nails are helpful during antimycotic follow-up treatments.
9. The most unreliable diagnostic method to identify and classify nail and foot mycoses is through culture set-up.
   A much more reliable approach is the cytological or histological examination of body tissue whereby special dyes are used so that even the smallest colonies of fungi become visible during their growing phase. Nowadays PCR analyses or immunoblots ensure accurate genome analyses of fungi samples.
10. About 70–80% of even severe cases of onychomycosis are curable or significantly improvable with well-tolerated oral medication therapies implemented at regular intervals.
11. Fungal foot infections are easily mistaken for common skin diseases, such as psoriasis, eczema, neurodermatitis, congenital keratinization disorder, etc., and can aggravate these significantly. Performing thorough mycology diagnostics is, therefore, crucial for any sign of a skin disorder in the foot area.
12. Sample collection for diagnostics are generally taken proximal and from deep inside the skin. Since fungi often spread over the entire surface of the sole of the foot, samples must be taken by gently scraping the sole surface!

The accurate fungi analysis must be performed by specialists who provide results that answer the following questions:

- Is a mycotic infection present?
- Is it a contamination case or a true infection?
- Are the fungi easy or difficult to treat? Additional information is needed regarding hyphae, spores, metabolism.
- Is a bacterial infection present?
- Did the applied antimycotic medication penetrate the nail or the skin?
- Did the applied treatment impair the fungi? Should the treatment be continued, intensified or changed?
- What kind of treatment recommendations are suitable based on the medical history, the extent of the infection and the findings?

Sample-taking–how to do it correctly:
Taking skin and nail samples must be done correctly to ensure accurate examination results. The most sophisticated examination methods are rendered useless if the samples are taken incorrectly. The following principles apply:

- Take the samples from deep inside the nail where the vital mycotic structures are located.
- Since fungi on the sole of the foot spread over the entire surface, gently scrape the surface to get accurate sample results. In case of extreme hornification, samples must be taken from deep inside the horny layers.

Prior to the start of any mycosis treatment, patients must be made aware of the following:

- type of mycosis (diagnosed by a physician)
- risk of contagion
- treatment process
- treatment duration
- the need for consistent patient cooperation

A highly successful method for treating mycotic nails (image 3.97)

Prior to every treatment, disinfect the nail plate and cover the surrounding area with sterile cloths (images 3.98 and 3.99).

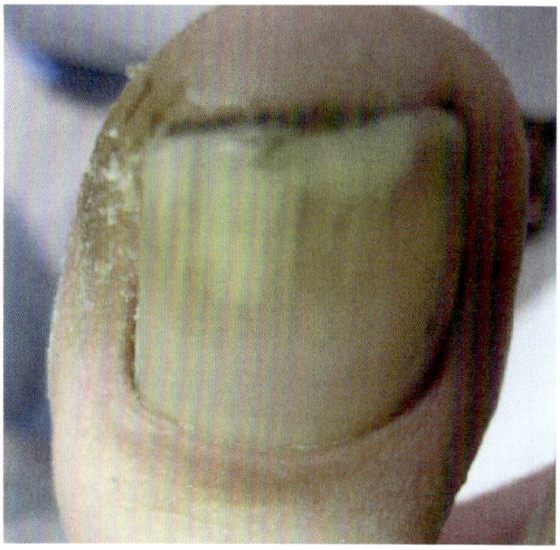

Image 3.97

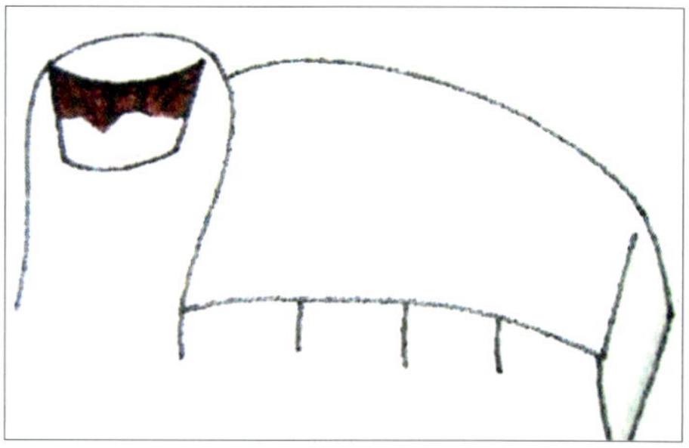

Image 3.98

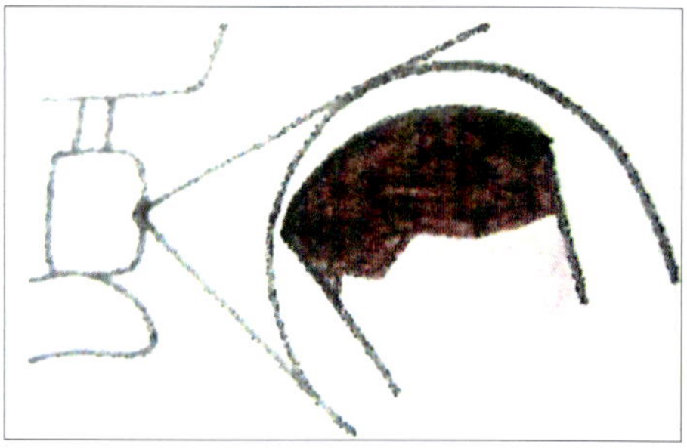

Image 3.99

Remove visible spots and stripes on the mycotic nail with a grinding tool (images 3.100 to 3.105).

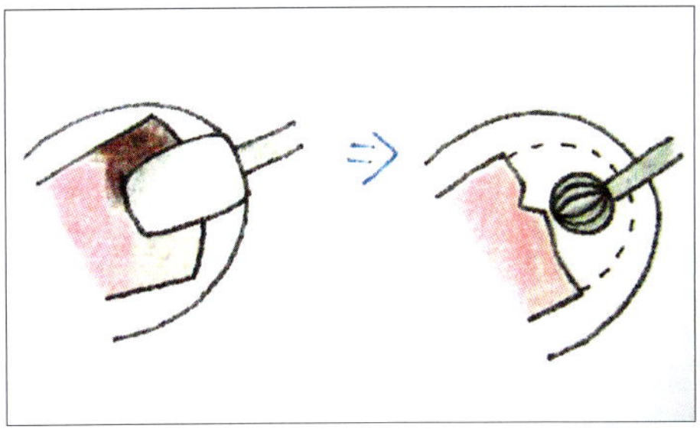
Image 3.100

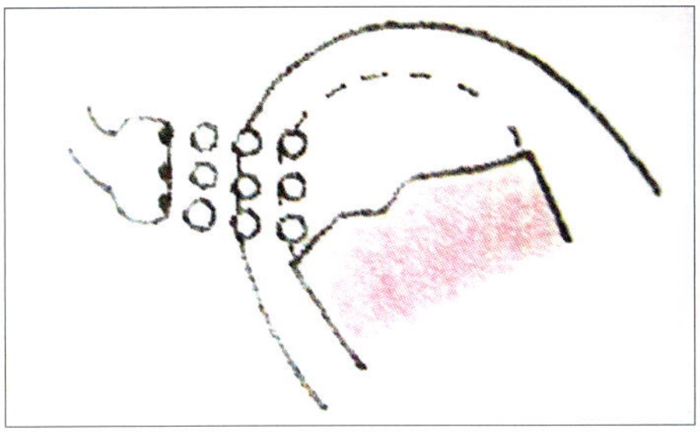
Image 3.101

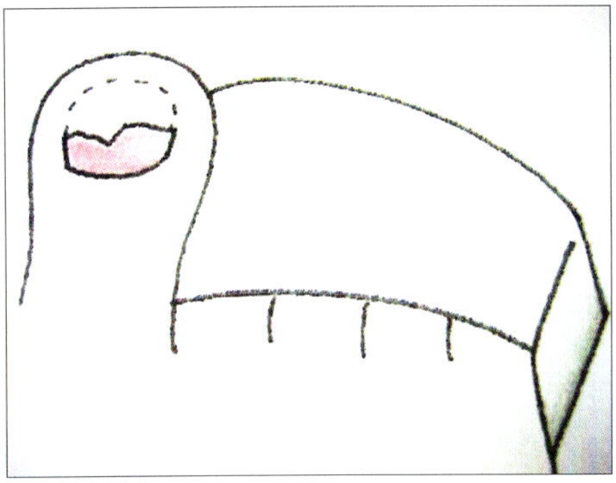
Image 3.102

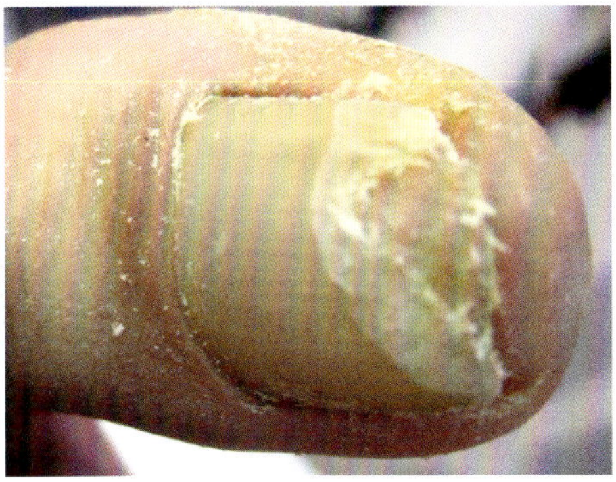
Image 3.103

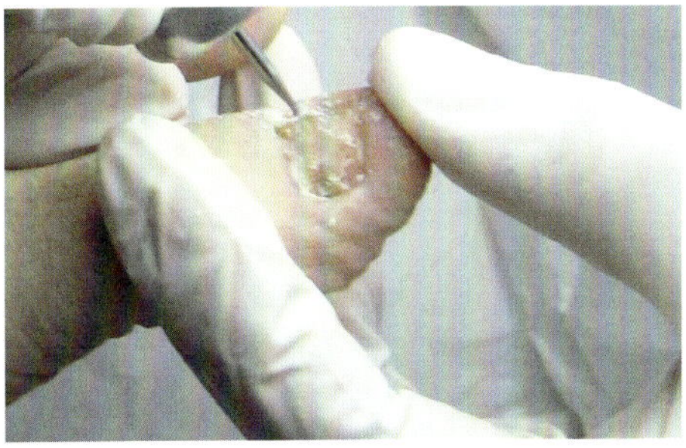
Image 3.104

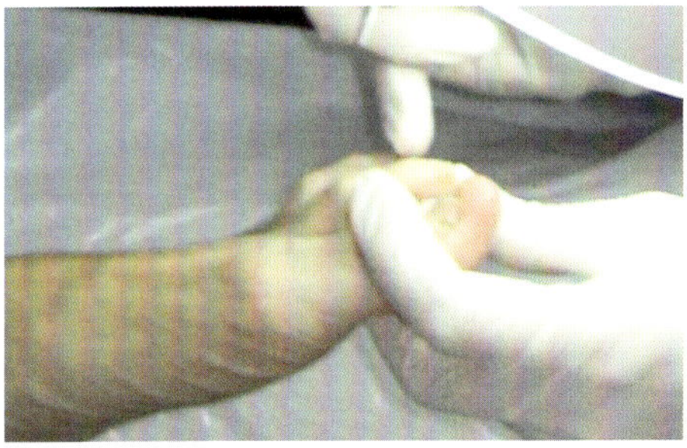
Image 3.105

Rinse the nail with a 3% hydrogen solution (images 3.106 to 3.109) using a disposable syringe and irrigation cannula to ensure thorough rinsing.

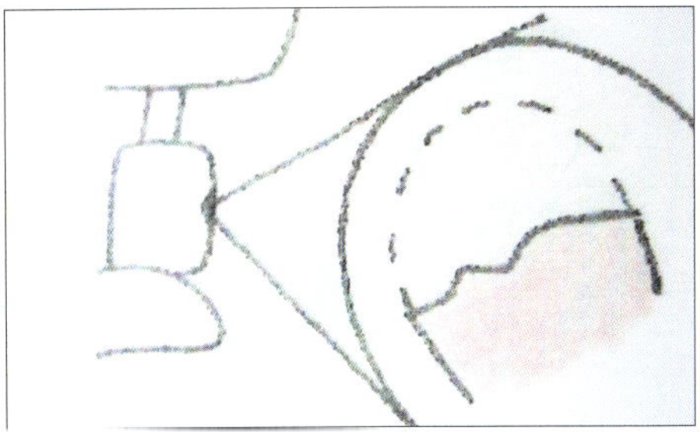
Image 3.106 Disinfect the nail

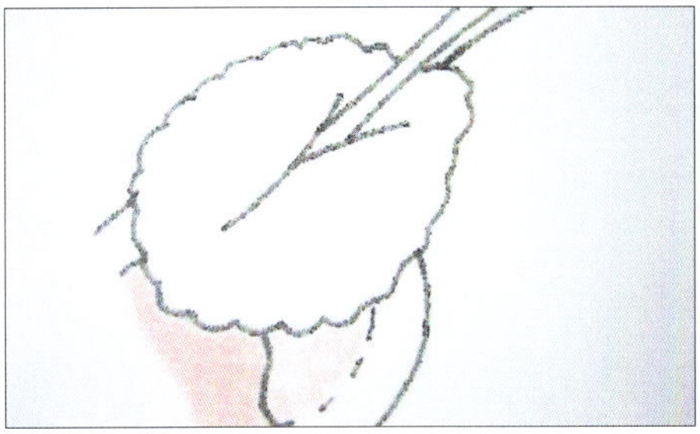
Image 3.107 Clean the nail

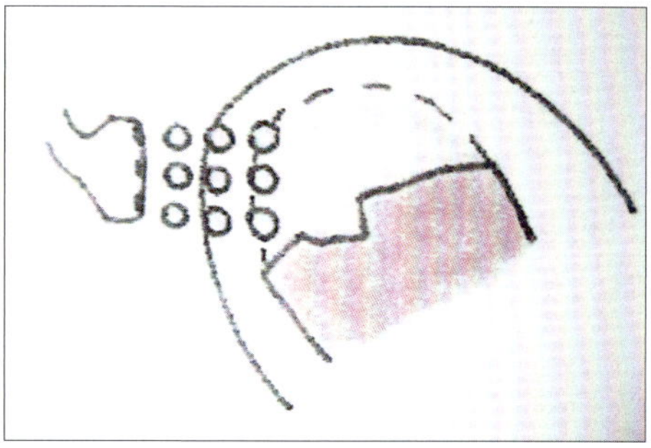

Image 3.108 Rinse with a 3% hydrogen peroxide solution

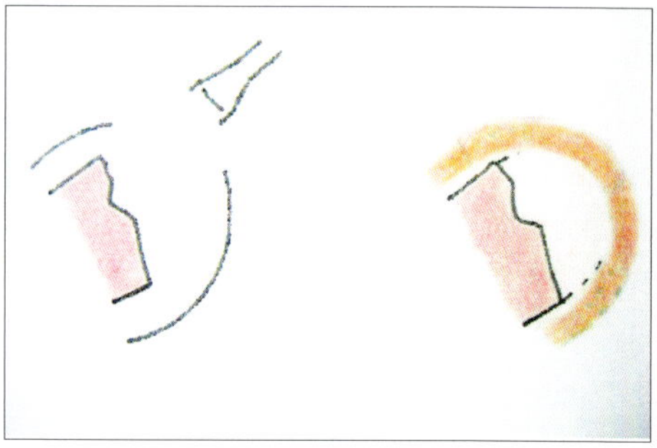

Image 3.109 Carefully remove loose nail particles

Occlusive dressing with an application of a 40% urea ointment (images 3.110 to 3.116).

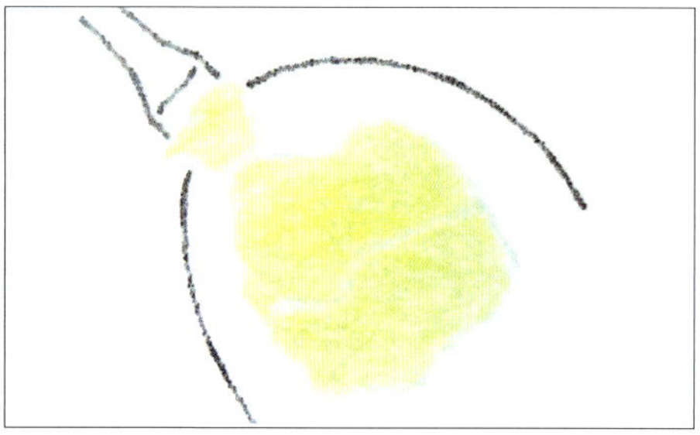

Image 3.110 Apply a 40% urea ointment on the nail

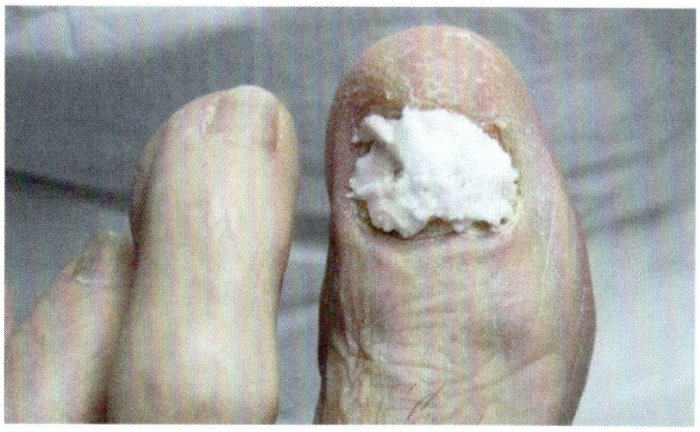

Image 3.111 Apply a 40% urea ointment on the nail

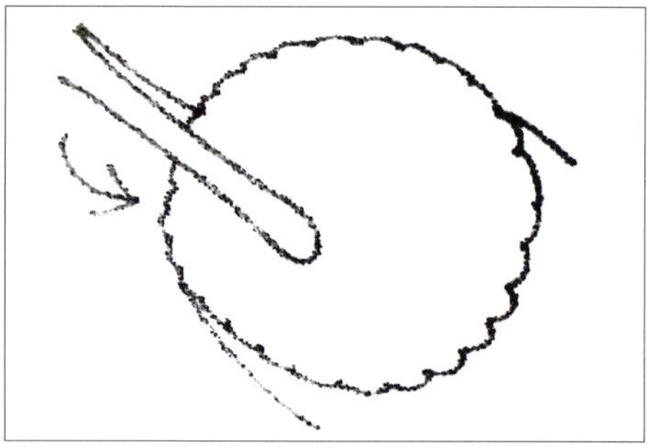

Image 3.112 Cover the nail with Copoline or a gauze compress

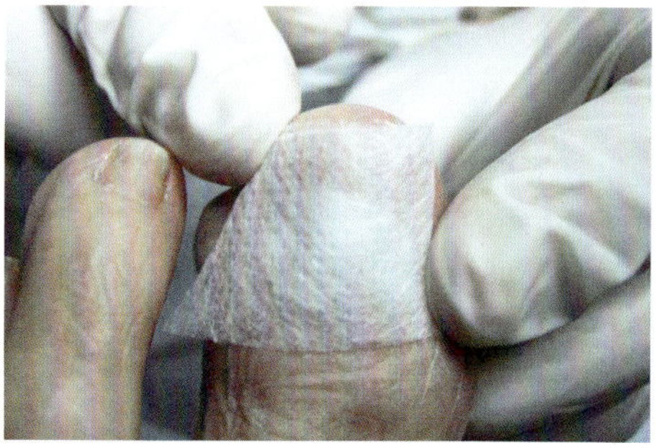

Image 3.113 Cover the nail with Copoline or a gauze compress

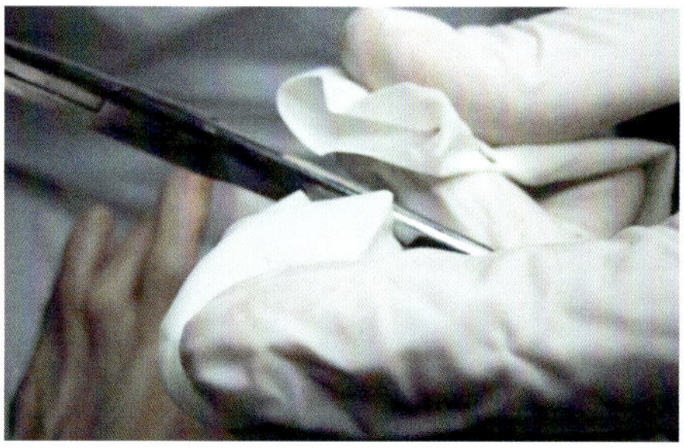

Image 3.114 Cut the tip of a glove in half

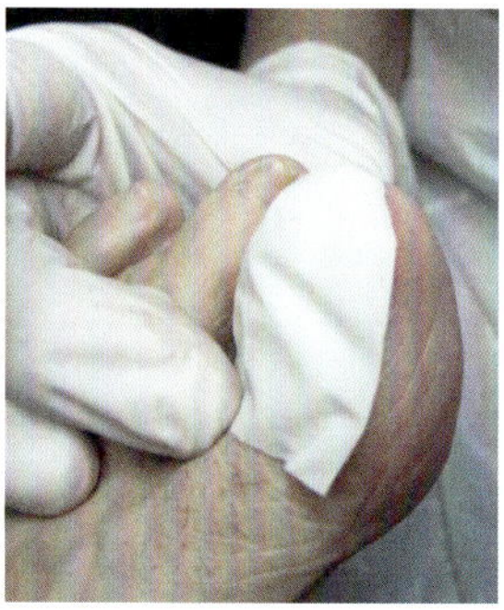

Image 3.115 Place the glove piece on the dress-ing

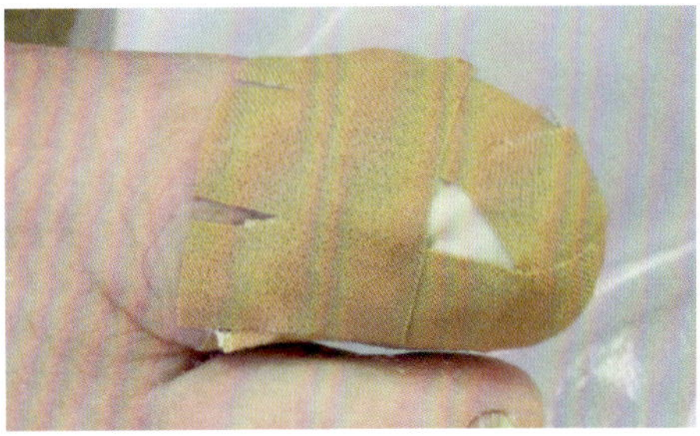

Image 3.116 Secure with Leucoplast

For an occlusive dressing you need a disposable glove, scissors, a spatula, a 40% urea ointment (prepared at the pharmacy), gauze compresses and Leukoplast (Leukosilk or a similar anti-allergic bandage for patients suffering from allergies). Cut the tip of the glove in half so that it only covers the nail, not the entire toe. Cut the gauze compress to fit the nail. Distribute the 40% urea ointment with a spatula over the entire nail area, apply the gauze compress, cover with the half glove tip and secure everything with Leukoplast or a similar bandage. The patient must ensure that the dressing does not get wet for the duration of the treatment. Schedule a follow-up visit two days later during which all loosened nail particles are removed with a nail nipper, excavator (double-end instrument), small grinding burs followed by thoroughly rinsing with a 3% hydrogen peroxide solution or octenisept (image 3.101).

Should there be still any sign of mycosis, repeat the above procedure until all infected nail particles can be painlessly removed. The aftercare involves an application of an antimycotic agent, such as Spirularin® nail serum, to be applied by the patient once or twice daily. To protect the nail bed the patient must wear a toe tip bandage.

Alternative method

Remmele offers mycotic nail removal products that are especially suitable for diabetic patients.

Cleaning the nail with propolis spray and applying propolis solution loosens even tough hornification and facilitates the swift and efficient removal of infected nail particles (images 3.117 and 3.118).

The infected nail parts are easily removed within three minutes and the use of Propolis solution reduces the risk of bacterial infection (image 3.119).

Seal the nail with Propolis solution before it undergoes additional treatment. Its extraordinary properties ensure that the skin stays elastic, water resistant and allows the skin to breath.

Removing infected nail particles increases the effectiveness of medicinal products that will be applied by the patient. Motivating the patient to consistently follow recommended aftercare procedures ensures successful treatment results.

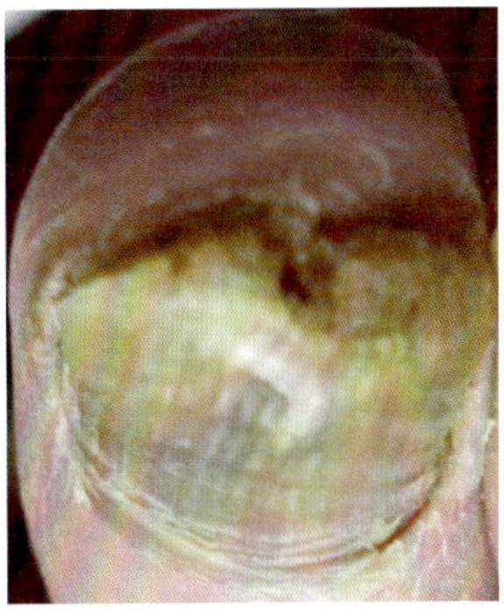

Image 3.117 TDO

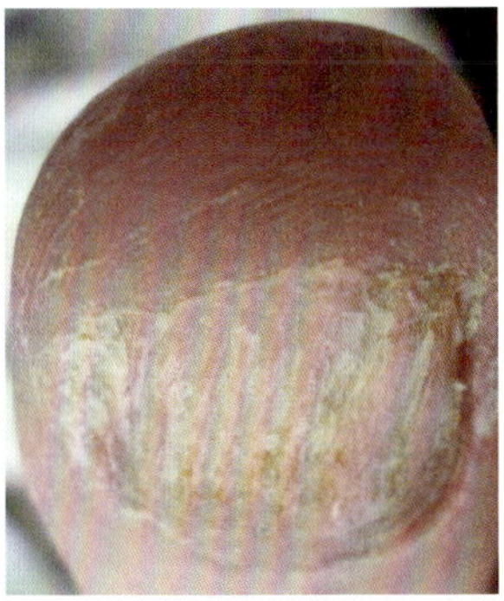

Image 3.118 Bloodless removal of a nail with propolis

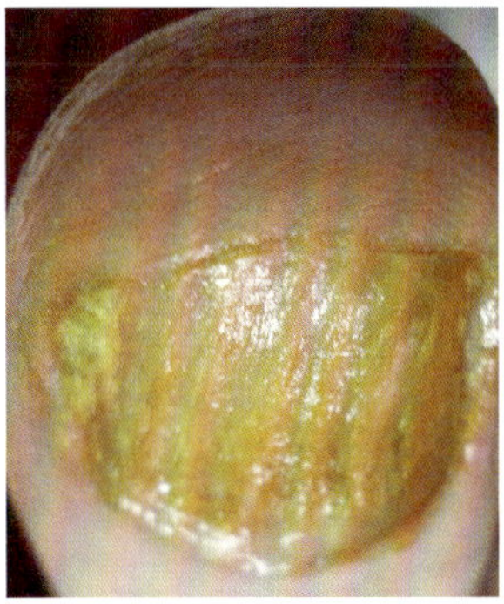

Image 3.119 Sealing the nail with propolis

(Image 3.117 – 3.119 Remmele Seibt)

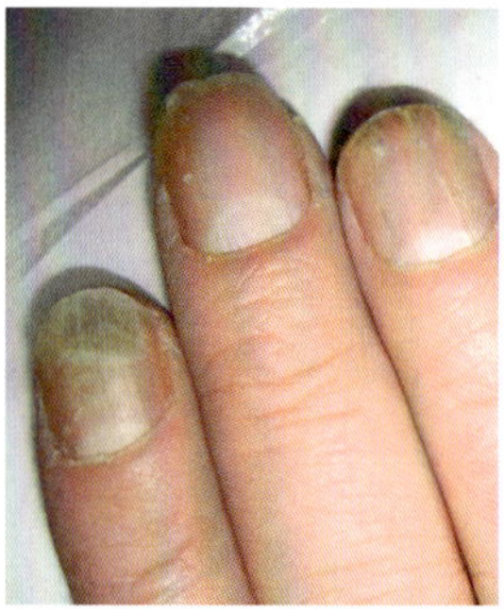

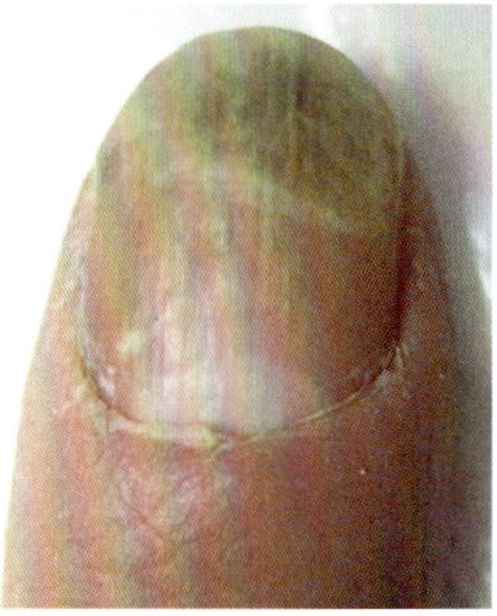

Images 3.120 and 3.121 DSO on a fingernail

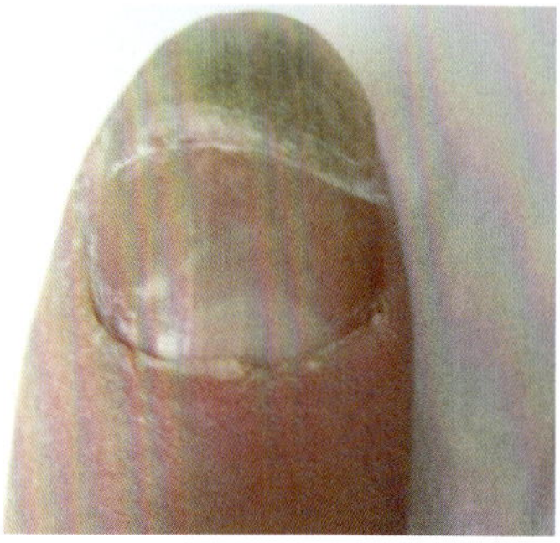

Image 3.122 Rosehead bur line separating the healthy nail part from the infected one

Additional treatment options for nail mycosis

Create a visible line with a rosehead bur separating the healthy part of the nail from the mycotic part and focus the antimycotic treatment on the infected part of the nail (3.120 to 3.122).

This method serves as a visual guideline to see if the mycosis has spread or if it has been controlled. The patient must continue the treatment to ensure successful healing results.

Should the patient refuse the grinding off of the infected nail part, then small holes are drilled into the nail with a rosehead bur; it is important that the holes along the transition line between healthy and infected nail are close together so that an antimycotic medication is most effective. Again, the patient's cooperation is important to prevent further spreading of the mycosis.

A new treatment option offers the **PACT® nail fungus therapy** which is a photodynamic antimicrobial therapy (www.hahnmedicalsystems.com). This revolutionary method of treatment involves the interaction of light with a photosensitive agent to effectively kill off microorganisms, such as bacteria and fungi, on skin surfaces and toenails. A special non-toxic dye (phenothiazine) is selectively stimulated with light at a wavelength of 6,300 nm so it kills off fungi by forming singlet oxygen without harming the skin. Stimulation is performed using the specially developed PACT® MED device, because light intensity, wavelength and light treatment time must be matched exactly to the dye gel to be effective.

Start by grinding off the mycotic parts of the nail (image 3.123). Should the patient disapprove, roughening the surface is also effective. Apply PACT® nail fungus gel to the affected nail generously so that the gel covers the entire nail and is allowed to act for approximately 10 minutes (image 3.124). Then treat with light using the PACT® MED light for 9.5 minutes (image 3.125).

Repeat the treatment two times leaving one or two days in between treatments. In cases of severe infection, use twice daily for several days.

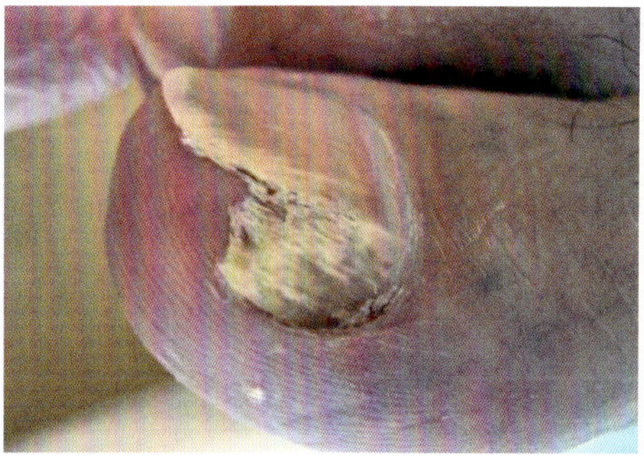

Image 3.123

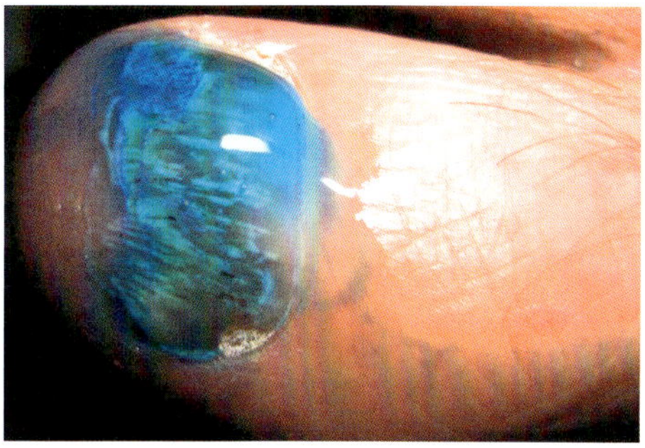

Image 3.124

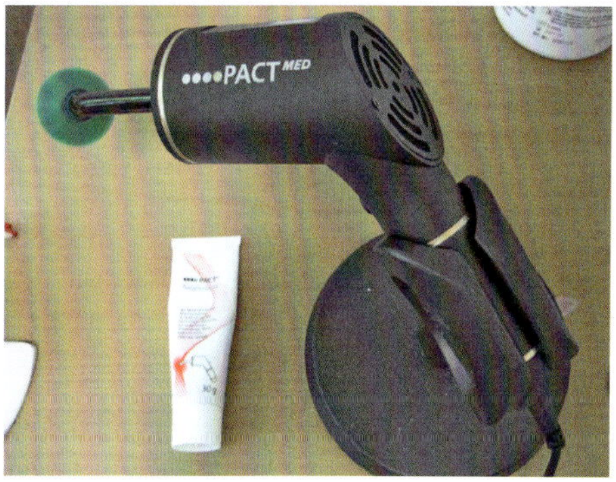

Image 3.125

End of treatment

The effectiveness can only be assessed after a lengthy period because the affected part of the nail must grow out (approx. 3 months). If the affected part of the nail fails to grow out and spreads towards the nail wall, the application should be repeated and prolonged if necessary.

It is recommended the PACT® nail fungus therapy be repeated every six months for 9.5 minutes as a preventative measure.

The patient must apply an antimycotic ointment (e.g., containing spirulina algae) after the first treatment to promote healing until a healthy nail has regrown. This can take up to several years in patients with a slow nail growth rate.

Hygiene instructions

Following proper hygiene guidelines is crucial. Use an approved disinfection agent to properly protect you, the patient and the other patients from contagion.

Always wear gloves, a face mask (preferably one with a filter) and a disposable apron or smock.

A nail infected with mould fungus must always be removed due to the high reproduction rate of that type of fungus. It is highly contagious and dangerous since mould spores can enter the lungs.

An antimycotic treatment will be effective only after the nail has been removed (image 3.126). Most OTC medications such as Clotrimazole, Itraconazole, Fluconazole and Bifonazole contain fungistatic azole.

The main substance of Spirularin nail serum, Peclavus Spirularin and CuraMar is the enzyme chitinase that derives from spirulina algae, a species of blue algae. This enzyme destroys the chitin of fungi and spores and kills them. The effect has been scientifically proven.

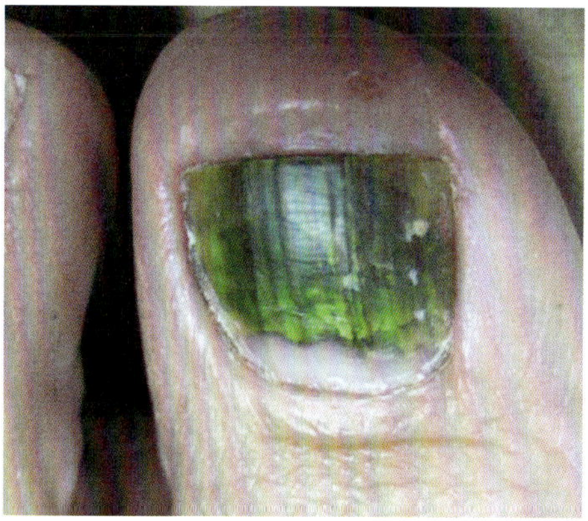

Image 3.126 Mould fungus

- **Spirularin nail serum**: Apply a small drop two times daily on all ten nails and the surrounding skin.
- **Peclavus spirulina lotion**: Apply a small drop two times daily on all ten nails and the surrounding skin. Do not use oily creams or nail oils.
- **Propolis solution**: Apply two to three times daily.
- **Gehwol med** nail protection pen: Apply two times daily.
- **Peclavus AntiMyx**: Apply two to three times daily and allow to be completely absorbed.
- **Allpresan** nail tincture: Spray the nail two times daily.
- **Arendt** nail tincture A6: Apply two times daily.
- **Sixtus** nail protection liquid or cream: Apply two times daily.
- **Mycored spray** (Caution: Can irritate the throat!), pipette bottle Mycored Forte Cream: Apply two times daily.
- **Camillen** Fudes solution
- **Yavatop solution:** Apply two times daily.
- **ProntoMan gel:** Apply two times daily.
- **Tea tree oil:** Apply morning and evening (Caution: May cause allergic reaction!).
- **Zalain nail patch:** Cut the patch to cover the entire nail. Replace once a week.

The following substances with an antimycotic effect are available as a medicinal product. They either destroy fungi or inhibit its growth:

- **Allylamine**: Naftifin and Terbinafin, fight skin and nail fungus, topical application.
- **Azole**: Bifonazole, Clotrimazole, Econazole and Isoconazole, topical application Fluconazole and Itraconazole, taken orally.
- **Hydroxopyridone-Derivate:** Ciclopirox and Octopriox, in nail polish, lotions and solutions, topical application.
- **Morpholine-Derivate**: Amorolfin, in nail polish, topical application.

Prophylaxis

Improving the condition of the skin is equally important. That includes eliminating hyperhidrosis (sweaty feet):

- Peclavus silver bath: promotes nail growth with organic silicon and zinc (e.g., Hair & Nails by Ocean Pharma)
- tap water iontophoresis.
- salt water foot bath: dissolve two teaspoons of table salt or preferably Dead Sea salt in one glass of water and add to a foot bath (plastic bucket or tub); one or two times daily.
- apple cider vinegar: effective during mycosis treatment and fights hyperhidrosis
- add 30 g sage and 30 g agrimonia root (available at the pharmacy) to two glasses of white wine and boil for 20 minutes; let cool and submerge the foot in this decoction several times.

Herbs with an antifungal effect:

- garlic (allium sativum)
- ginger (zingiber officinale)
- liquorice root (glycyrrhiza glabra)
- honey myrtle (melaleuca, different species)
- camomile oil
- echinacea (different species)
- orangeroot (hydrastis)
- lemon grass oil
- oregano oil
- cinnamon
- antimycotic tea blends: fennel, peppermint, cinnamon, orange, black currant, sage, thyme, spearmint
- dill, estragon, basil, red clover, lemon
- saffron root

To restore the skin's acid protective layer skin function lotions with an antimycotic substance have been proven to be very effective (e.g., Spirularin gel, Spirularin mousse, Peclavus foot cream, tea tree oil, Peclavus sensitive lotion, Silver foot cream, Remmele's Propolis balm, Allpresan pedicure antimycotic mousse, Gehwol foot care green, Akilëine anti-transpirant cream, Callusan Fresh, Sixtus foot balm Forte plus, Peclavus foot cream sensitive, foot balm with eczema protection, Pedibaehr cream mousse with clotrimazole).

Improving blood circulation to promote cell growth is just as important as strengthening the immune system. However, a well-balanced diet, preventing micro traumas caused by improper footwear, wearing clean socks, changing towels and bath mats frequently, wearing bath sandals even in the water, taking contrast baths, sauna visits, reduced sugar intake, proper foot care, drying between the toes, applying sheep wool between the toes, foot exercises and applications with antimicrobial cinnamon oil and bark are equally important to combat mycosis and promote healing.

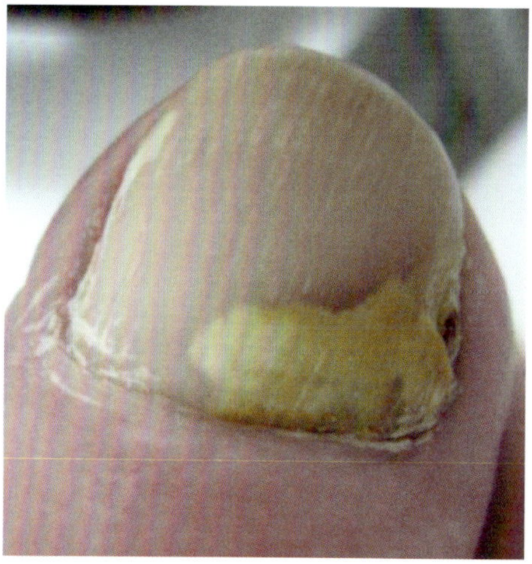

Image 3.127 PSO

Patient case

A 73-year-old patient with cardiac insufficiency and large oedemas on the lower legs suffered from proximal subungual onychomycosis (PSO). The infected nail was removed followed by an application of CuraMar lotion twice daily. After four weeks, the infection was under control and ten months later a healthy nail had regrown. Conclusion: A mycotic infection is curable with consistent treatment (images 3.127 to 3.132).

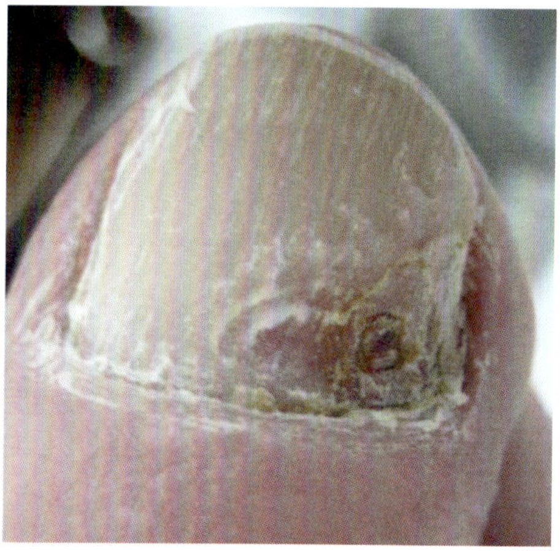

Image 3.128 After the removal of the infected nail parts

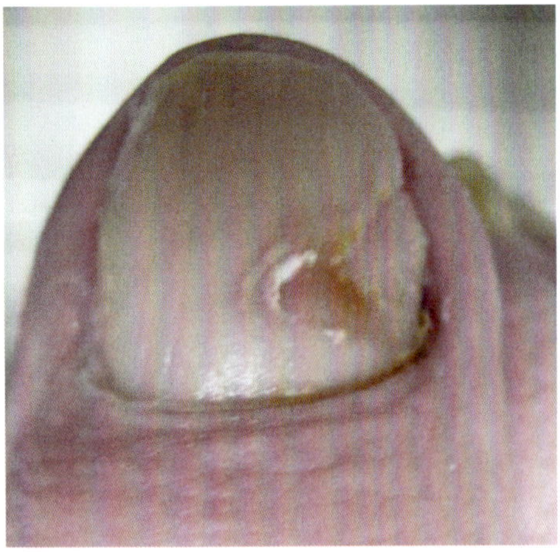

Image 3.129 After a four-week treatment with CuraMar lotion

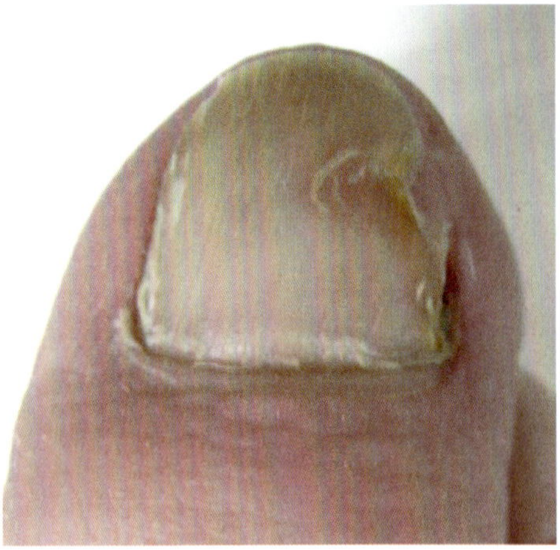

Image 3.130 After six months' consistent treatment with CuraMar lotion

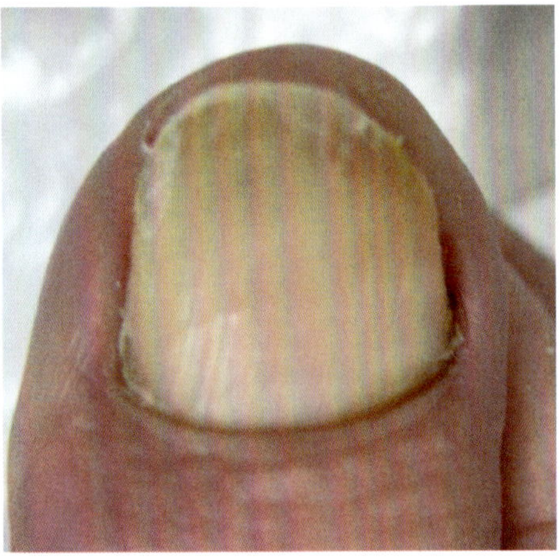

Image 3.131 and 3.132
After ten months, the nail has completely regrown

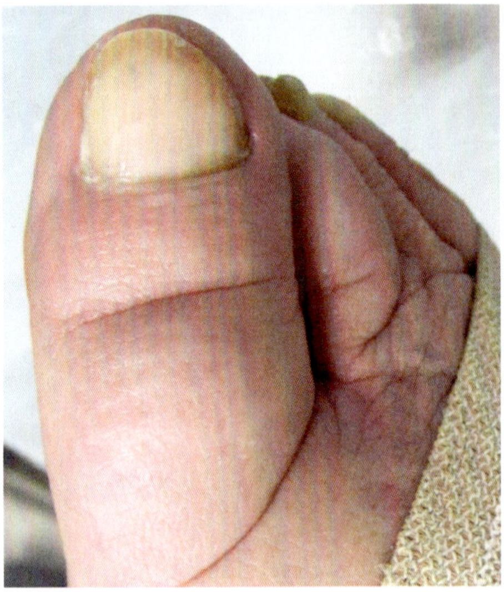

Image 3.132

Patient Questionnaire

Foot and nail fungus
Are you at risk?

Have you noticed skin changes on your feet in the last four weeks?

☐ Yes ☐ No

Is the area between your toes itchy?

☐ Yes ☐ No

Do you feel a burning sensation in certain areas of your feet or/and is the skin red?

☐ Yes ☐ No

Did you notice a change in colour of one or more nails?

☐ Yes ☐ No

Did you notice small spots in your nails?

☐ Yes ☐ No

Do you use disinfection sprays in public pools?

☐ Yes ☐ No

Do you wear bath sandals in public pools or in the sauna?

☐ Yes ☐ No

Do you frequently stay in hotels (more than ten times a year)?

☐ Yes ☐ No

Do you dry the area between your toes after showering or bathing?

☐ Yes ☐ No

Did any family member suffer from mycotic nail or foot infection?

☐ Yes ☐ No

We will gladly assist you with filling out this questionnaire and answer all your questions foot health and health maintenance.

Information for the patient

Nail mycosis
Often diagnosed too late and widespread

It is considered the wolf in sheep's clothing of fungal infections: nail mycosis. Harmless looking changes in the colour of toe and finger nails are often the first sign of one of the most stubborn mycotic infections of the skin. Most people misread the first symptoms believing that it is a small injury caused by wearing improper footwear or the result of irritating nail polish. This misconception can have serious consequences: allowing the infection to spread can destroy the nail, resulting in nail loss.

More than just an esthetic flaw

Nail mycosis is a highly contagious and irritating infection because the nail plate does not only protect the sensitive tips of toes or fingers but serves also as a protection shield for spreading fungus. Once pathogens have colonized the nail area, a radical and thorough treatment is the only option to destroy them.

Various fungus species (filamentous fungi, yeast and mould fungi) trigger a nail infection, the same fungi that cause mycotic foot and skin infections; toenails are four times more often affected than fingernails as a result of an incorrectly performed foot fungus treatment.

Many people are not aware that they have a mycotic infection since it is usually painless at the beginning. The first signs are believed to be minor harmless injuries and are left untreated allowing the fungus to destroy larger parts of the nail.

One in five people is affected by nail mycosis

17% of the adults in western industrial societies, approximately ten million men and women, suffer from mycotic nail infections making it a widespread health issue. In some segments of the population the percentage is significantly higher. Circulatory disorders often seen in the elderly and diabetics pose an increased risk of mycotic foot and nail infection.

The following individuals must be especially cautious when it comes to the health of their nails:

- people over 50
- people infected with nail mycosis
- diabetics
- people suffering from circulatory disorder on their hands and feet
- athletes who expose their feet to extreme mechanical strain

We gladly assist you with all your concerns regarding foot health and health maintenance.

3.6 Psoriasis nails

Definition
Nail changes due to psoriasis (images 3.133a to 3.135)

Appearance
- pitted nails (shallow, pinhead-size dents located on the nail surface)
- onycholysis (mostly in the centre of the nail) with a yellowish margin (oil stain)
- irregular thickening of the nail plate, the dorsal layer of the nail is brittle and loose
- white patches
- crumbling nail substance
- onycholysis semilunaris
- increased or decreased curvature of the nail
- beading
- subungual hyperkeratosis

Cause
Psoriasis is a systemic disorder.

Pathogenesis
Psoriasis is an immunologically inflammatory skin disease which can have a genetic component and is sometimes brought on by certain risk factors. The affected skin is red and sometimes itchy and can be covered with silver or whitish scales. Normally it only affects certain areas of the body. It is especially common on the elbows and knees, on the lower back and on the scalp and it can affect individual nails or all nails.

Differential diagnosis
- onychomycosis
- onychauxis

Complications
- nail damage caused by incorrect treatment
- clavus formation caused by pressure and friction
- decay of the entire nail plate
- nail infection (secondary infection)
- micro-abscesses

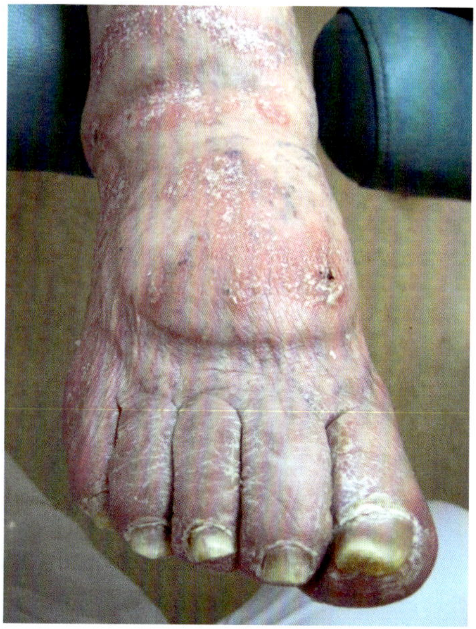

Image 3.133 a Psoriatic foot with psoriatic nails

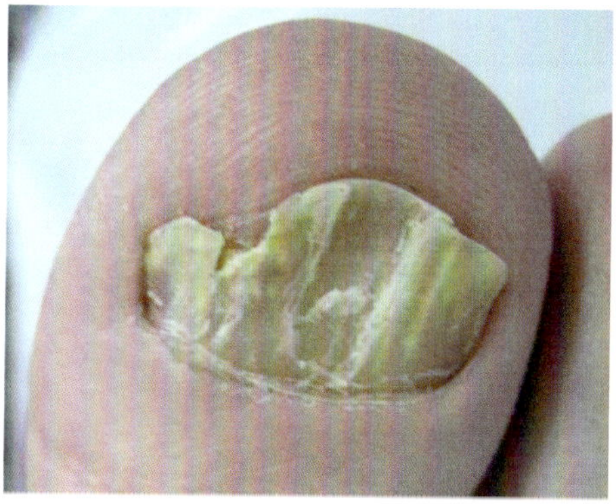

Image 3.133 b Psoriatic nail with onychomycosis, onychorrhexis, onychoschizia and onycholysis

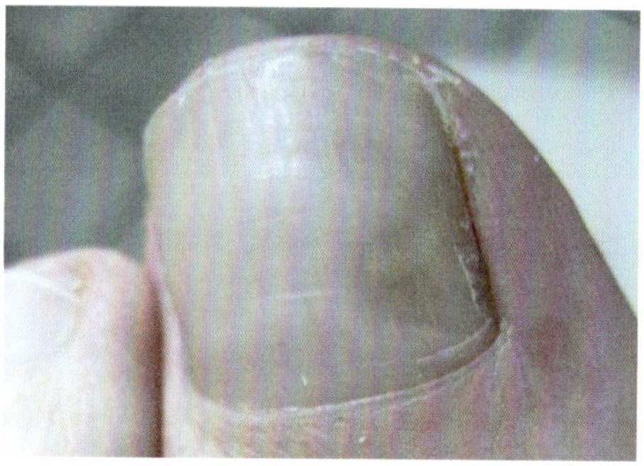

Image 3.134 Oil stain nail

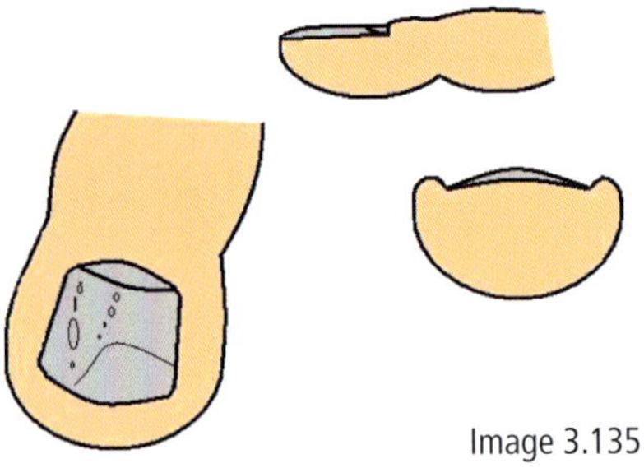

Image 3.135

Treatment

Careful filing or grinding of the nail surface is sufficient to prevent brittle nail particles from getting caught on clothing. If necessary, a nail prosthetic can be applied. In case onychomycosis is present, it must be treated first. Bamboo, common horsetail, zinc and organic silicon taken orally strengthen the nail.

Prophylaxis

- avoid additional irritation
- professional foot care
- mycosis phrophylaxis
- Peclavus nail groove filler
- sea salt foot baths (add 1 tbs. of salt to a foot bath)

3.7 Koilonychia
(Greek: koilos = hollow)

Definition

Hollow nail or spoon nail. Abnormally thin nails which have lost their convexity, becoming concave in shape (drop test) and which may be brittle and chip or break easily (images 3.136 and 3.137a and b).

Appearance

Gradually flattening nail plate that develops into a concave shape. The nail surface appears polished. Iron deficiency causes the nail to become thin and soft.

Causes

- chronic iron deficiency
- circulatory disorders (Raynaud's disease)
- vitamin deficiency (vitamin B2 and C).
- trauma
- genetic factors
- anemia
- incorrectly performed orthonyxia treatment
- diabetes mellitus
- psoriasis

Treatment

In young children koilonychia is often a temporary condition. In adults, the nail usually regenerates itself once an iron or vitamin deficiency has been cured and glucose levels are normalized. Trimming the

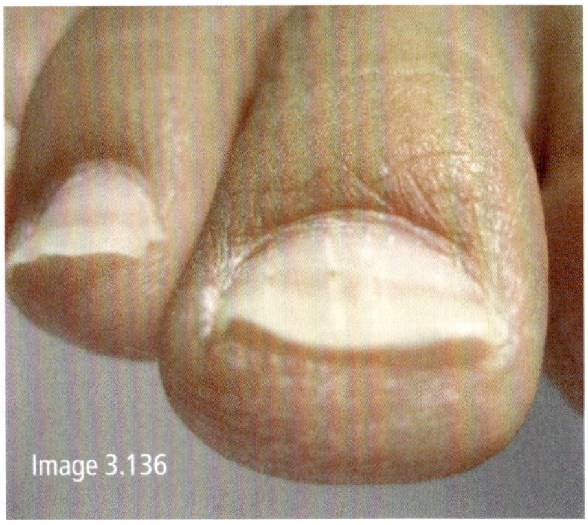

Image 3.136

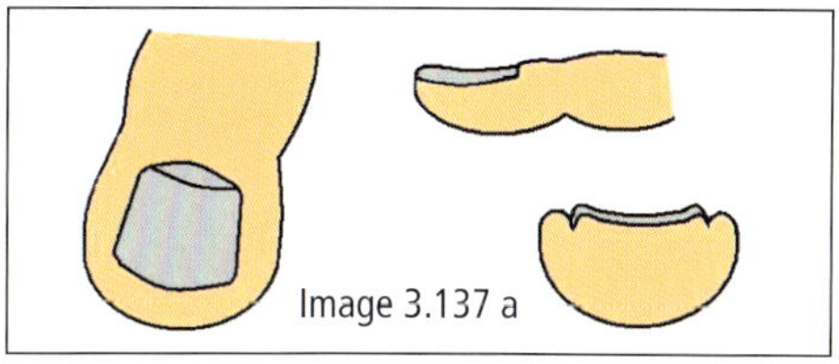

Image 3.137 a

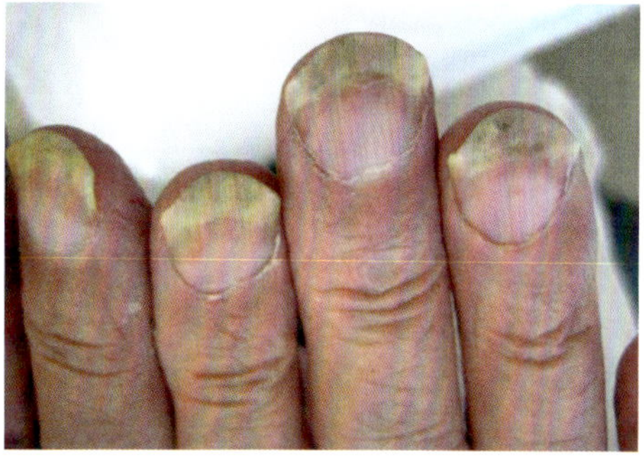

Image 3.137 b Psoriatic fingernails with koilonychia

nail edges regularly and correcting the tension and position of nail braces also achieves treatment success.

Prophylaxis

- healthy nutrition
- blood circulation stimulation

3.8 Leukonychia
(Greek: leukos = white)

Definition

White discolouration of the nail (images 3.138 to 3.141).

- leukonychia totalis = entire nail plate
- leukonychia punctata or striata = small dots or stripes

Causes

- minor trauma
- altered light reflection caused by impaired hornification
- small blisters in the nail substance
- heredity
- loosening of the nail plate
- contact with concentrated table salt
- symptom of poisoning
- incorrect cutting

Appearance

White discolouration of the nail spreading towards the distal edge. The nail becomes brittle and cracks.

Differential diagnosis

Onychomycosis, onycholysis and onychoschizia.

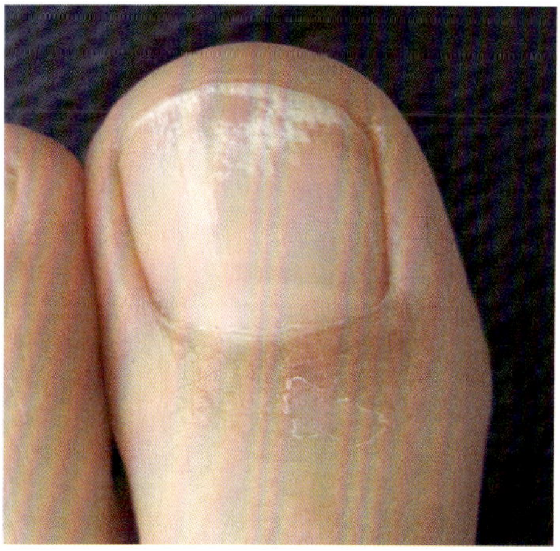

Image 3.138

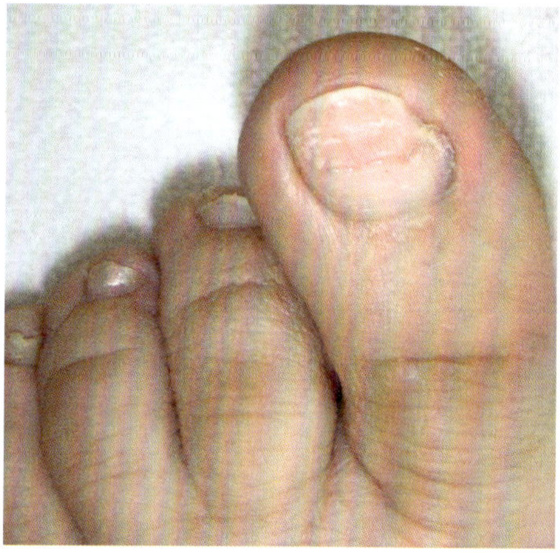

Image 3.139

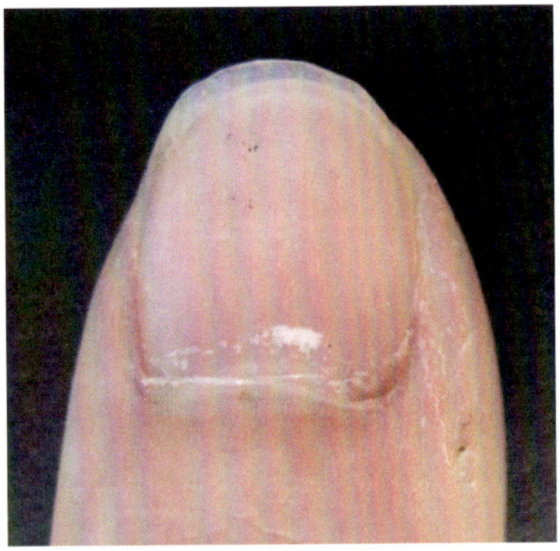

Image 3.140

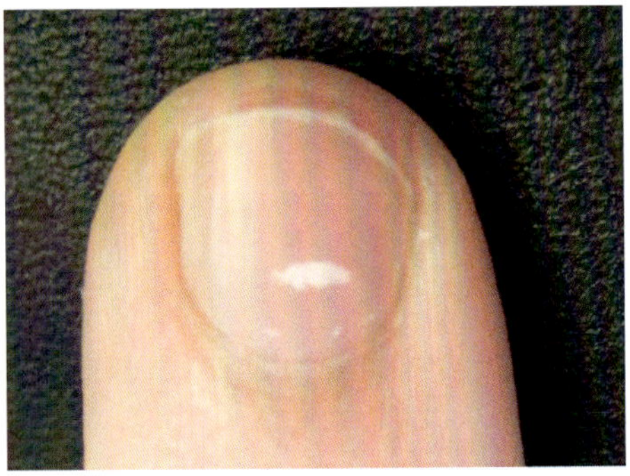

Image 3.141

Treatment

- not treatable
- treatment not necessary since the nail is otherwise healthy
- trimming the nail edges regularly
- stabilizing the nail with a prosthetic

3.9 Onychauxis
(Greek: onyx = nail, claw, auxis = growth)

Definition
Thickening of the nail without signs of deformity (images 3.142 to 3.146).

Causes
The condition is more commonly seen in older adults due to poor blood circulation in the feet causing nail growth to slow down.

Differential diagnosis
Subungual hyperkeratosis

Complications
Onychomycosis

Treatment
Filing or grinding the nail plate is only recommended if the thickened nail plate causes discomfort when wearing footwear since it makes the nail vulnerable to microorganism penetration. Furthermore, it weakens the nail leading to unguis convolutus or even unguis incarnatus.

Prophylaxis
Foot exercise to improve blood circulation.

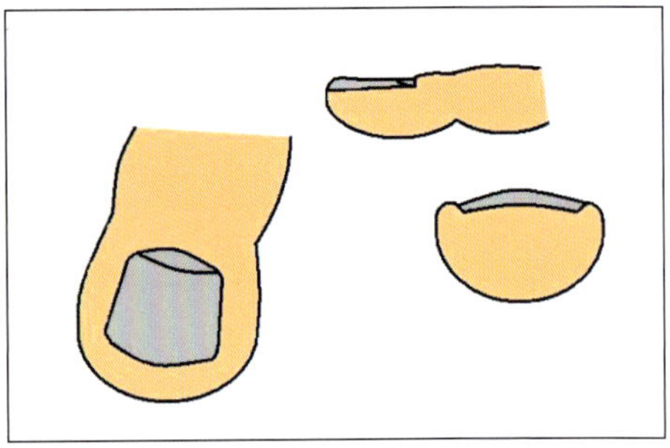

Image 3.142

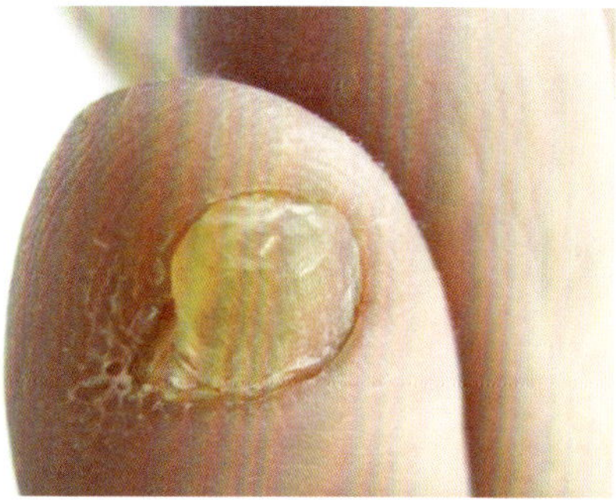

Image 3.143
Onychauxis with beginning onychophosis

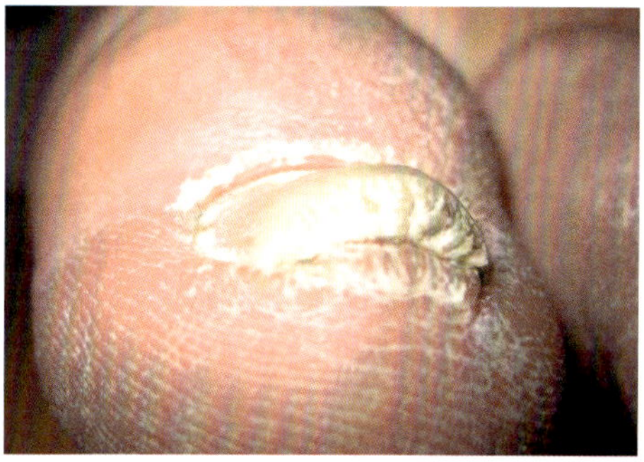

Image 3.144
Onychauxis with beginning onychomycosis

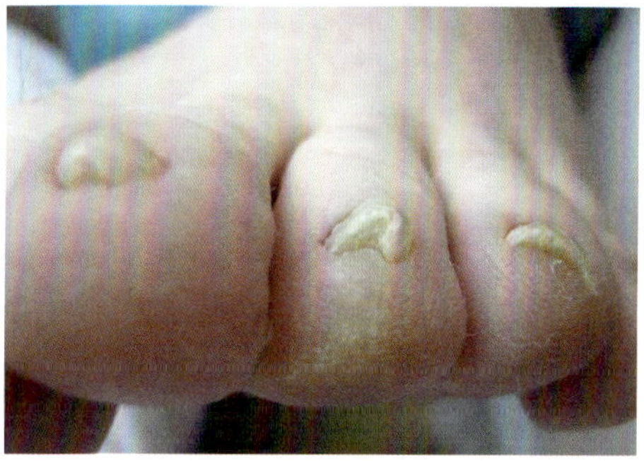

Image 3.145 Onychauxis with unguis convolutus

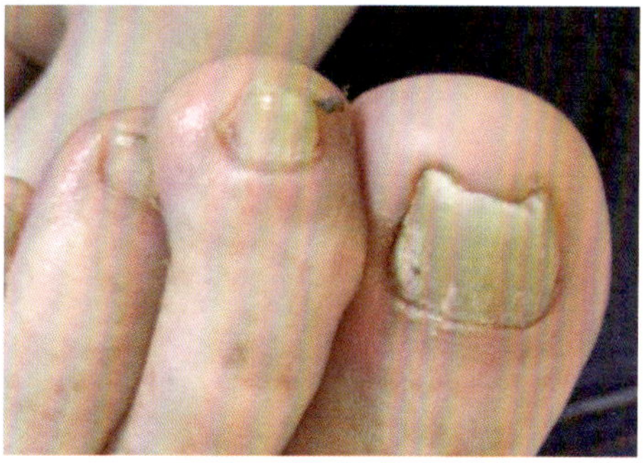

Image 3.146

3.10 Onychogryposis

(Greek: grypos = curved)
Claw nail
(images 3.147 to 3.154)

Definition
The nail resembles a claw or ram's horn and grows upwards almost completely detaching from the nail bed. The condition is often caused by trauma to the nail. The underside of the claw nail displays thick horn substances and dead epithelial cells. The nail often has a yellowish or brownish colour.

Epidemiology
Elderly people more commonly have this condition as the blood supply to the nails diminishes with age. Older weaker patients living alone (maybe single patients) often lack the strength to trim their nails properly. Only present in younger patients as a result of post-traumatic growth deformity.

Causes
Trauma or injury but also poor blood circulation and nerve damage can cause this condition. A familial presence is very rare.

Pathogenesis
The thick twisted nail grows upwards, often detaching from the nail bed.

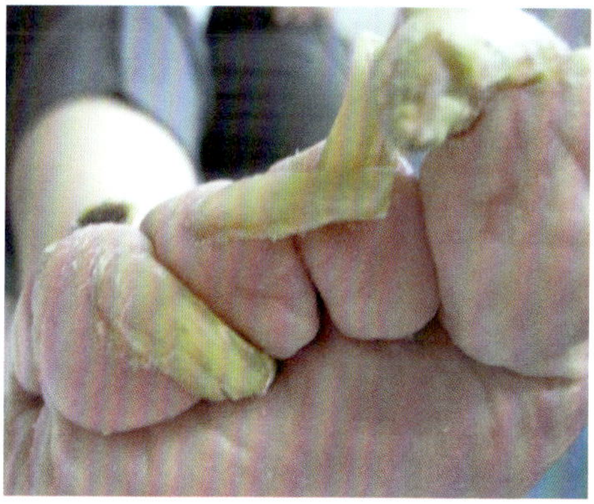

Image 3.147

Differential diagnosis
Pachyonychia

Complications
Onychomycosis, bacterial infection of the nail bed

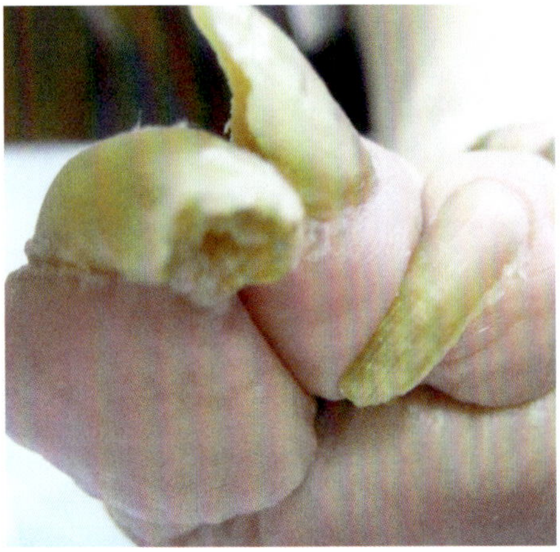

Image 3.148

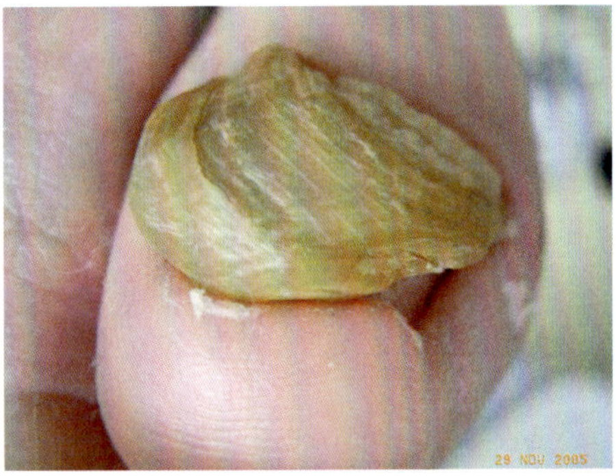

Image 3.149 Source: Rathenow

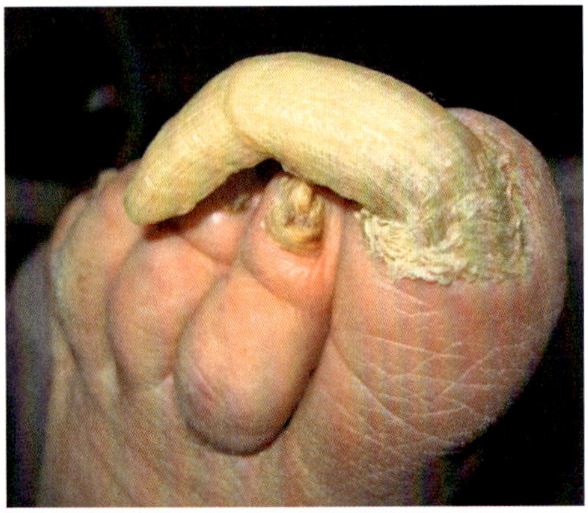

Image 3.150

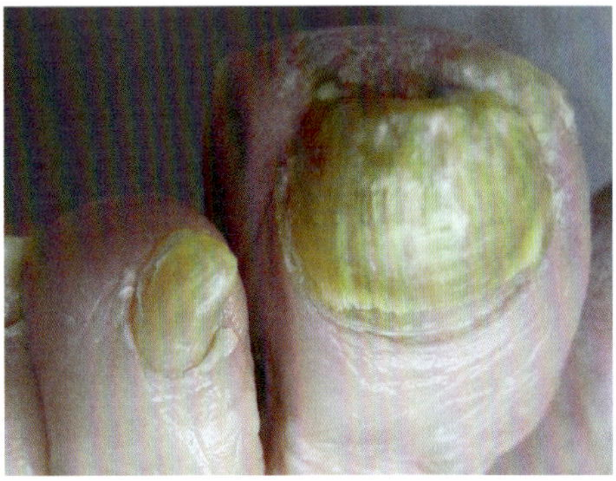

Image 3.151

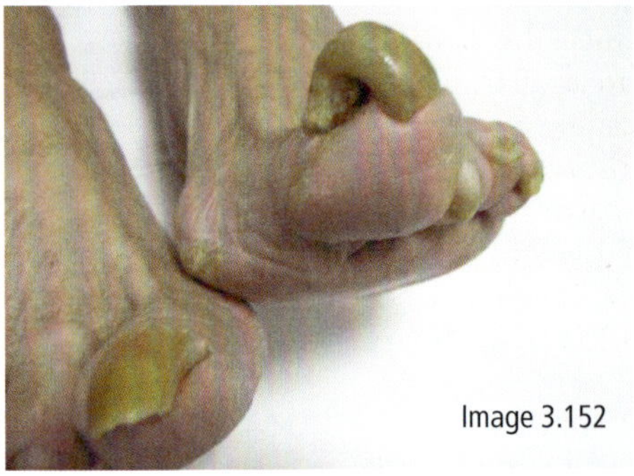

Image 3.152

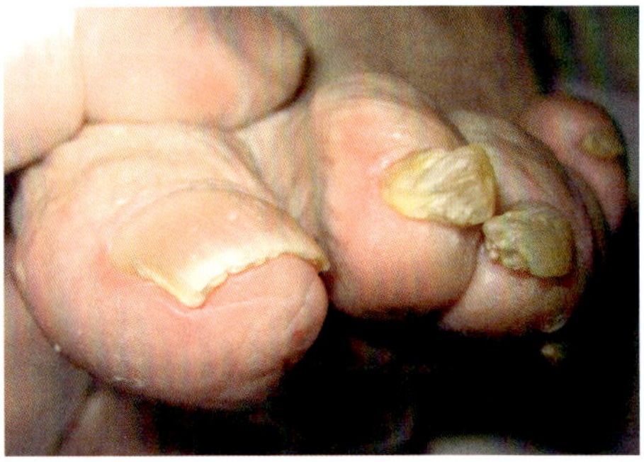

Image 3.153

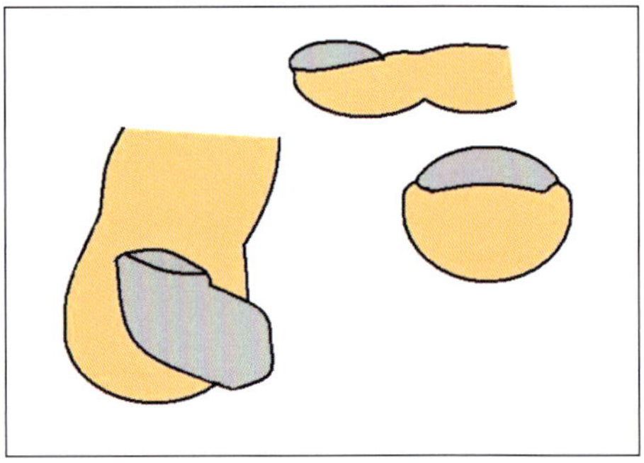

Image 3.154

Treatment

With a fissure cutter or diamond disc (image 3.157) define the new nail margin by cutting into both sides of the nail (image 3.156). Then cut the remaining part of the nail with a nail nipper. Cut the nail short enough so that it no longer protrudes past the tip of the toe. Remove nail bed hyperkeratosis only after softening it with a keratolytic agent such as Prontoman spray. Reducing the nail thickness with a carbide cutter, a rough diamond grinder or a cap grinder is also possible (image 3.158). This has to be done with caution though since the nail is often mycotic and can break apart fairly fast. A prophylactic procedure and an assessment by a dermatologist is, therefore, recommended. If no mycosis is present, a nail prosthetic can be applied to protect the nail bed. Otherwise the mycosis must be treated first (images 3.155 to 3.164).

Prophylaxis

- cut and grind the nail plate to a normal thickness, reduce any thick parts with a carbide cutter
- mycosis prophylaxis with one of the following: Spirularin nail serum, Peclavus Spirularin lotion, Antimyx protection pen, Peclavus after care tincture, Silver foot spray, foot baths with sea salt, Peclavus silver foot bath and nail oil
- foot exercise to improve blood circulation

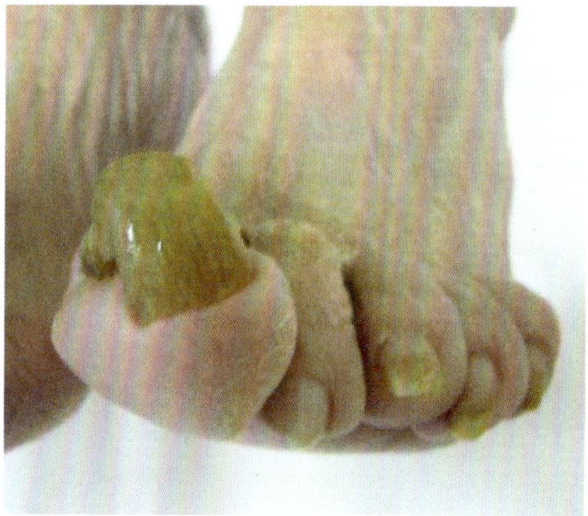

Image 3.155 Onychogryposis before the treatment

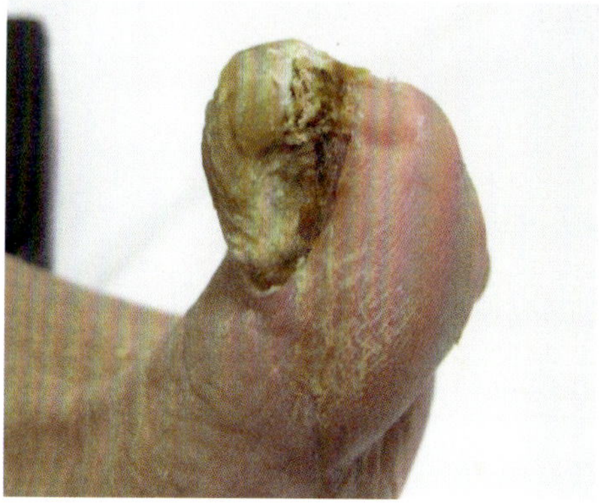

Image 3.156 Reducing the nail thickness

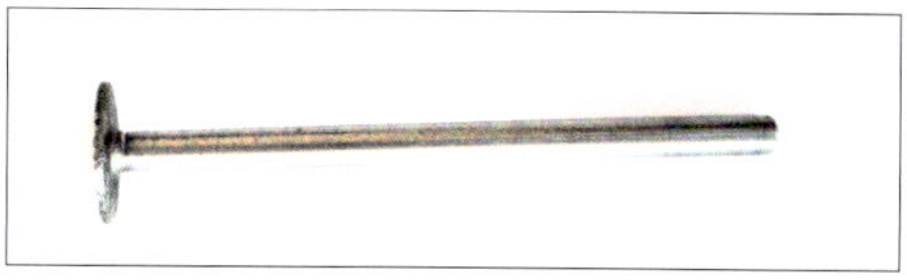

Image 3.157 Groove cutter for grypotic nails

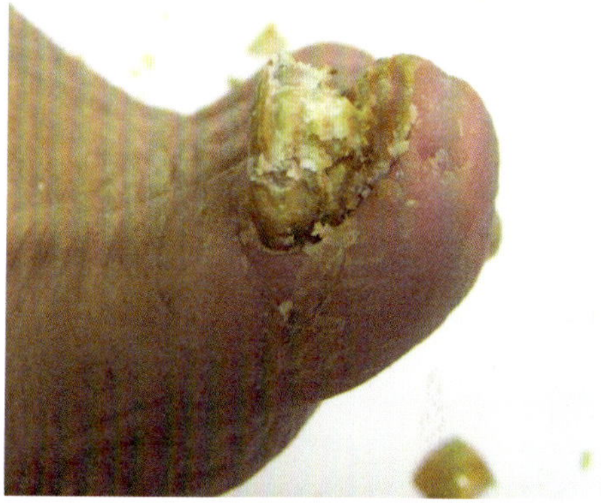

Image 3.158 Reducing the nail thickness

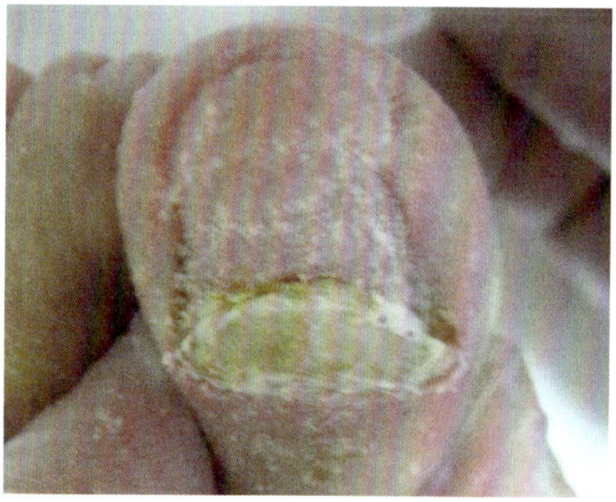

Image 3.159 The prepared nail

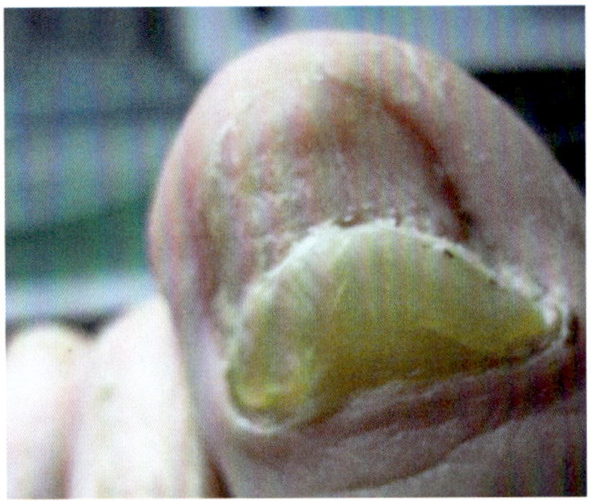

Image 3.160 After two months

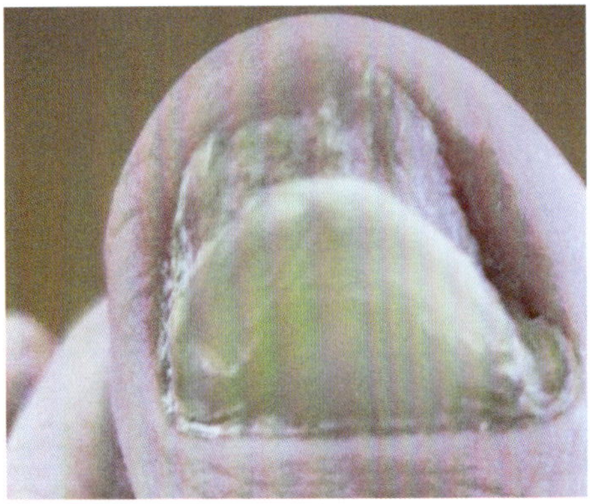

Image 3.161 After four months

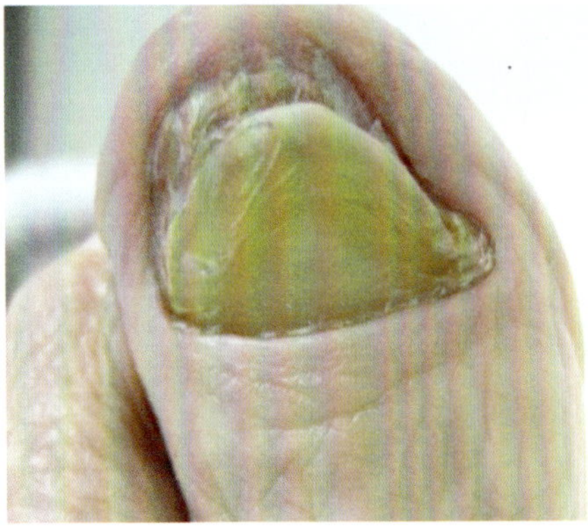

Image 3.162 After six months

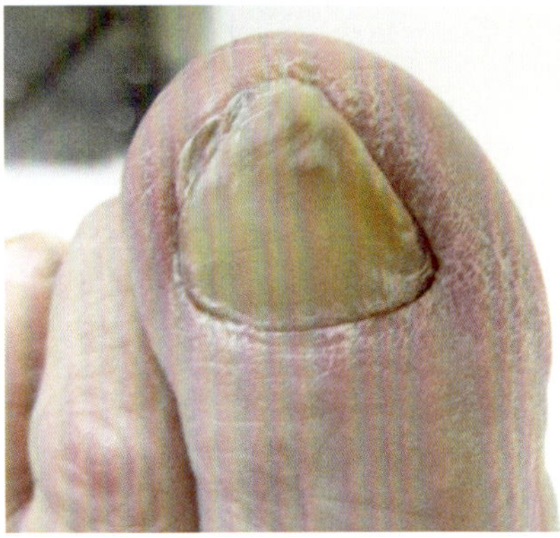

Image 3.163 After one year. The patient is 95 years old. The nail still has the tendency to thicken but there is no sign of mycosis.

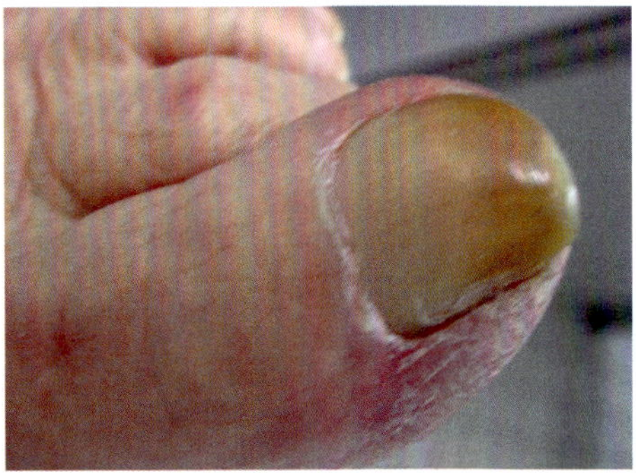

Image 3.164 After two years

3.11 Pachyonychia
(Greek: pachys = thick)

Definition
Nail bed development disorder with hypertrophic papillae and solid horn substance whereby the nail plate itself is thin (images 3.165 to 3.167).

Causes
- trauma caused by prolonged pressure from adjacent hammer or claw toes
- frostbite
- heredity

Symptoms
Usually affects one or two nails.

Pathogenesis
The horizontal papillae of the nail bed are abnormally hypertrophied with a solid horn substance formation between the papillae ridges. The nail plate is thin and smooth.

Differential diagnosis
Onychogryposis

Complications
Nail mycosis, bacterial infection of the nail bed.

Treatment
Do not file or grind the nail plate since it is already very thin. Unlike in the case of onychogryposis, carefully remove hornification buildup. Sometimes pachyonychia is misdiagnosed as onychogryposis (images 3.168 to 3.170). Grinding or filing can result in spot bleeding and is painful for the patient. Treat the bleeding immediately with sterile wound compresses and apply a toe tip dressing. Once the wound has healed, a transparent nail prosthetic can be applied.

In some cases, a nail brace has been proven to be helpful in flattening the nail bed, but foremost pressure from hammer or claw toes must be eliminated with cor-

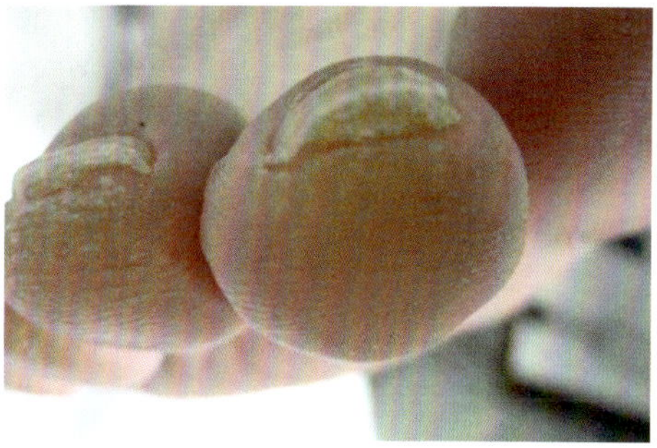

Image 3.165

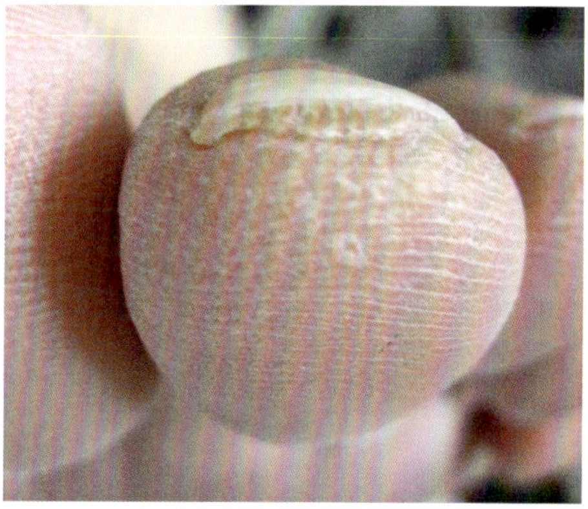

Image 3.166

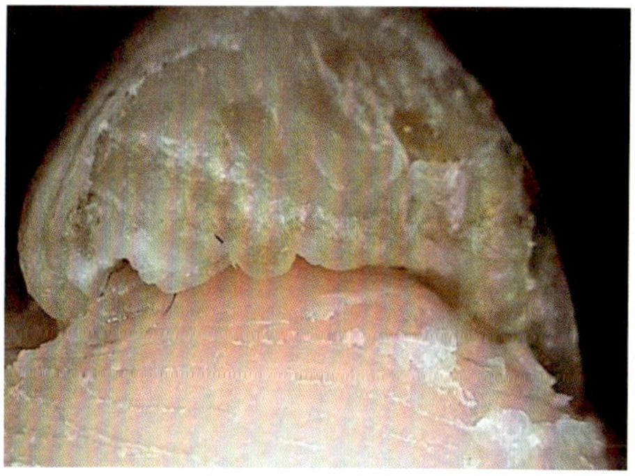

Image 3.167

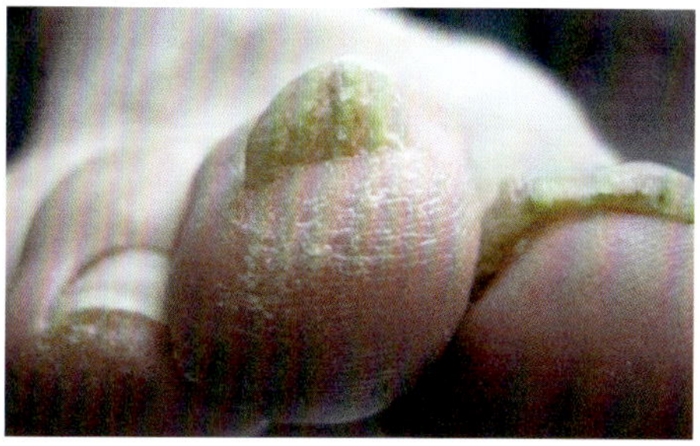

Image 3.168 Pachyonychia

rective orthoses and properly fitting footwear. Taping hammer and claw toes to reduce pressure on the affected nail causes the hornification in the nail bed to regress. For long-term results and to see improvement, avoid pressure on the nail.

Prophylaxis

- wide shoes
- foot exercise to strengthen foot muscles
- orthoses to correct toe deformities
- in certain cases, if the patient suffers from pain, a surgical procedure is the only option

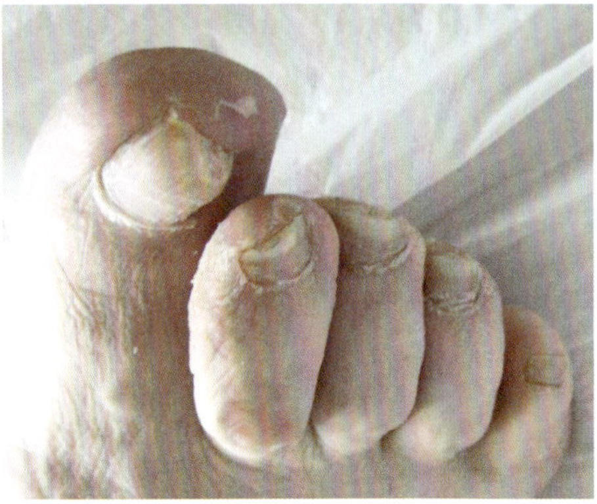

Image 3.169

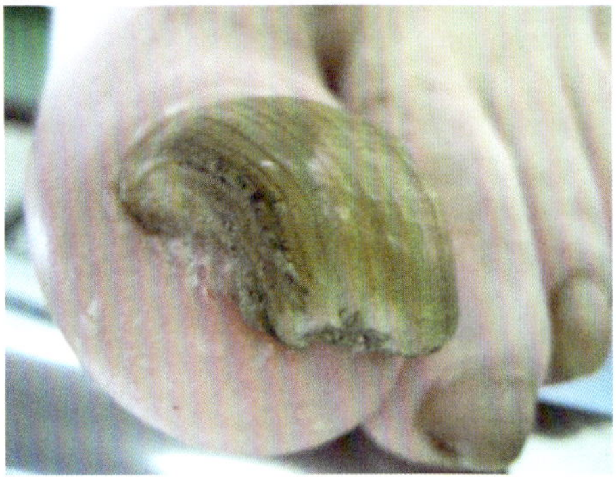

Image 3.170 Onychogryposis

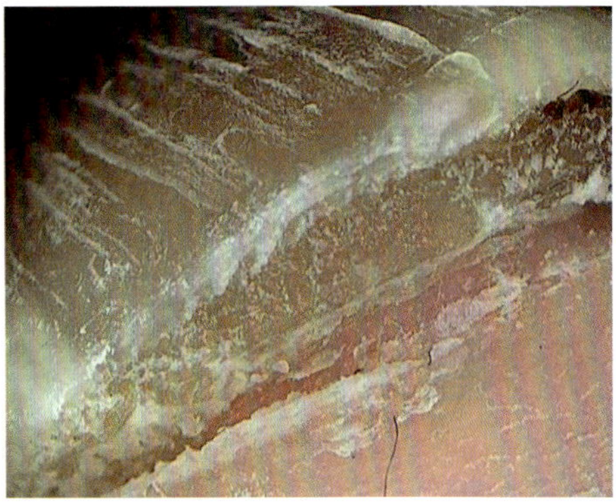

Image 3.171 Pachyonychia

3.12 Onychodystrophy
(Greek: dys = flawed, trophe = nutrition)

Definition

Changes in the nail's colour, shape and texture. Onychodystrophy is a congenital or acquired nail growth disorder (images 3.172 to 3.176).

The following nail disorders fall under onychodystrophy:

- onychogryposis
- onychoatrophy
- platonychia (flat nail)
- koilonychia (spoon nail)
- claw nail
- brachyonychia (racquet nail)
- median canaliform dystrophy (midline furrow nail)
- onychorrhexis and onychoschizia (split nail)
- hourglass nails and drumstick fingers (clubbing)
- pitting, Mee's lines
- trachyonychia (sand paper nail)
- beading
- beau's lines
- leukopathy, leukonychia, milk glass nails
- nail discolouration
- onychomycosis
- onychauxis
- onycholysis
- paronychia
- pachyonychia
- unguis inflexus and retroflexus

Causes

- various auto-immune disorders
- epidermolysis bullosa
- Reiter syndrome
- onychomycosis
- psoriasis
- Sezary syndrome
- verrucae vulgaris
- nail matrix disorder
- mechanical, chemical or thermic causes
- medication
- metabolic disorders
- lichen ruber disorder
- bacterial and viral diseases
- arterial circulatory disorder
- hyperkeratosis in the nail bed
- gout
- malnutrition
- hormonal disorders
- febrile illnesses
- kidney diseases
- incorrect nail cutting
- psychological disorders
- ageing
- blood diseases
- cardiovascular diseases

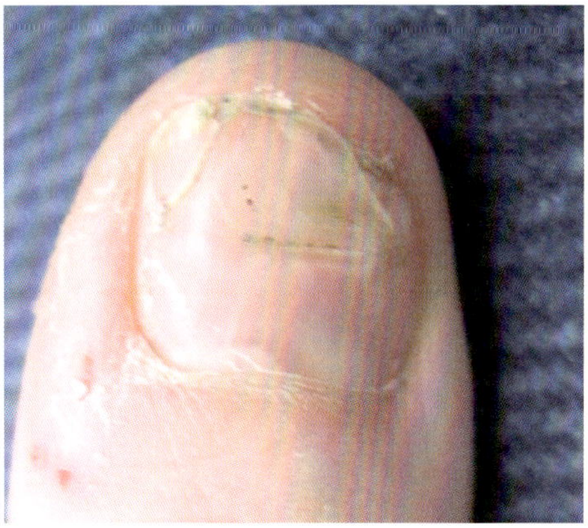

Image 3.172 Combat injury

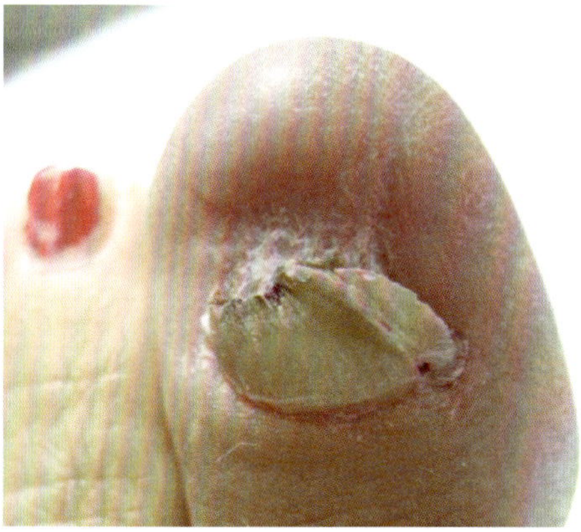

Image 3.173 Nail removed several times surgically because of unguis incarnatus

Pathogenesis
Depending on the disorder.

Differential diagnosis
See causes.

Complications
Depending on the disorder. Incorrect treatment will worsen the condition.

Treatment
Treat according to the cause of the disorder and degree of damage.

Prophylaxis
- avoid additional irritation
- frequent professional foot care as a preventative measure

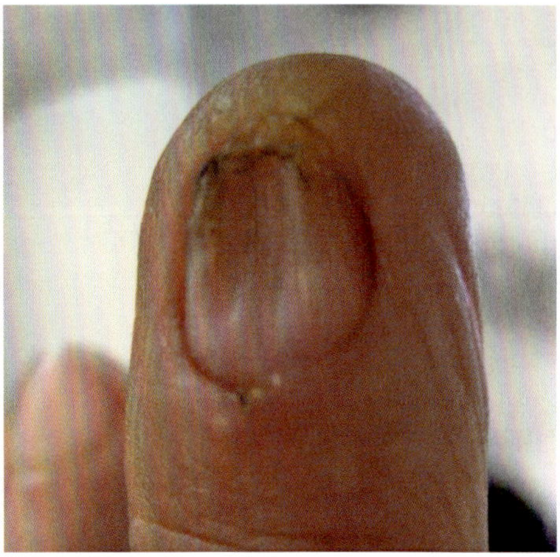

Image 3.174 Onychodystrophy

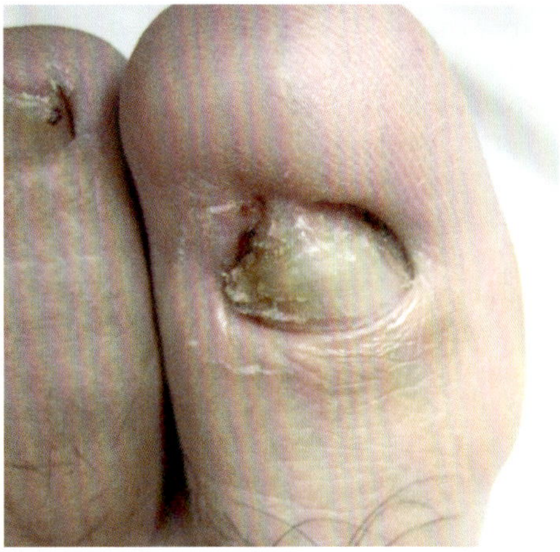

Image 3.175 Congenital nail disorder

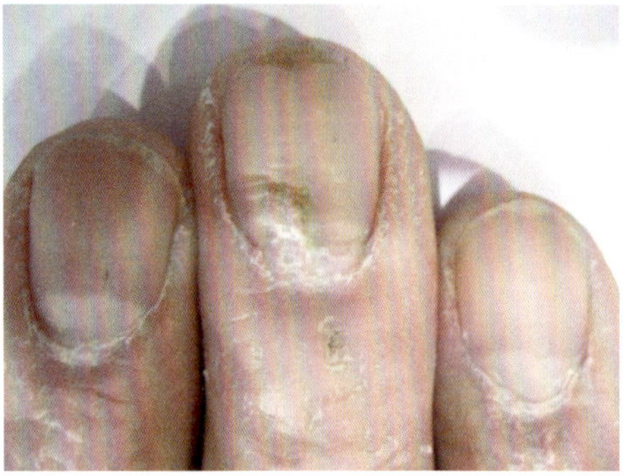

Image 3.176 Burn injury

3.13 Unguis inflexus

Definition

Longitudinal overcurvature of the free nail margin. The nail grows over the tip of the finger or toe in ventral direction (images 3.177 to 3.180).

- curvature of a nail over the ball of the toe
- strong convex curvature

Causes

- impaired nail growth, e.g., onychogryposis
- tight footwear
- abnormally shortened terminal phalanx (tip of the toe) caused by trauma or atrophic disease such as progressive scleroderma

Pathogenesis

- impaired nail growth affected by an arterial blood circulation disorder causing a longitudinal curvature of the nail
- nails that are too long
- progressive scleroderma (inflammatory disease of the blood vessels, the skin's connective tissue and the inner organs) affecting the nail fold
- tight footwear

Differential diagnosis

Hourglass nails, usually the result of heart disease (image 3.164).

Complications

Onycholysis, subungual inflammation, onychomadesis.

Treatment

- Keep the nail relatively short.
- In case of impaired nail growth, remove hyperkeratosis.
- To prevent additional hyperkeratosis build-up, apply a nail prosthetic.

Prophylaxis

Verify the sock size (see chapter 2) and ensure that socks and shoes fit correctly.

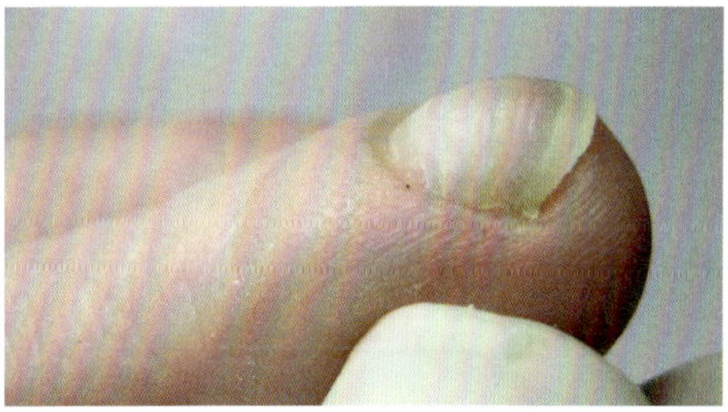

Image 3.177

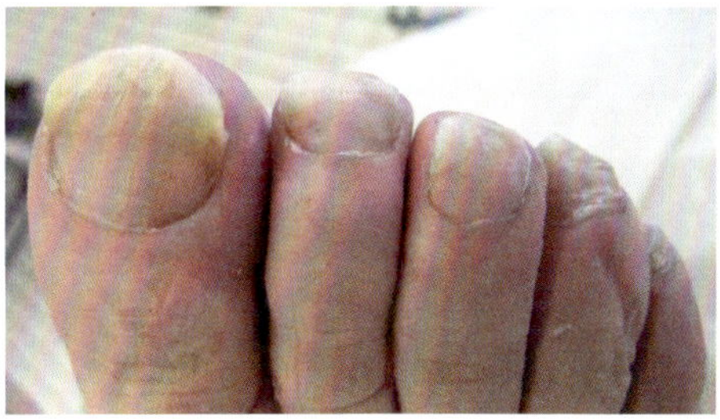

Image 3.178

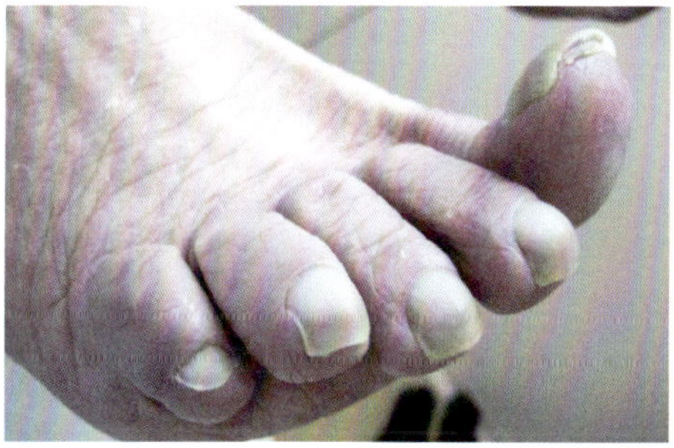

Image 3.179 Unguis inflexus caused by an arterial blood circulation disorder

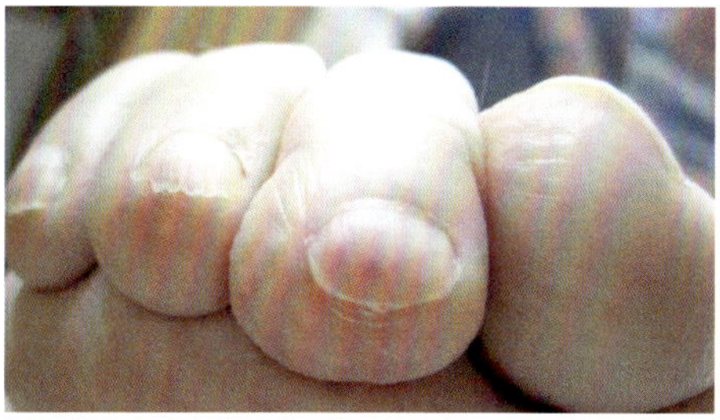

Image 3.180 Unguis inflexus on a claw toe

3.14 Unguis retroflexus

Definition
Dorsal curvature of the nail (images 3.181 to 3.185)

Causes/symptoms/appearance
- ill-fitting footwear, shoes or socks that are too small
- the nail plate substance is not affected

Complications
Onycholysis, onychomadesis, subungual inflammation.

Treatment
Treat symptomatically. Keep the nail short to prevent further deformity, round off the nail edges so that the nail does not get caught on shoes, socks or bed sheets risking loosening of the nail. Glide with the finger over the nail edges and the apex from distal to proximal to ensure that there are no rough edges.

Remove loose hyperkeratosis from under the nail. If necessary, correct the toe deformity using the taping technique.

Prophylaxis
- wearing properly fitting shoes and socks
- foot exercise

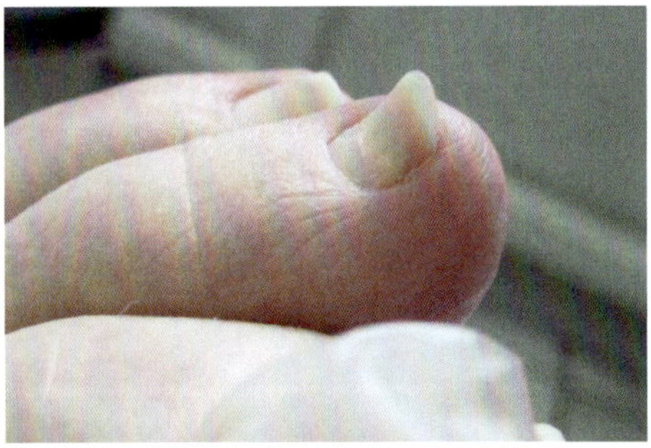

Image 3.181

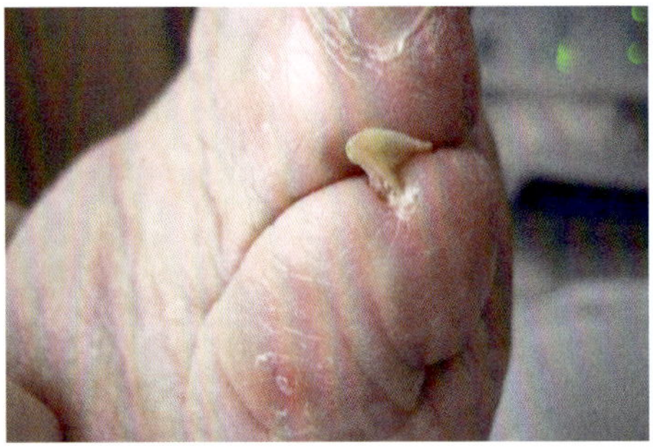

Image 3.182 Unguis retroflexus caused by wearing ill-fitting socks over a long period

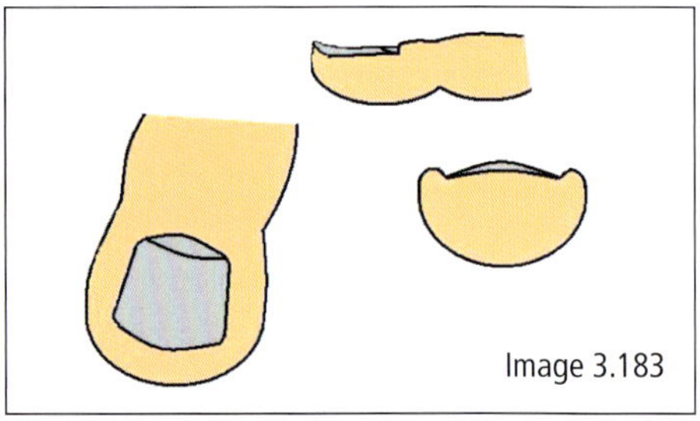

Image 3.183

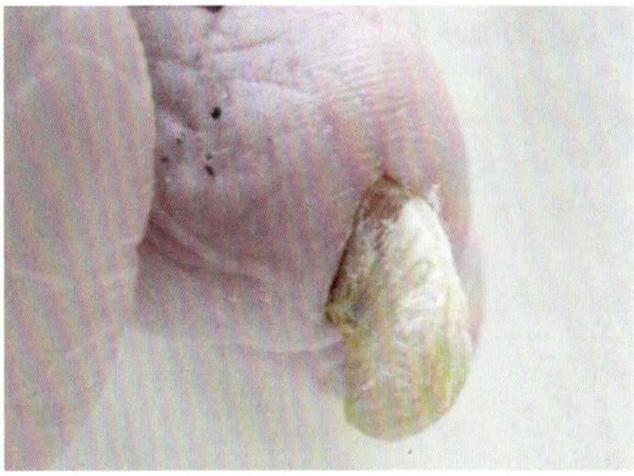

Image 3.184

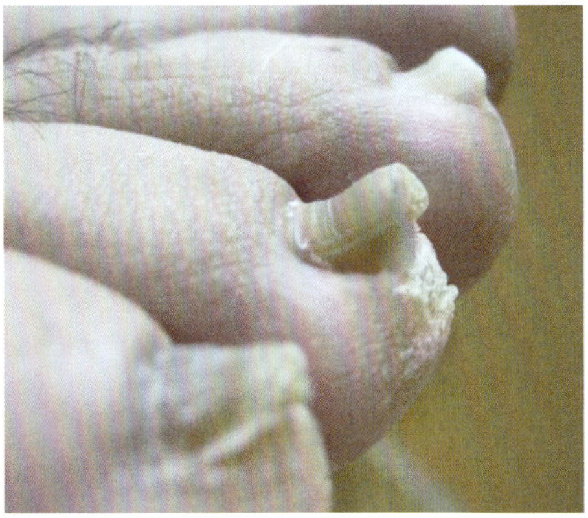

Image 3.185 Unguis retroflexus with pachyonychia caused by a hammer toe

3.15 Onychorrhexis/ Onychoclasis

Definition
Longitudinal splitting and decaying of the nail (image 3.186 to 3.192).

Causes
- abnormal groove formation caused by lichen ruber
- hepatopathy
- inner secretory disorders
- deposit dermatoses
- anemia
- trauma to the nail plate or matrix
- vitamin B deficiency
- gout
- using alkaline and anti-grease cleansing lotions on the feet
- noxious chemical agents
- radiation and heat damage
- nutritional and hormonal disorders with associated skin diseases

Special variant
Split nail (onychodystrophia canaliformis). The nail splits in half lengthwise.

Complications
Onychomycosis, onycholysis.

Treatment
After disinfecting the nail, smooth the nail surface with a fine diamond bur or corundum stone removing any loose nail particles. Disinfect the nail again and apply a nail prosthetic to prevent microorganisms from penetrating the nail's surface. The prosthetic must be transparent to notice any changes in the nail such as the development of a subungual hematoma, the formation of a subungual clavus or signs of onychomycosis. Damage to the nail bed caused by improperly removed nail parts always poses a risk of infection.

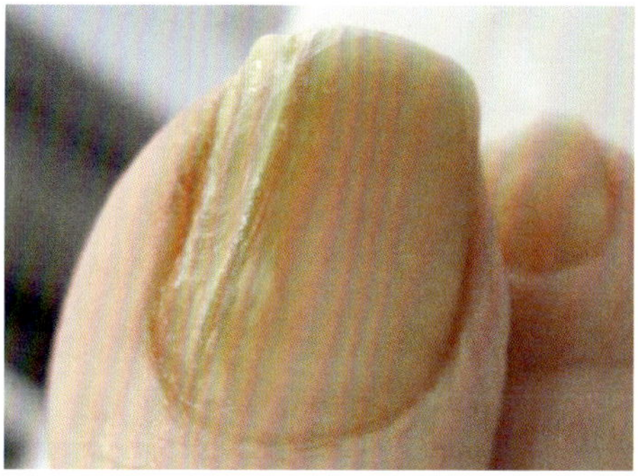

Image 3.186

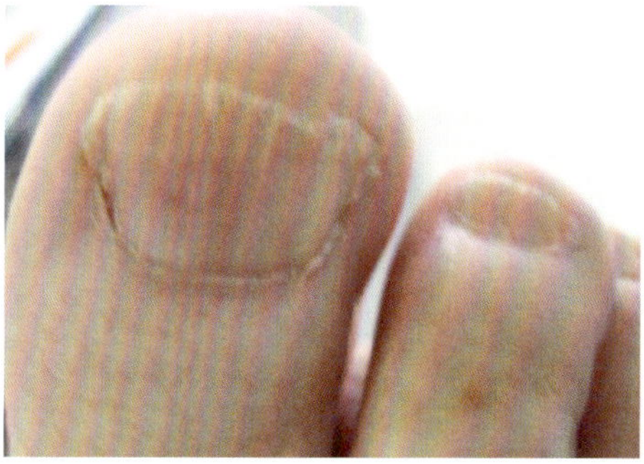

Image 3.187

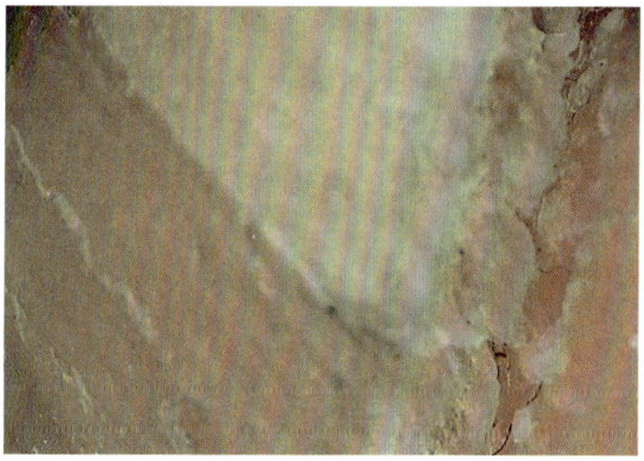

Image 3.188

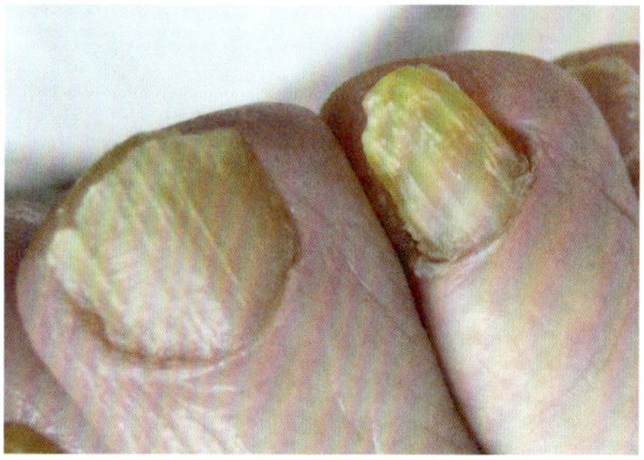

Image 3.189

Prophylaxis
- regular application of nail tinctures or nail serums
- frequent oil baths to promote healthy nail growth
- trauma preventio
- avoidance of alkaline solutions and degreasing agents
- vitamin deficiency treatment
- promoting healthy nail growth with organic silicon (found in high concentration in common horsetail and bamboo), vitamin B6, zinc, manganese (supports the connective tissue and bone growth), calcium (strengthens hair, nails, bones and the connective tissue)

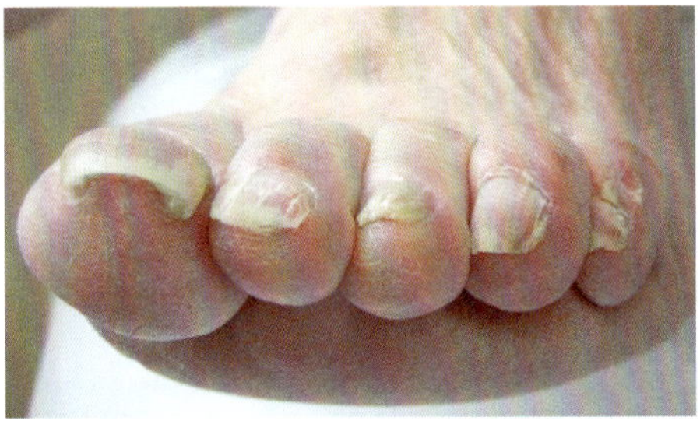
Image 3.190

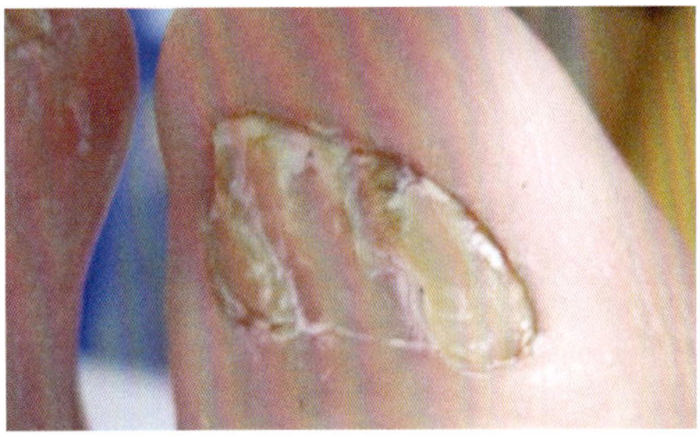
Image 3.191

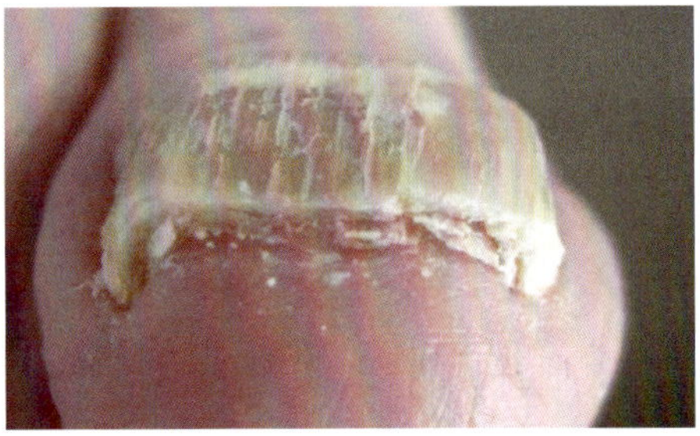
Image 3.192

3.16 Onychoschizia
(Greek: s-chísis = splitting)

Definition

Lamella-like flaking of the dorsal nail layer that starts at the free nail margin (images 3.193 to 3.195).

Causes
- chemicals, e.g., alkaline solutions and cleaning detergents
- mineral deficiency and metabolic disorders

Pathogenesis
Frequent exposure to harsh chemicals removes oil and softens the horny layer allowing water to penetrate and causing it to swell up.

The alternating water absorption and release in the upper horn cell layers impairs the interlamellar connection causing individual nail layers to detach.

Differential diagnosis
Psoriasis.

Complications
- unguis incarnatus
- bulging of the nail wall
- nail wall callositas
- clavus formation
- onychomadesis

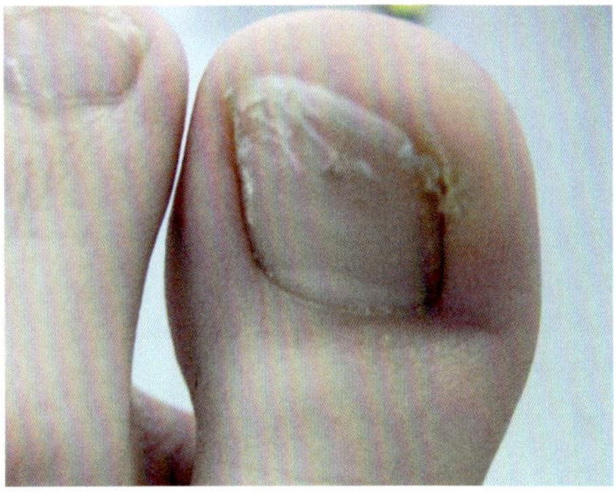
Image 3.193

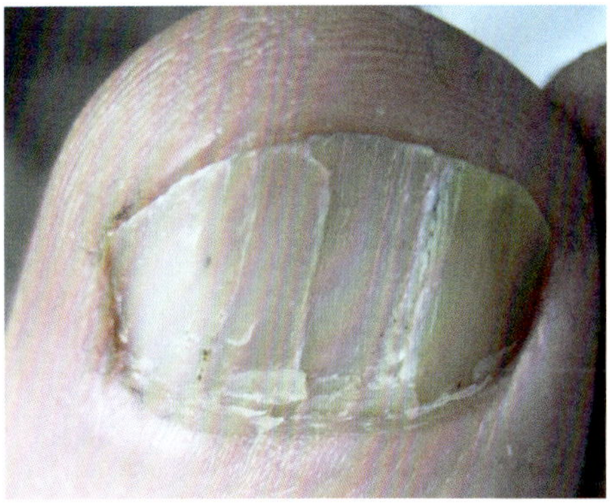

Image 3.194

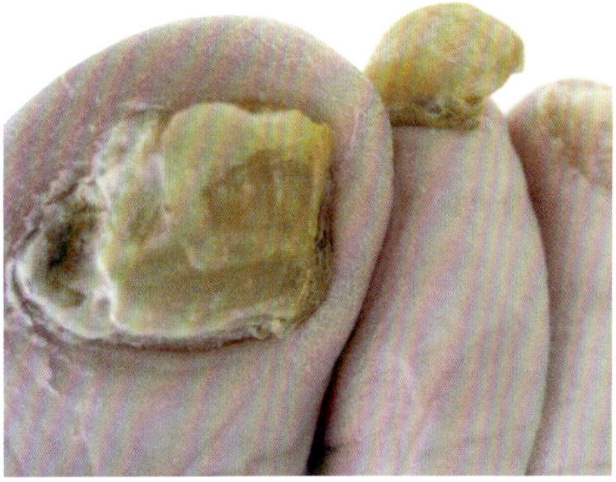

Image 3.195

Treatment
Smooth the nail surface with a fine diamond bur or corundum stone and apply a nail prosthetic to even out the nail surface, but only if onychomycosis has been diagnosed. In case mycosis is present, perform a mycosis prophylaxis prior to applying the nail prosthetic.

The mineral deficiency must be treated by a physician. Regularly applying nail oil or olive oil helps regenerate the nail.

Prophylaxis
- metabolic disorders: treatment by a physician
- good nutrition
- avoid exposure to degreasing and softening alkaline cleaning agents
- consultation regarding properly fitting shoes and socks
- wear gloves while handling alkaline solutions
- promoting healthy nail growth with organic silicon (found in high concentration in common horsetail and bamboo), vitamin B6, zinc, manganese (supports the connective tissue and bone growth), calcium (strengthens hair, nails, bones and the connective tissue).

3.17 Onychoatrophy

Definition
A faulty underdevelopment of the nail plate, in which the nail is thinned and smaller (images 3.196 to 3.198).

Causes/symptoms/appearance
Cause unknown.

The nail plate is paper thin and brittle. Commonly seen in older patients and patients with heart insufficiency and arterial blood circulatory disorders.

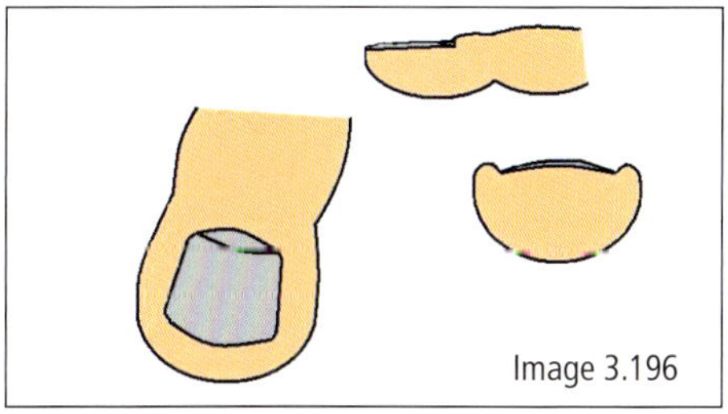

Image 3.196

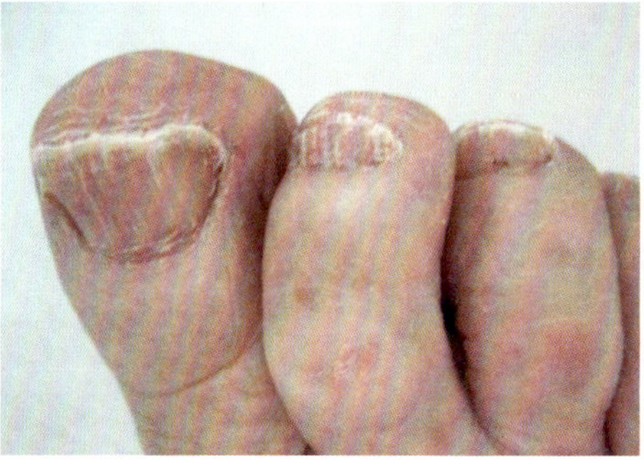

Image 3.197

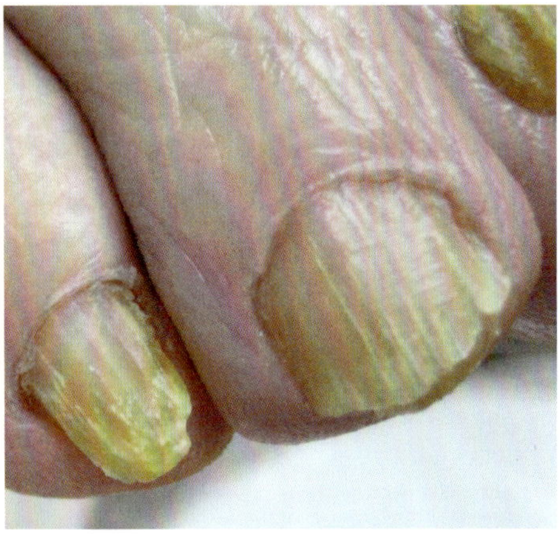

Image 3.198 Onychoatrophy with onychorrhexis

Complications

Onychomadesis, onychomycosis.

Treatment

Remove loose nail parts with a corner nipper or a fine diamond bur to prevent them from getting caught on socks. Glide with the finger over the nail edges and the apex from distal to proximal to ensure that there are no rough edges. This preventative measure is important to avoid injuries and onycholysis. If there are no signs of mycosis, the nail can be strengthened with nail prosthetics such as nail filler, BS nail or by using light curing techniques.

3.18 Onychomadesis (nail loss)

Definition

Complete shedding of the nail (images 3.199 to 3.203). Onychomadesis is also known as alopecia unguium.

Causes

- epithelium inflammation, trauma, arterial disorders, febrile infections, scarlet fever, sepsis, influenza, pneumonia, blistering diseases, chemotherapy, alopecia areata, psoriasis, drug-induced toxic epidermal lysis, bullous dermatoses, medication exanthema, intense X-ray radiation, acute paronychia or severe psychological stress, but can also be idiopathic
- dominant genetic disorder (e.g., associated with the abnormal enamel formation of teeth)
- progressive shedding of the nail beginning at the proximal end: the nail gradually detaches from the nail matrix; the hereditary condition results in nail loss and nail dystrophy, it can affect several nails simultaneously
- complete nail loss with scarring of the nail bed may be caused by permanent damage to the matrix (e.g., trauma-in-

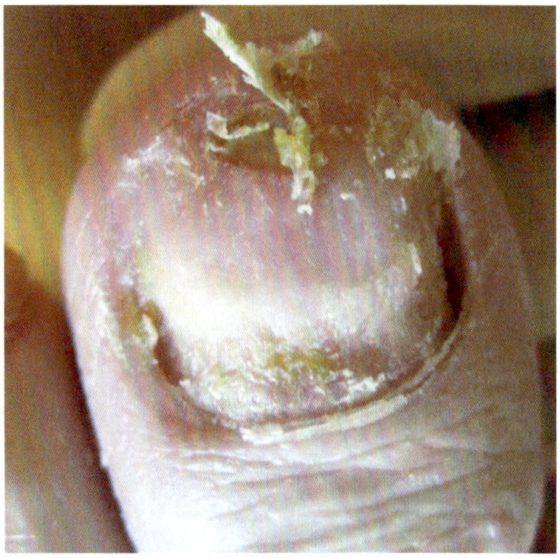

Image 3.199 Exposed nail bed

duced, later stages of lichen ruber planus unguium, epidermolysis, bullous dermatoses or severe PAOD)

Complications
Onychomycosis, subungual hematoma.

Treatment
The wound care must be documented. Always use sterile dressings such as Ligasano white for the nail bed. Consult with a physician. Once the infection has completely healed, protect the nail bed and the regrowing nail with an artificial nail. However, keep in mind that an artificial nail only adheres to a newly grown nail or an existing one, not to skin (see chapter 6).

Prophylaxis
- prevent trauma caused by ill-fitting footwear
- strengthening of the immune system

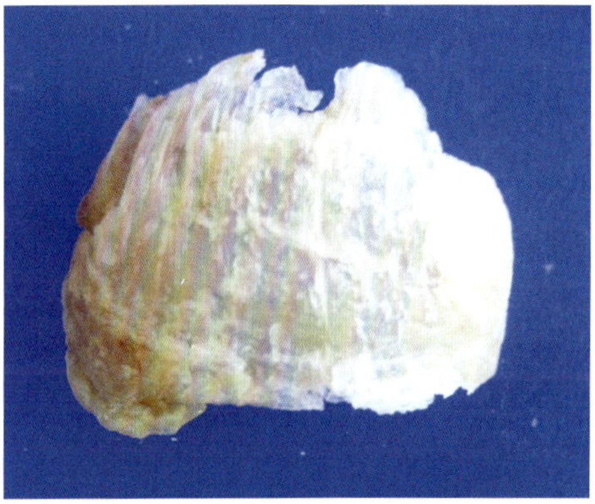

Image 3.200 Detached nail of a diabetic patient

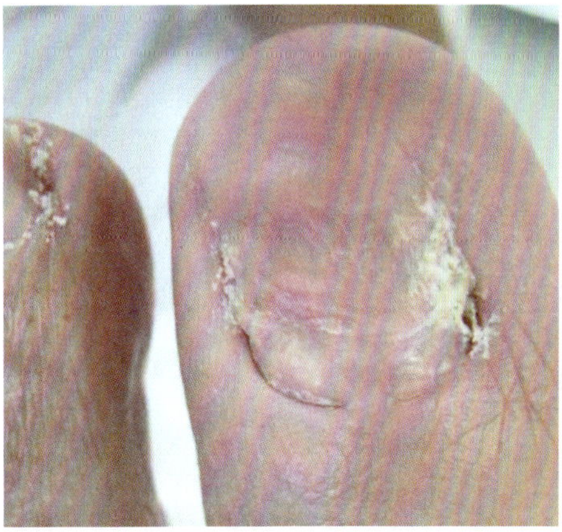

Image 3.201 Onychomadesis after multiple surgical nail removal procedures

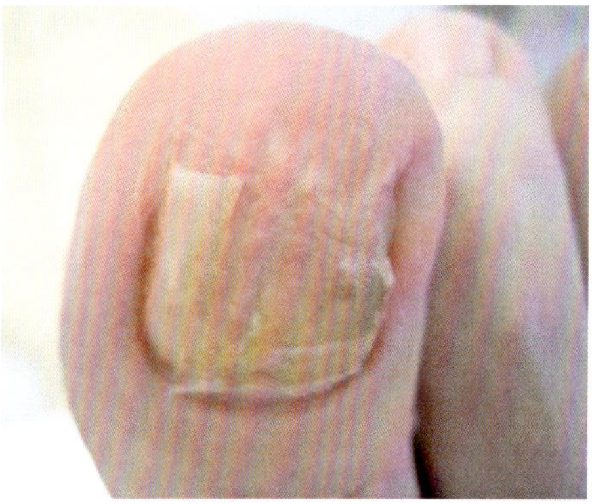

Image 3.202

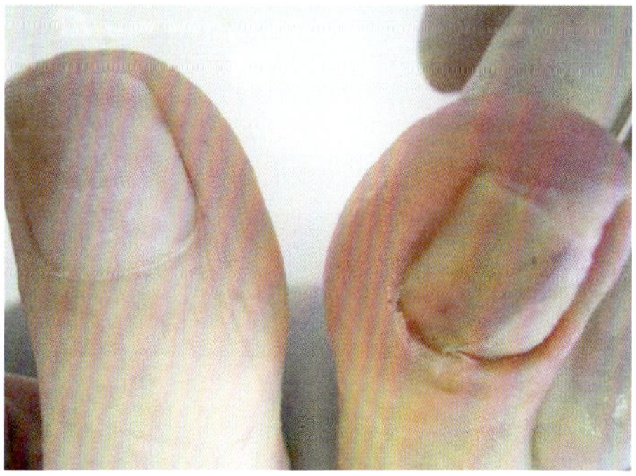

Image 3.203

3.19 Onycholysis

Definition

Detachment of the nail plate from the nail bed (images 3.204 to 3.208).

Epidemiology

Onycholysis often occurs with other nail diseases but also with systemic diseases of the inner organs.

Onycholysis is associated with onychia, onychomycosis, onychogryposis, psoriasis and injuries to the nail bed caused by trauma. The lysis can be accompanied by bleeding and serous secretion. See onychomadesis.

Causes

- arterial blood circulatory disorders
- thyroid disorders
- common metabolic disorders
- skin diseases (less common) such as contact dermatitis
- medically-determined skin rash
- partially detached nail plate
- different injuries and trauma
- chemicals such as alkaline solvents or cosmetics
- static issues: foot deformities such as splayfoot can cause toe deformities such as hammer and claw toes, digitus subductus (toe lies over the neighbouring toe) and hallux valgus subjecting the nail to permanent (maybe constant) pressure

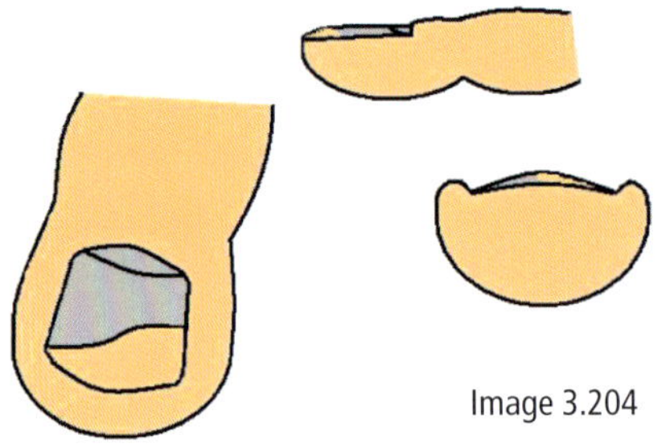

Image 3.204

Appearance

When the nail starts to separate from the nail bed, the raised part looks white, as there is only air between the nail bed and the nail. This is often accompanied by excessive hornification build-up underneath the raised nail plate.

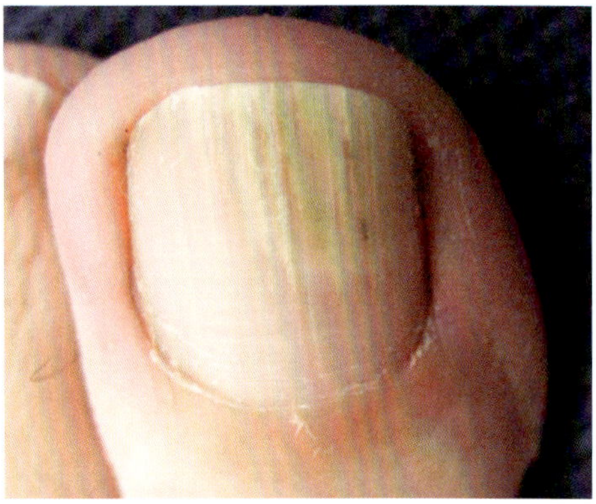

Image 3.205

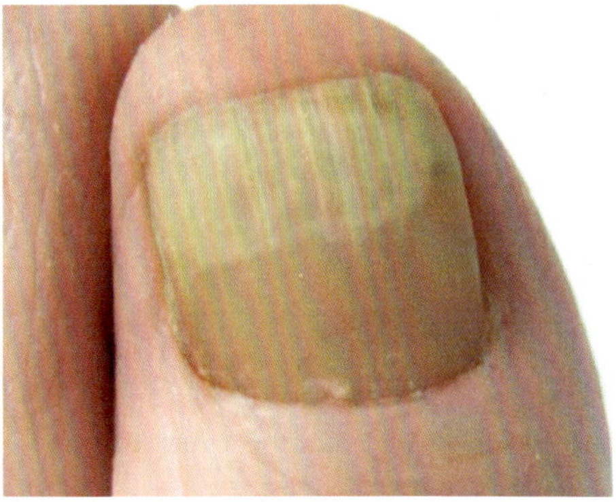

Image 3.206

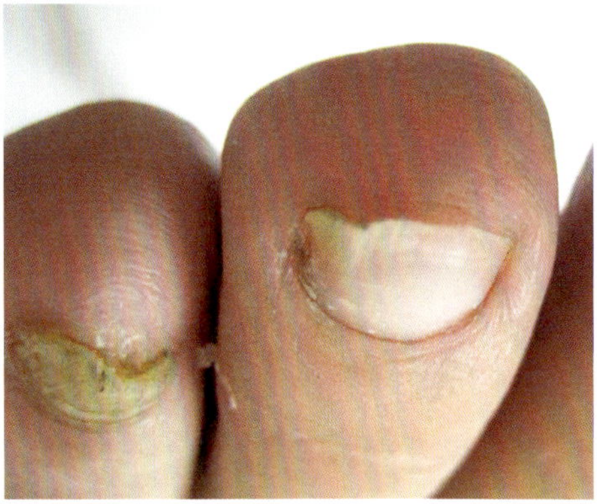

Image 3.207

Onycholysis semilunaris is a special form of onycholysis whereby the nail detaches in a crescent-shape at the distal end. This is often seen after long exposure in water or soap solutions.

Differential diagnosis
Often accompanied by other nail diseases such as mycosis, onychogryposis or psoriasis.

Complications
Development of mycosis, a nail growth disorder or the abnormal thickening of the nail. Once the nail has been completely removed, the nail bed regenerates itself.

Treatment
- Prevent the nail from separating further from the nail bed. By eliminating pressure on the nail, onycholysis sometimes heals by itself.
- To expose underlying subungual granulation tissue, subungual clavus or onychomycosis, remove parts of the nail completely with nail scissors or nail nippers and use a fine diamond bur for detailed work.
- A suitable nail prosthetic can be applied if there are no concerns from the physician's side.
- Eliminate pressure applied on the nail as a result of a foot or toe deformity.
- Carefully rinse the onycholysis using a disposable syringe and a cannula with an antimycotic or a disinfecting solution. Do not use an excavator or probe deep under the nail since this can enlarge the lysis.
- Promote blood circulation with foot exercise, baths and creams.

Prophylaxis
- properly fitting footwear
- mycosis prophylaxis
- improvement of the acid protective layer of the skin
- blood circulation stimulation
- pressure relief if toe deformities are present
- orthoses
- interdigital wedge
- do not apply braces
- professional foot care
- foot exercise

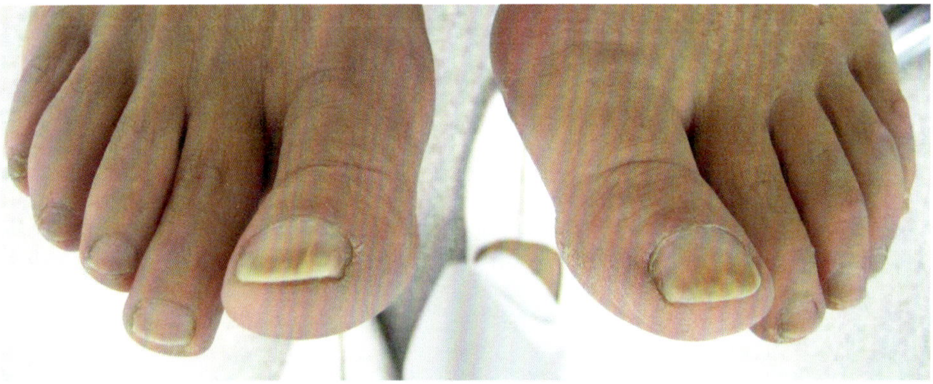

Image 3.208

3.20 Onychophosis

(Greek: phos = clear, light, osis = condition

Definition

Wax-like callus build-up on the nail fold.

Causes/symptoms/appearance

Ill-fitting and too tight footwear forces the toes to overlap. All areas of the nail fold can be affected. The hard hornification texture of the epidermis resembles scar tissue and cannot be mistaken for a clavus or callosity.

Complications

Clavus formation in the sulcus.

Treatment

- Remove the callus skin with products containing urea or salicyl acid.
- Relieve pressure on the nails.
- The treatment is often long. It is important to eliminate its causes.

Prophylaxis

Eliminate all causes.

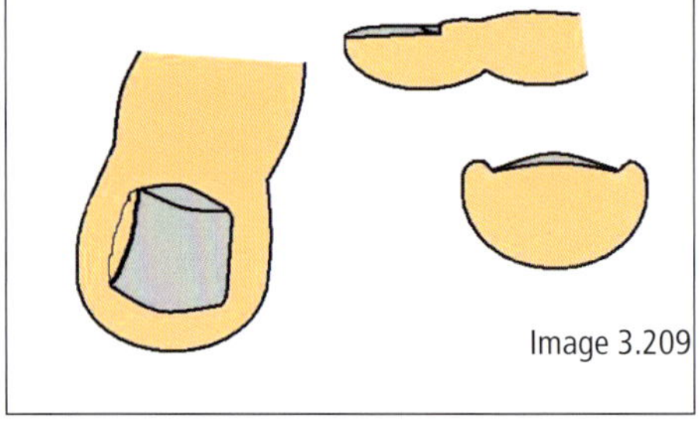

Image 3.209

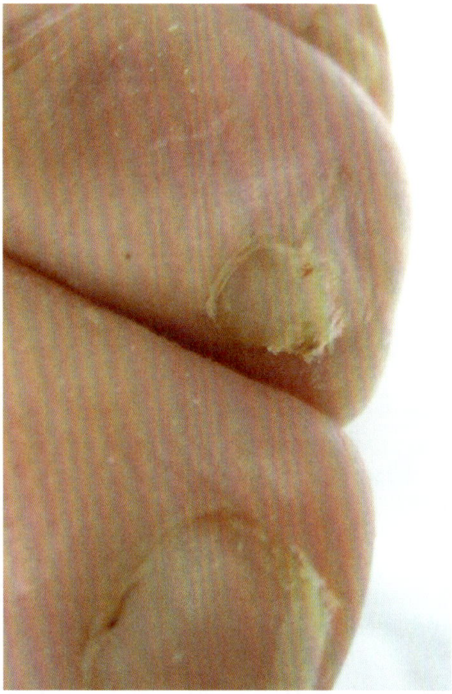

Image 3.210

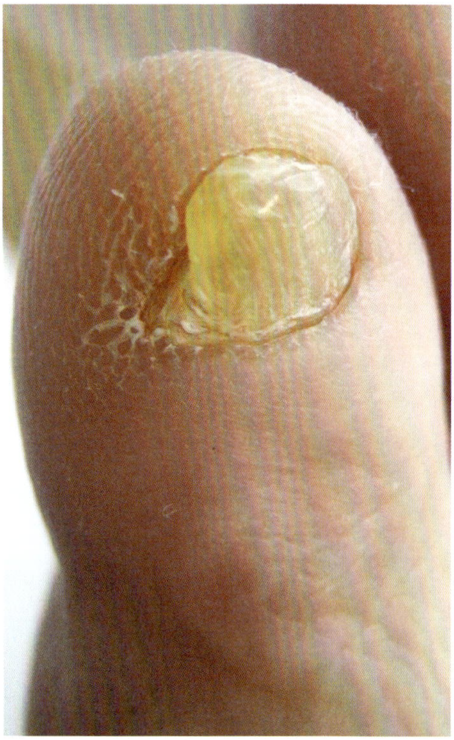

Image 3.211

3.21 Beau's lines

Definition
Deep horizontal ridges.

Causes
- cevere physical stress
- serious sudden illness
- surgery
- psychological stress
- arterial circulation disorder
- zinc deficiency
- tight footwear

Complications
- lysis
- onychomycosis due to the partial splintering of the nail substance

Treatment
- Eliminate all causes.
- Do not try to grind off the ridges since it will interfere with the nail's static. The upper layer of the nail is the hardest and removing it can lead to unguis convolutus and allow the penetration of microorganisms such as fungi.
- File and smooth the edges of the nail to ensure that the nail does not get caught on socks or blankets.
- If necessary, apply a nail prosthetic.
- Consultation regarding properly fitting shoes and socks.

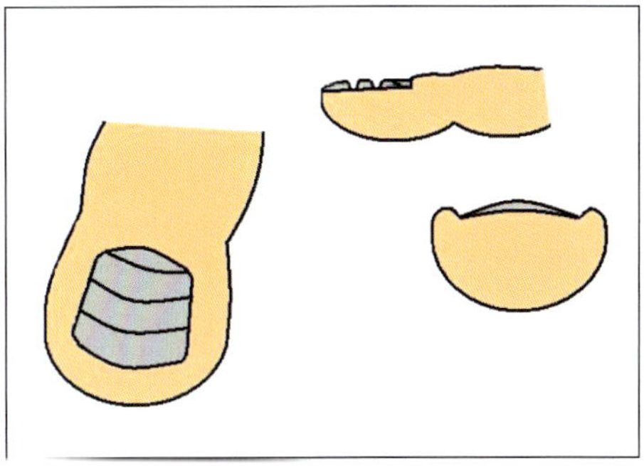

Image 3.212

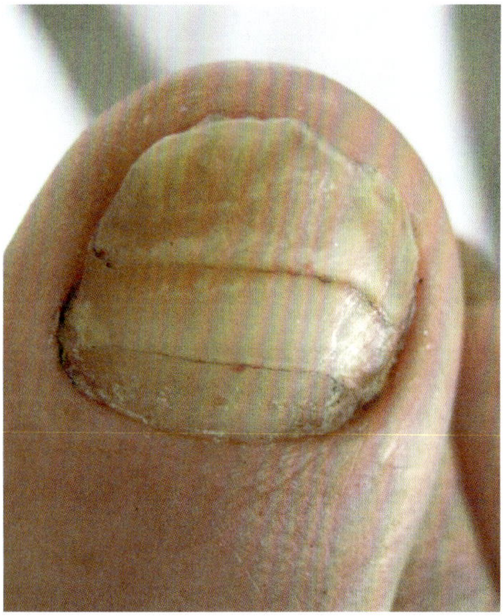

Image 3.213

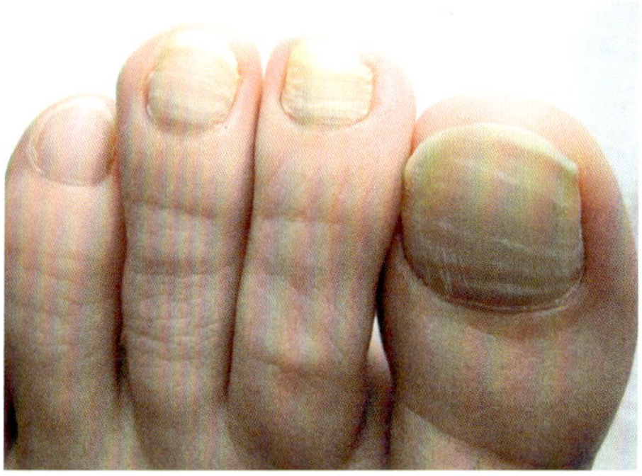

Image 3.214

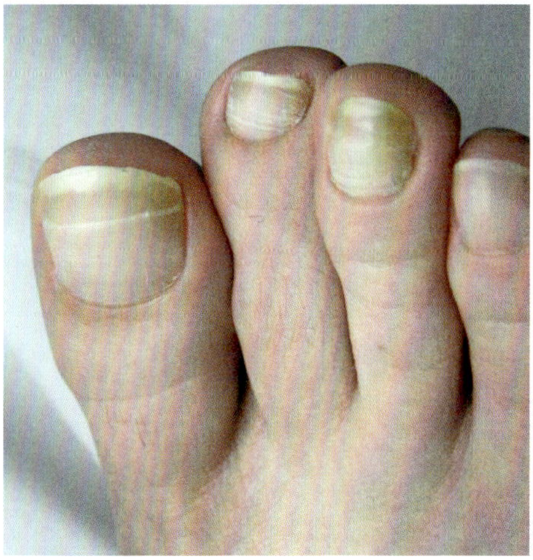

Image 3.215

3.22 Subungual hematoma

Definition

Also known as nail hematoma. A hematoma located under a fingernail or toenail (images 3.216 to 3.225).

Causes/symptoms/appearance

It is usually caused by traumatic pressure (e.g., when a car door slams on a finger, by knocking the toe on a door frame or hiking with improper footwear).

Complications

Damaging the nail matrix and the nail bed results in onychodystrophy and permanent onycholysis which can lead to a mycotic infection.

Differential diagnosis

A tumor under the nail.

Treatment

It is a harmless yet often painful injury. The healing process can be accelerated with a nail trephination. For this procedure, the tip of a cannula is held into an open flame until it is red hot. The hot tip is then placed on the nail above the hematoma without adding pressure. The intense heat melts a tiny hole into the nail where the blood is pooled, allowing it to drain. Once the pressure is relieved, most patients get immediate relief.

A thin sterile rosehead bur can also be used instead of a cannula. The nail must be bandaged afterwards and throughout the whole process it is crucial to follow sterile guidelines. It is also important to inform the patient that the unusual procedure is completely pain-free.

To distinguish a subungual hematoma from a tumor under the nail, carefully draw a thin line on the nail below the dark discoloured area with a fissure grinding instrument. After one month, verify if the line is still below the dark discoloured area or if it has moved up while the dark area stayed in the same place or got even larger. If the latter is the case, the patient must be immediately referred to a dermatologist with an accompanying document.

Prophylaxis

Wearing properly fitting and protective footwear is the best preventative measure to avoid subungual hematoma. Prior to engaging in a mountain hike, for example, the distal free nail margins must be shortened so that the nail does not rub on the shoe during walking.

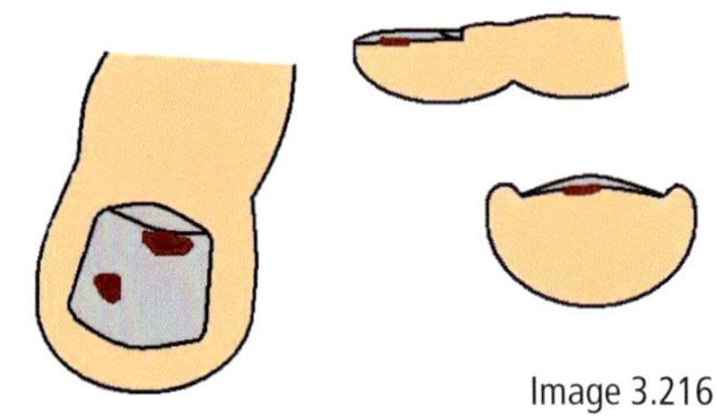

Image 3.216

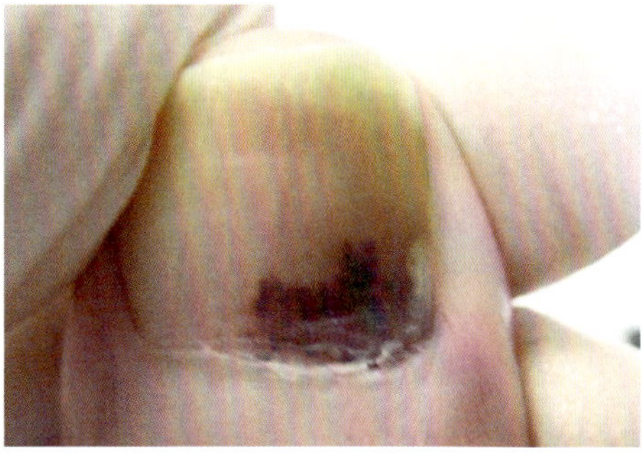

Image 3.217 Subungual hematoma

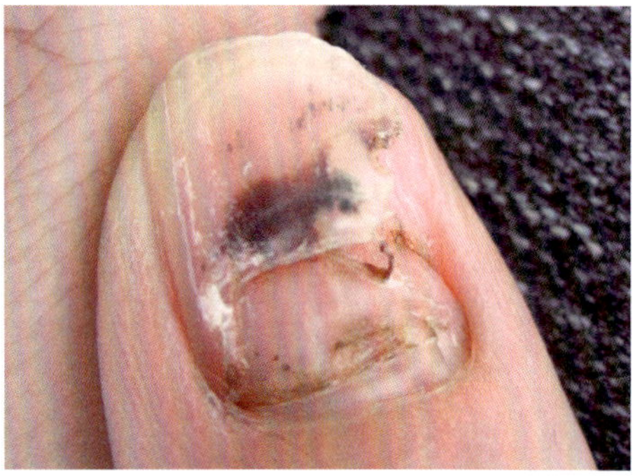

Image 3.218

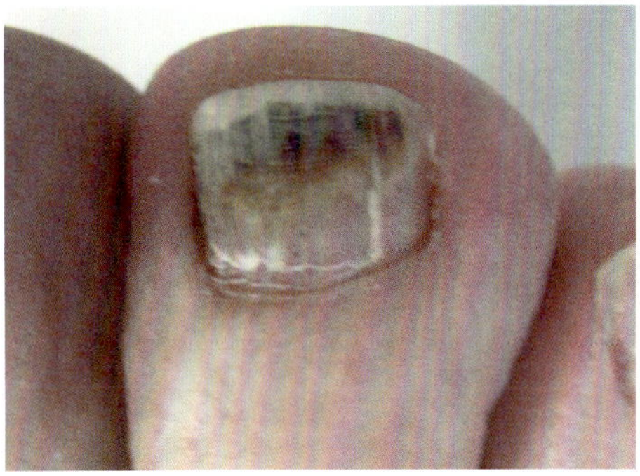

Image 3.219

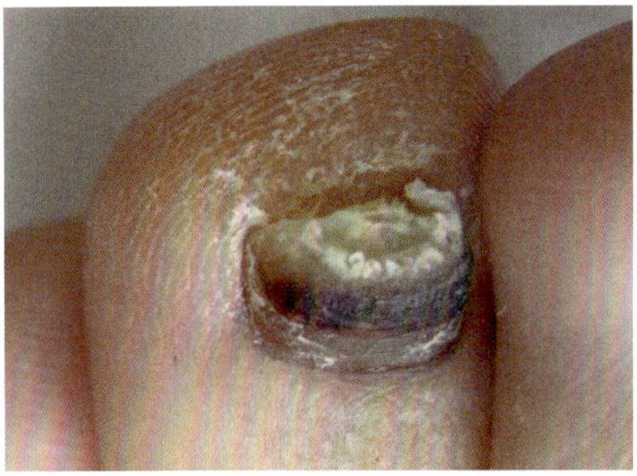

Image 3.220 Subungual hematoma with pachyonychia

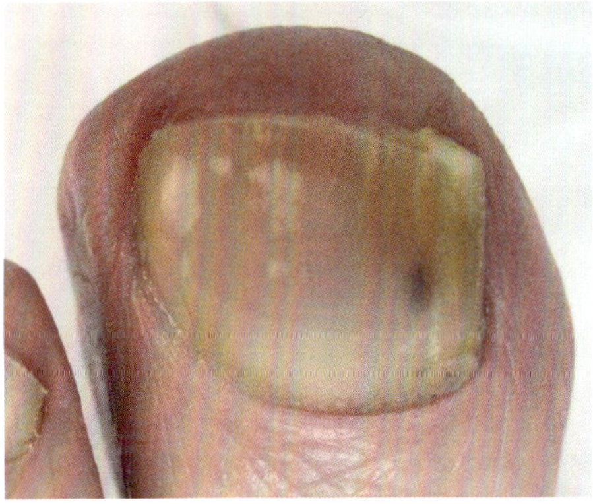

Image 3.221 Tumour or hematoma? Difficult to distinguish.

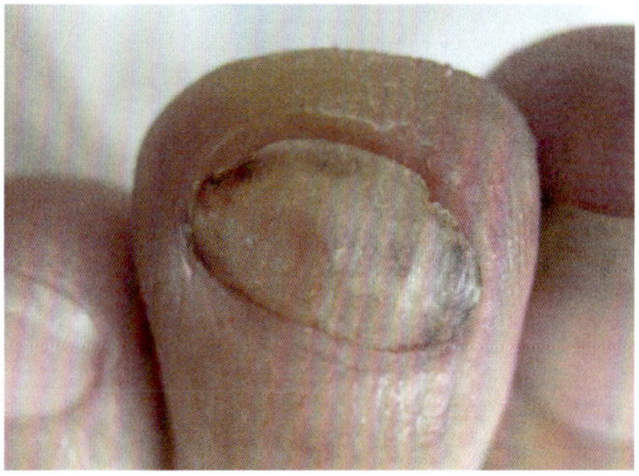

Image 3.222 An older hematoma after a marathon

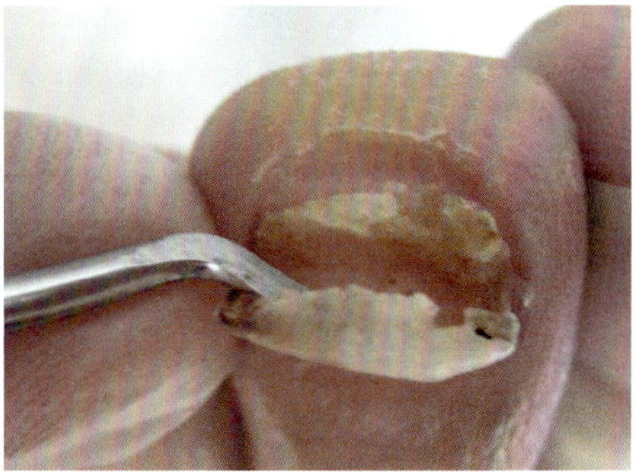

Image 3.223 Detaching nail

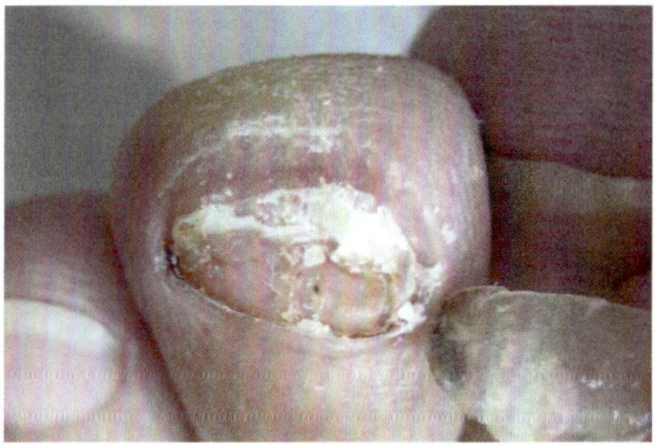

Image 3.224 The new nail is growing

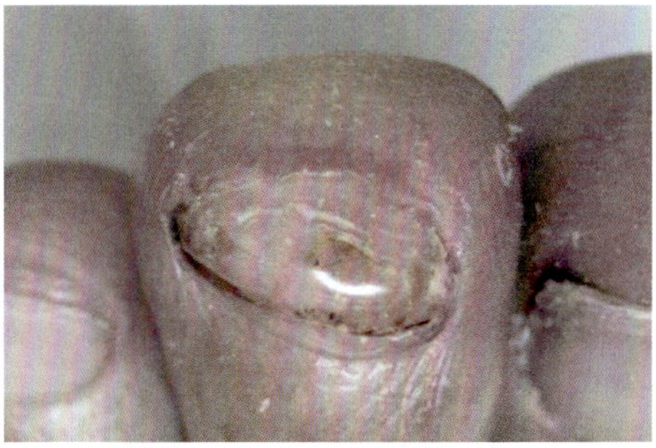

Image 3.225 Strengthening the new nail with a nail prosthetic

3.23 Onychia

Definition
Onychia is known as an inflammatory reaction in the nail bed with the induction of microorganisms such as bacteria, fungi and viruses (images 3.226 and 3.227).

Causes/symptoms/appearance
Strong constantly applied pressure (e.g., wearing shoes that are too tight) or a subungual clavus are often the cause for developing onychia.

Complications
Serous secretion under the nail promotes the development of granulation tissue. The surrounding tissue cannot "breath" and at worst the infection moves deeper and affects the bone.

Treatment
Wound care procedures must always be documented in writing. A complementary image can be added.

Using sterile instruments is of utmost importance.

> Cooperation with a physician is crucial!

After thorough disinfecting (e.g., octenisept) the area, use sterile instruments to expose the centre of the inflammation. Apply an etching agent, such as albothyl 3%, on the granulation tissue. Do not use on diabetic patients or patients with wound healing dysfunction and then use only as instructed by a physician. This procedure promotes faster wound healing than a purely medicinal treatment. Remove an infected clavus under the nail plate with a rosehead bur and a scalpel. The subsequent wound care involves the application of disinfecting ointments and tinctures and an air-permeable bandage, such as instructed by a physician. To promote faster healing in a wound pocket use a sterile tamponade such as Ligasano

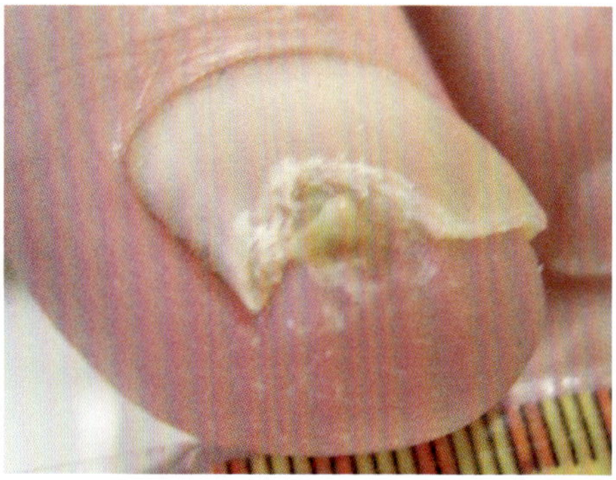

Image 3.226 After removing part of the nail
Source: Brigitte Rathenow

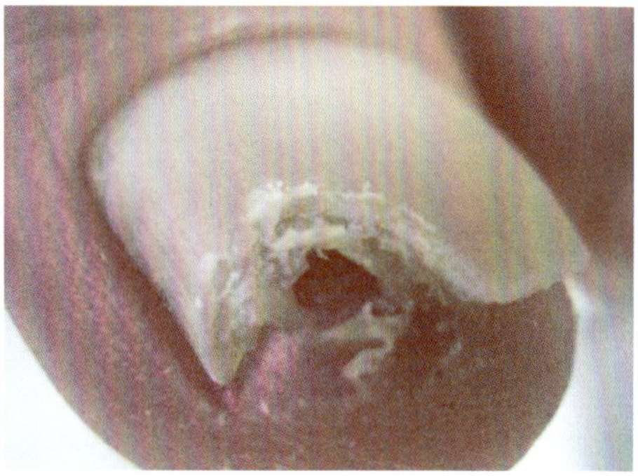

Image 3.227 After disinfecting the noticeable wound canal
Source: Brigitte Rathenow

white. Schedule a follow-up visit for the patient within 24 to 48 hours.

However, eliminating the cause for onychia is the prerequisite for successful healing.

Prophylaxis
Avoid any kind of strong and constant pressure on the nail, such as wearing footwear that is too tight.

3.24 Subungual granulation tissue/ Ulcers

Definition

A sponge-like, highly vascularised yet less fibrous tissue beneath the nail plate (images 3.228 to 3.231).

Causes/symptoms

Often the result of a trauma, such as a blow, strong pressure or cut injuries or wearing shoes that are too small and too tight.

Granulation tissue develops when constant pressure is applied to an already injured and inflamed nail bed with serous secretion.

Complications

The warm and moist environment provides a perfect breeding ground for microorganisms, such as bacteria, fungi and viruses. Patients suffering from an immune deficiency or an arterial circulatory disorder are especially vulnerable.

Treatment

Consult with a physician and follow his/her instructions.

Wound care procedures must be documented in writing. A complementary image can be added for additional clarification.

Disinfect the wound and surrounding area with an approved disinfection agent such as octenisept. Following proper hygiene guidelines is of utmost importance. Carefully remove the developed onycholysis with a sterile nail nipper or grinding instrument. Rinse the open wound thoroughly with octenisept, then cover the wound with a sterile compress such as Ligasano white; then apply a toe cap dressing and Ligasano green ensuring that the nail is properly protected from pressure (image 3.231).

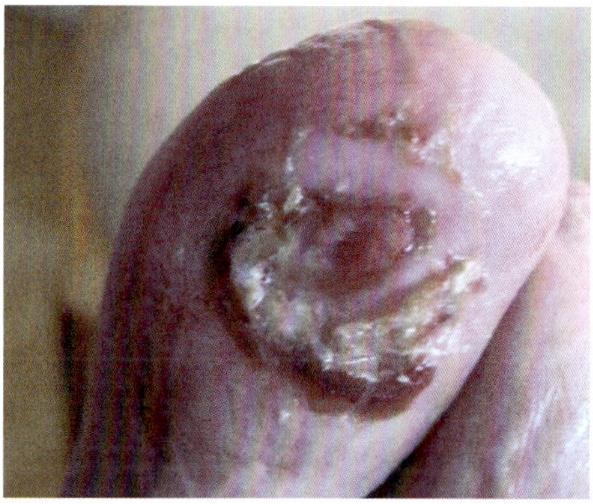

Image 3.228 Loose nail plate

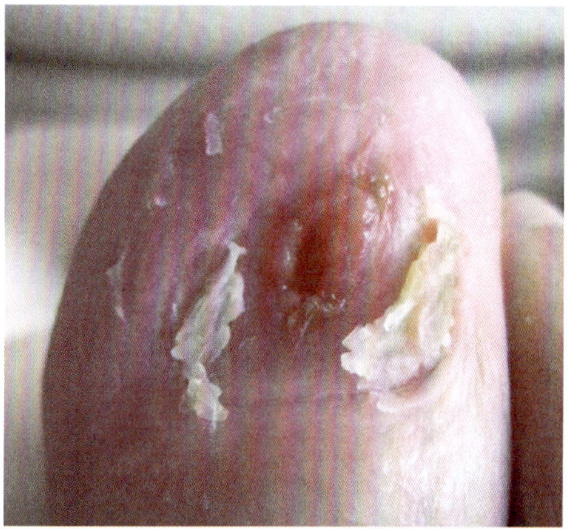

Image 3.229 After thorough wound disinfection

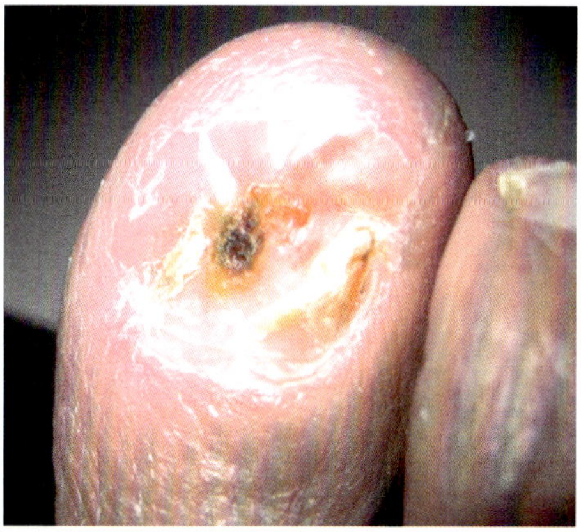

Image 3.230 14 days after treatment by a physician

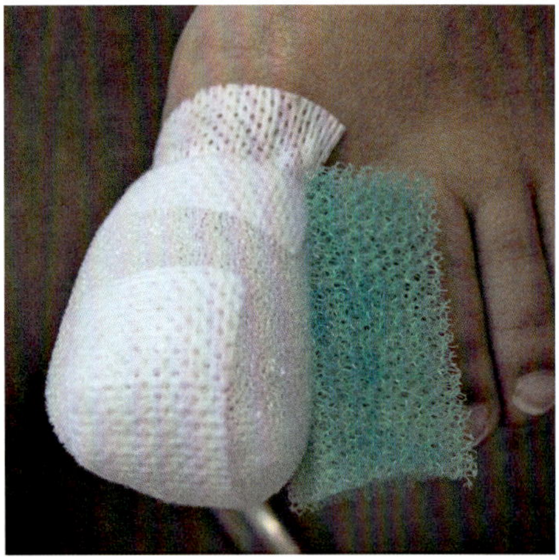

Image 3.231 Additional toe cap dressing with preparation for pressure relief with Ligasano green

After treatment by a physician, continue the wound care by applying medicinal products with a drying effect, such as alginates or zinc oxide. The sterile wound dressing must be changed daily. Once the wound is completely dry, apply a sterile dressing with colourless wound and healing ointments. An ozone steam application, the use of a high frequency bar or laser therapy are all known to accelerate healing. Once the granulation tissue has healed completely, protect the nail bed with a thermo-moulded nail plate.

3.25 Subungual exostoses

Definition

Bony overgrowth underneath the nail. (Images 3.232, 3.233)

Causes/symptoms/appearance

The subungual exostosis commonly affects the big toe. It is often seen in adolescents and is caused by repeated trauma to the toe. In the initial stage, the skin underneath the nail is thick and very solid. In some cases, serous secretion is present. The developing pain is similar to pain inflicted by unguis incarnatus.

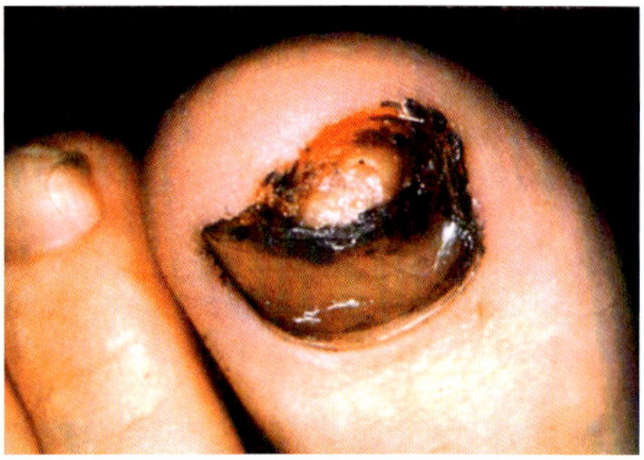

Image 3.232 Subungual exostosis underneath the nail plate of the big toe

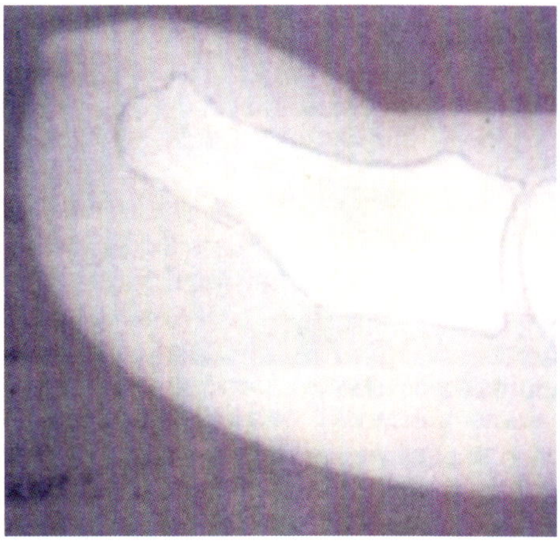

Image 3.233 X-ray image of a subungual exostosis

Images 3.232 and 3.233 Source: Klaus Grünewald, Theorie der medizinischen Fußbehandlung, tome 1, 4th edition 2012, Verlag Neuer Merkur

Complications

In its progressive stage (image 3.234), the nail can be destroyed by an infection caused by microorganisms.

Treatment

Apply sterile dressings, document the wound care procedure and refer the patient immediately to a physician. It is recommended the physician be briefed in the presence of the patient.

Surgery at an early stage prevents permanent damage to the nail bed and nail growth. If the condition progresses, damage is unavoidable (images 3.234 to 3.236).

Prophylaxis

Protecting the toe from pressure and trauma.

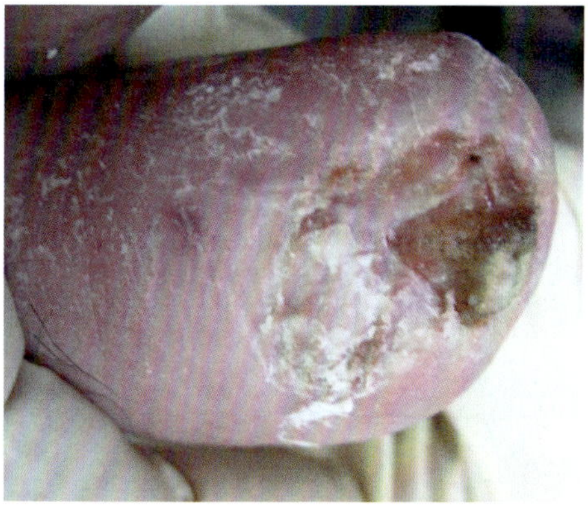

Image 3.234 After the removal of the loose nail, the bone of the distal phalanx is exposed

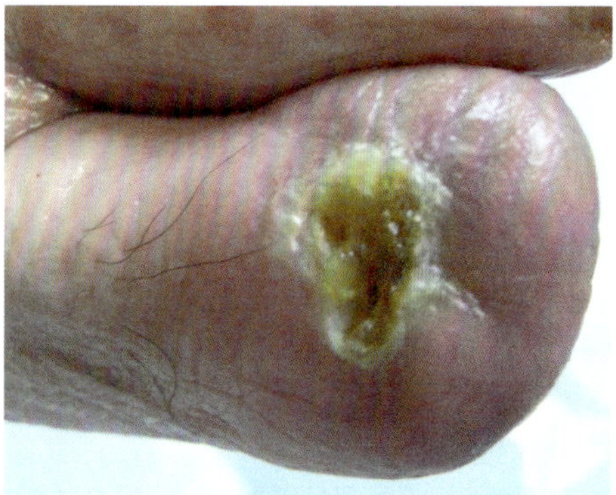

Image 3.235 After surgical removal of the bone

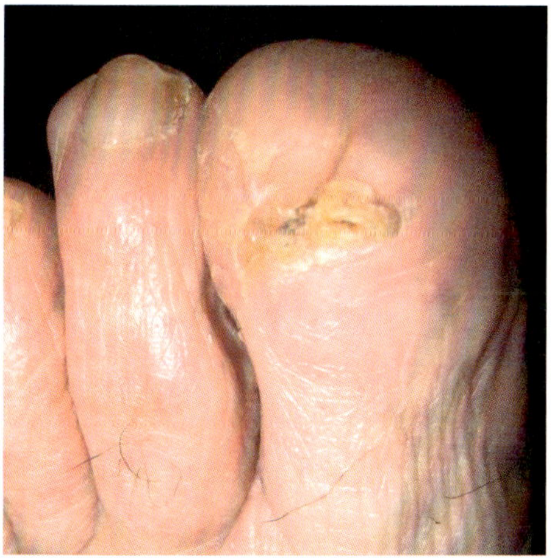

Image 3.236 After the wound has healed a new nail fragment has regrown

3.26 Subungual clavus

Definition

Clavus formation under the nail plate (image 3.237).

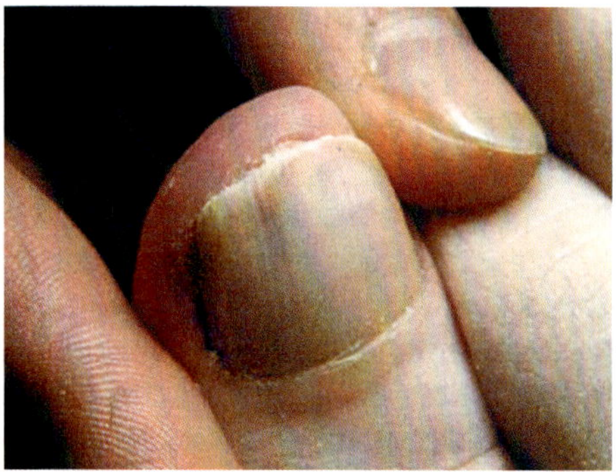

Image 3.237 Subungual clavus with brown discolouration due to a hematoma

Causes/symptoms/appearance

Subungual clavus is caused by shoes that are too tight and foot and toe deformities, such as hallux rigidus or hallux valgus. It develops when the nail is exposed to chronic irritation (pressure and friction). It is diagnosed by shining a flashlight on the nail. It has a dark, round or oval shape and does not get lighter when pressure is applied to the nail plate.

Differential diagnosis

Subungual melanoma is rarely painful.

Complications

Onycholysis, subungual granulation tissue.

Treatment

Expose the subungual clavus by carefully cutting or grinding the affected nail area (image 3.238). Cut out the core of the clavus with a cutting bur (caution: high injury risk!) or apply a mild etching tincture on the clavus combined with friction protection.

A nail prosthetic with a padded liner (images 3.239 to 3.245) or the Impro-system provide pressure relief. Advise the patient to wear properly fitting shoes that do not constrict the foot. They must be wide and long enough and should not be too tight on top. Wearing custom-made orthoses has also been proven to be effective. In some cases, surgery to correct the position of the toes is inevitable. If a hallux rigidus is the cause, then taping a not too stiff hallux rigidus provides additional relief. Apply the base of the tape at the apex plantar then gently pull the tape in plantar direction towards the MTJ 1.

Prophylaxis

- specific foot exercise and orthoses
- properly fitting shoes
- properly fitting socks

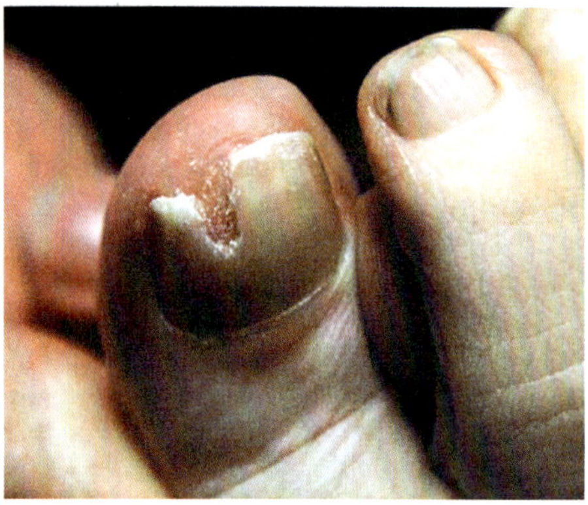

Image 3.238 Final condition of a treated subungual clavus (see image 3.237)

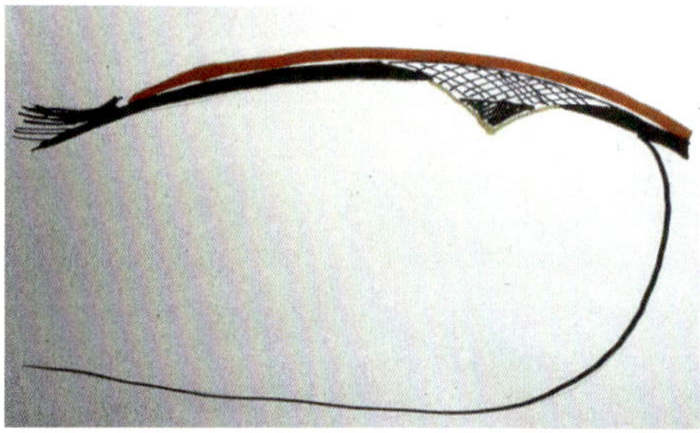

Image 3.239 Padded lining and sealing after the subungual clavus has been removed

Images 3.237 and 3.238 Source: Klaus Grünewald, Theorie der medizinischen Fußbehandlung, tome 1, 4th edition 2012, Verlag Neuer Merkur

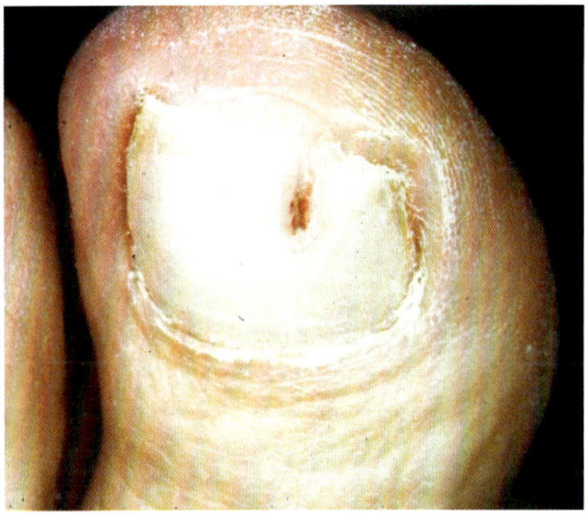

Image 3.240 Removal of the subungual clavus

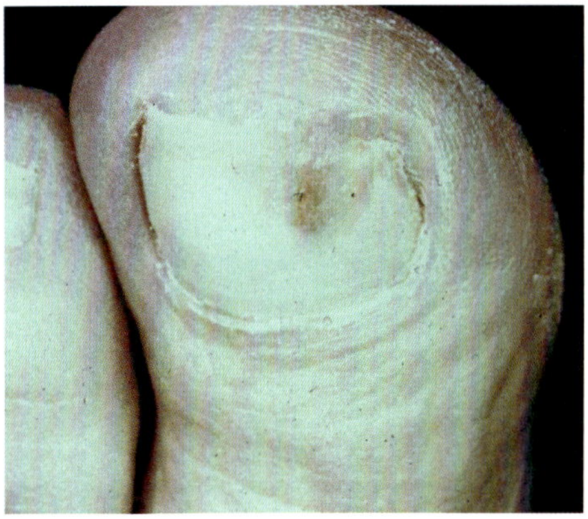

Image 3.241 Filling with BS filler

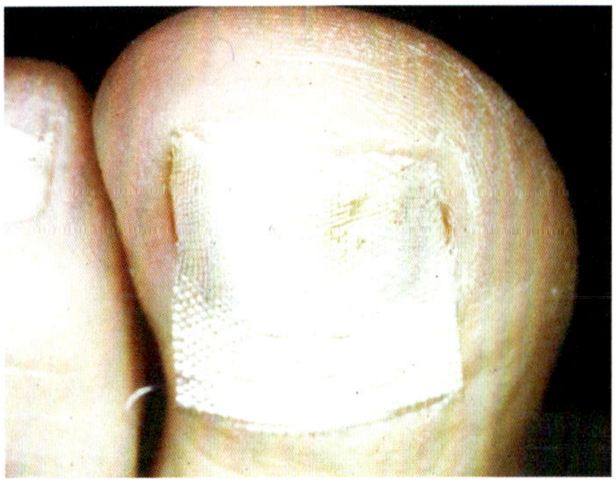

Image 3.242 Applying the BS stripe

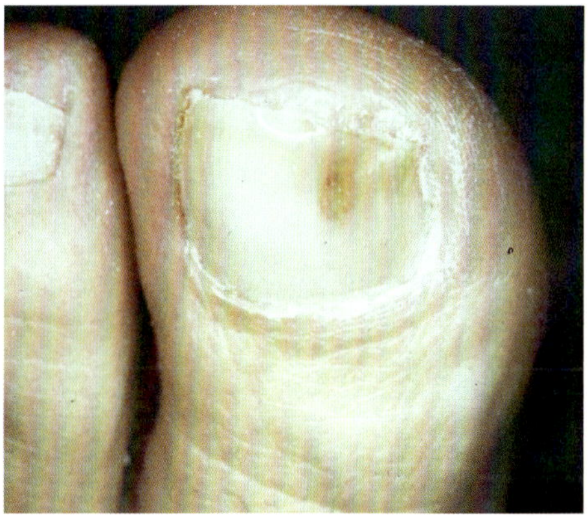

Image 3.243 BS liquid application

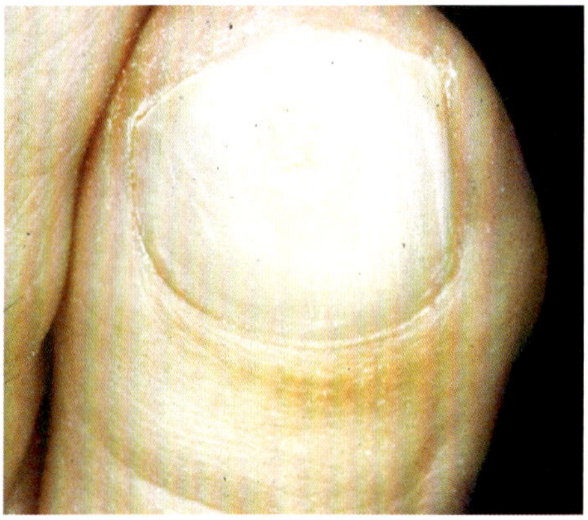

Image 3.244 Cut or grind off protruding BS parts

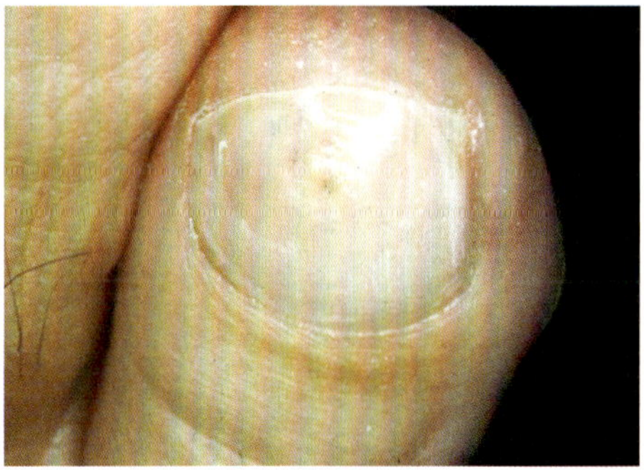

Image 3.245 BS nail – Bernd Stolz

3.27 Subungual hyperkeratosis

Definition

Excessive hornification of the nail bed with onycholysis (detachment of the nail from the nail bed, images 3.246 to 3.249).

Causes/symptoms/appearance

- circulatory disorders
- eczema
- psoriasis
- excessive pressure and friction on the nail

Once onycholysis occurs, the nail bed produces stratum corneum excessively to protect itself from infection.

Complications

Onychomycosis, onychogryposis.

Treatment

Carefully remove the hyperkeratosis build-up from under the nail. Applying special callus-softening solutions beforehand facilitates the removal. Hyperkeratosis with its high water absorption tendency creates a warm and moist environment under the nail which promotes onychomycosis. It is, therefore, important to check the nail regularly for symptoms. To effectively treat onychomycosis and to subsequently remove the clavus under the nail plate, remove the affected part of the nail with a grinding bur or a nail nipper. Once the core of the clavus has been successfully removed, ensure that the area is properly protected from pressure (see chapter 3.26).

Prophylaxis

- foot exercise to improve blood circulation
- properly fitting footwear
- correcting toe deformities with orthoses provided the toe's movement is not impaired
- mycosis prophylaxis

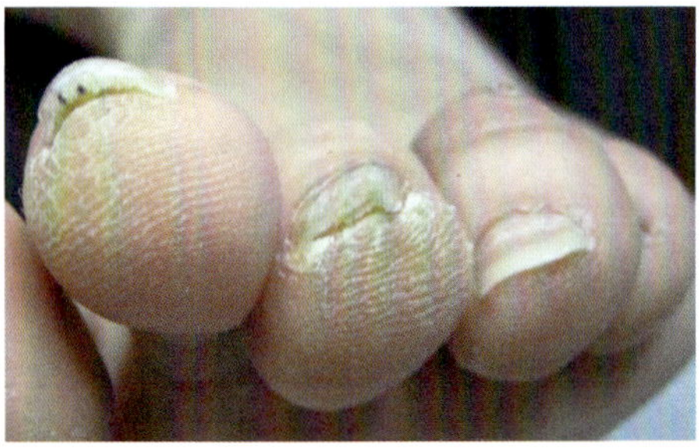

Image 3.246

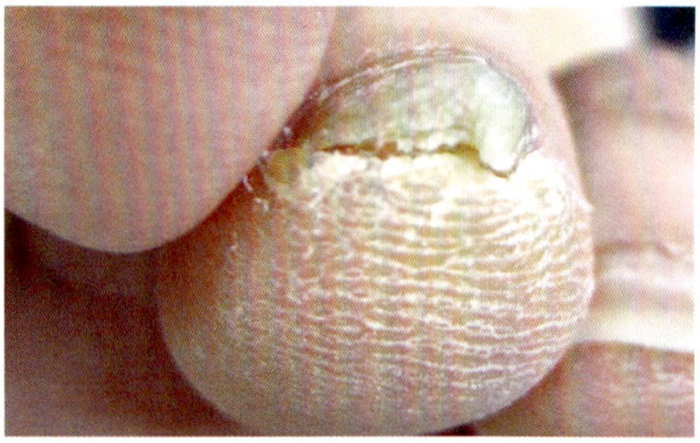

Image 3.248

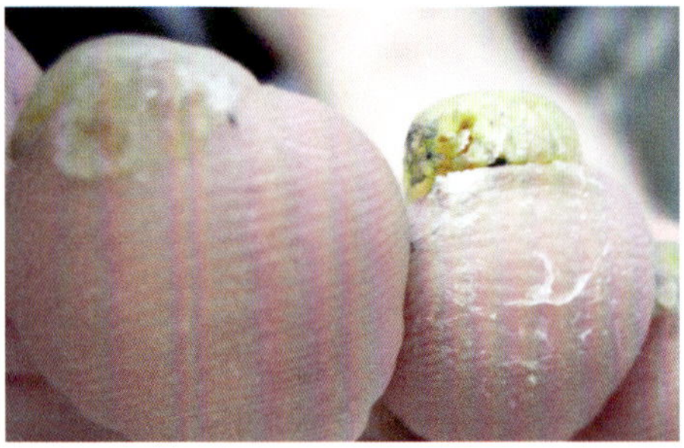

Image 3.247

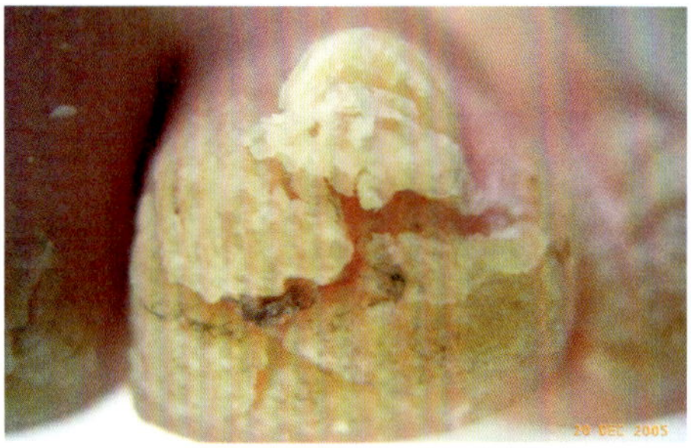

Image 3.249

3.28 Trachyonychia
(Greek: trachys = rough)

Definition
Sandpaper nails (images 3.250 and 3.251).

Causes/symptoms/appearance
Trachyonychia causes the nail to become thin and to display a spoon-like deformity. The nail plate is rough, dull, displays small dents and resembles sandpaper due to the whitish-grey scales. Damage to the matrix is believed to trigger trachyonychia.

Differential diagnosis
Endogenous eczema, psoriasis, lichen ruber, alopecia areata and the effect of certain chemicals can have a similar appearance.

Complications
Fungi penetration through the scale-like nail surface.

Treatment
Carefully smooth out the nail edges with a diamond disc. Ensure that all sharp nail particles are removed so that the nail does not get caught in socks or blankets. In some cases, a physician injects medication in the area surrounding the matrix; this, however, is a very painful and lengthy treatment approach.

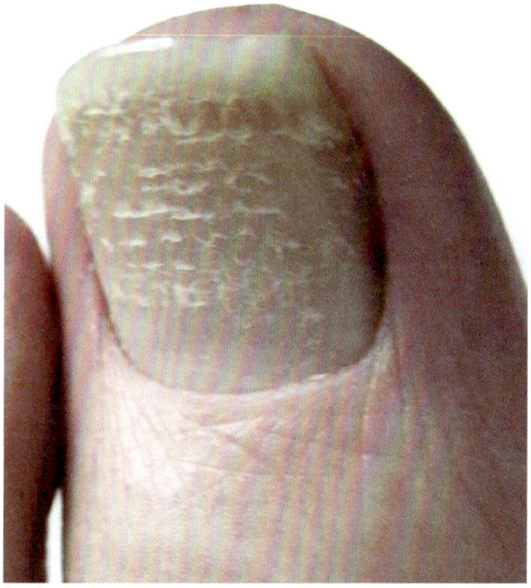

Image 3.250

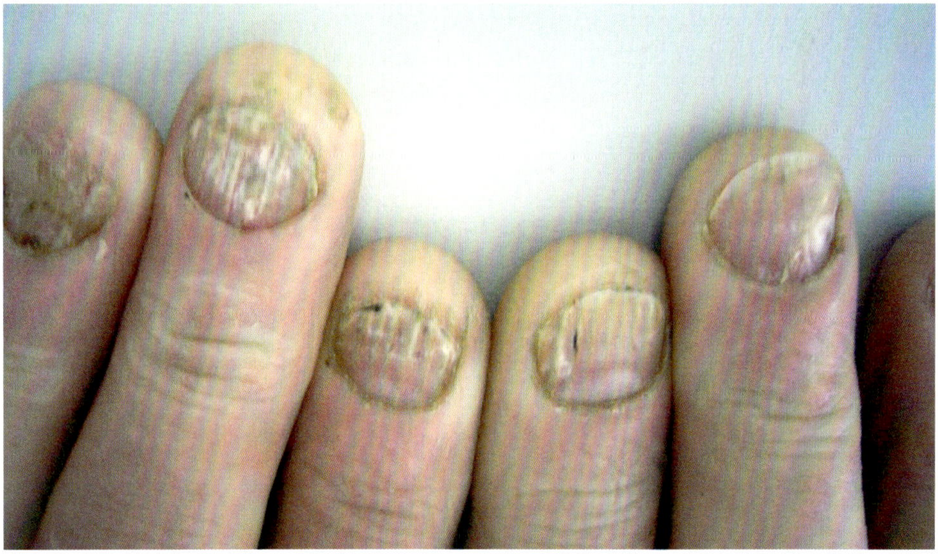

Image 3.251

Source: Brigitte Rathenow

3.29 Pterygium

(Greek: pteryx = wing,
Lat.: coniungere = connecting)

Definition

Abnormal overgrowth of the cuticle up to the free nail margin (images 3.252 to 3.256).

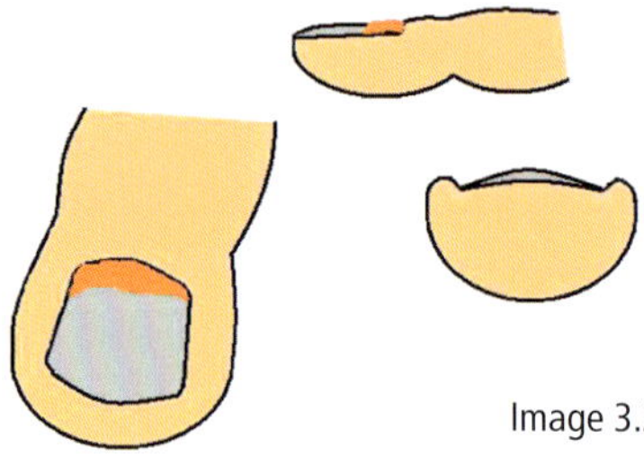

Image 3.252

Causes

dorsal:
- congenital
- bullous dermatoses (e.g., scarred pemphigoid)
- burn injuries
- dyskeratosis congenita
- graft-versus-host-reaction (gvhr)
- lichen ruber planus (most commonly)
- onychotillomania
- radiodermatitis
- Raynaud's disease
- PAOD

ventral:
- congenital
- familial
- idiopathic
- peripheral neuropathy
- Raynaud's disease and systemic scleroderma
- trauma
- mostly found on the small toe

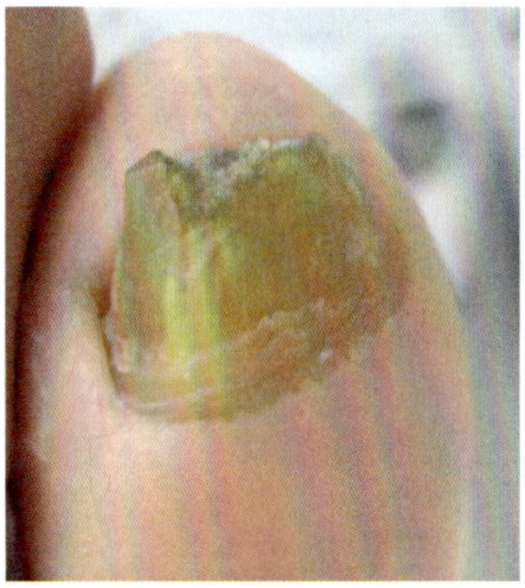

Image 3.253

Complications

An atrophied nail plate and, in extreme cases, it can lead to the partial or complete destruction of the nail matrix.

Treatment

Apply a swelling agent such as Prontoman spray or Peclavus nail-softening tincture on the cuticle and gently push back the overgrown cuticle. Sand off the upper cuticle layer or cut it off with a cuticle nipper without damaging the nail plate. Do not remove too much of the cuticle since it protects the matrix from microorganism invasion.

Prophylaxis

Frequently pushing back the cuticle and applying nail oil, nail serum or olive oil keeps it soft and flexible.

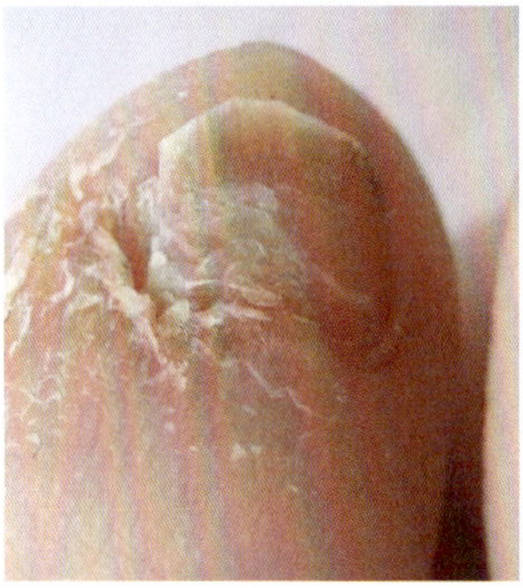

Image 3.254

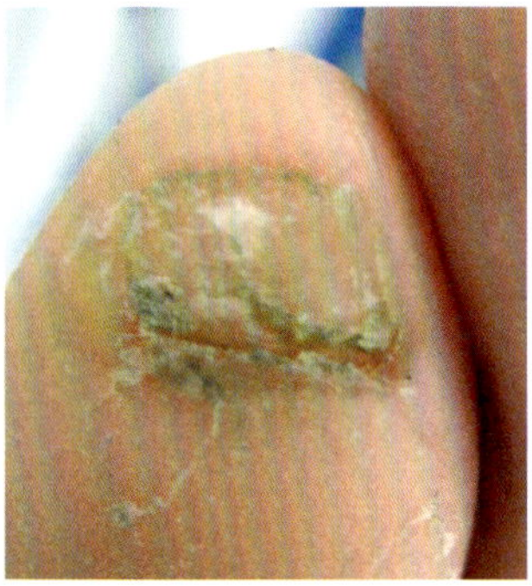

Image 3.255

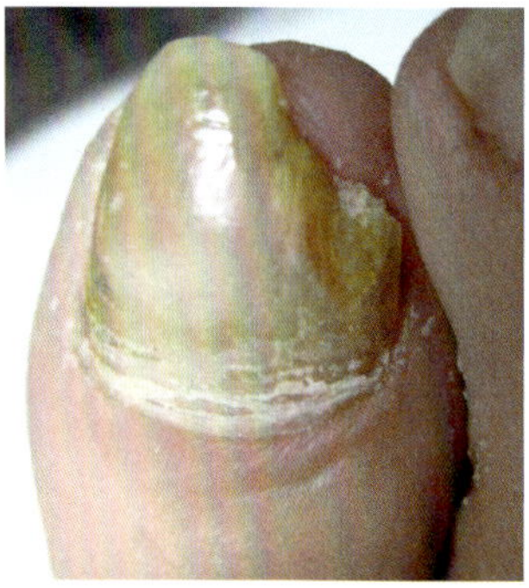

Image 3.256

3.30 Brachyonychia (racquet nail)

(Greek: brachýs = short)

wDefinition

The nail is abnormally short (images 3.257 and 3.258).

Causes/symptoms/appearance

The simple form of this condition is characterized by an abnormally short nail while the distal fingernails or toenails have a normal shape.

Congenital brachyonychia predominantly affects the fingers and most often only the thumb.

The nails are abnormally short and wide and the finger or thumb resembles a tennis racquet.

Complications

The simple form of this condition can cause bulging of the nail bed.

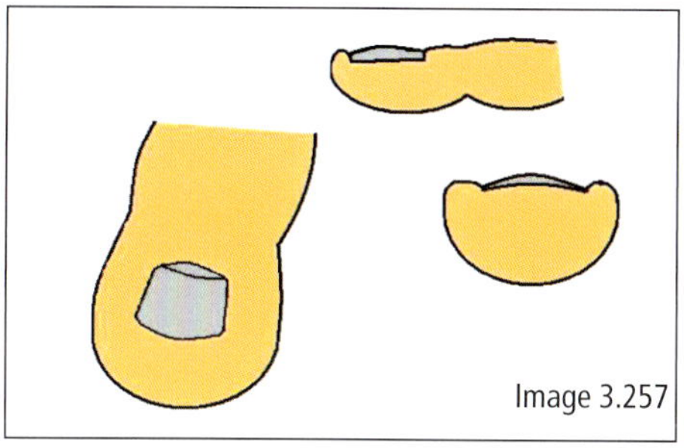

Image 3.257

Treatment

Do not cut the nails too short. If necessary, apply a nail prosthetic to prevent bulging. Congenital brachyonychia can, in most cases, only be corrected surgically.

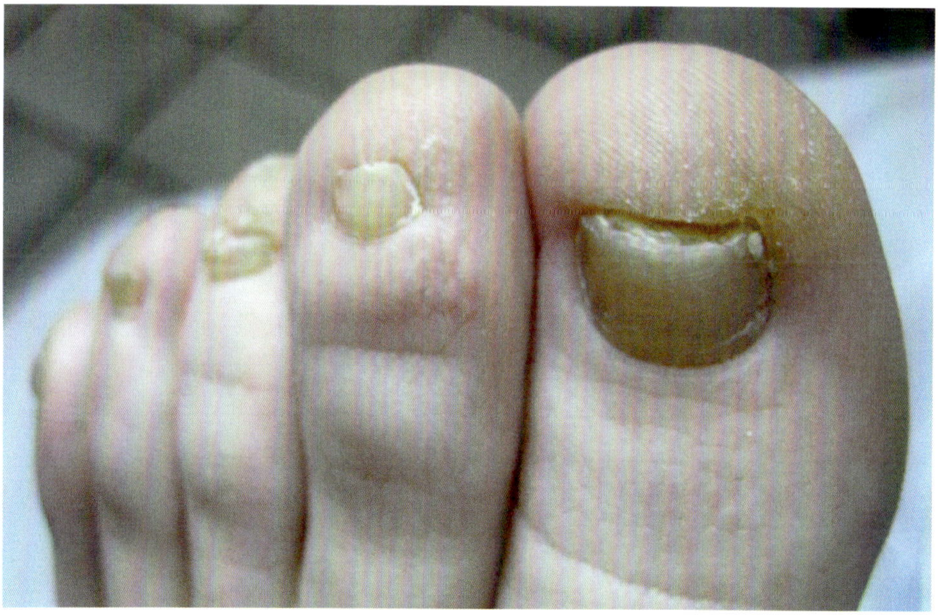

Image 3.258

3.31 Scleroderma
(Greek: sklẽros = hard)

Definition
Scleroderma is a disease of the connective tissue featuring thickened skin (images 3.259 and 3.260).

Causes/symptoms/appearance
The cause of scleroderma is not known. It is a rare disease and with its rheumatic inflammatory characteristics it belongs to the group of collagenoses. Collagens are important components of the connective tissue. Without them, the connective tissue hardens and loses its elasticity and functionality. Connective tissue is not only found in the skin. Blood vessels, the inner organs, simply all the tissue with a blood supply is composed of connective tissue. Almost all patients diagnosed with scleroderma (>90%) suffer from Raynaud's syndrome (paroxysmal circulatory disorder of the fingers or toes triggered by cold temperatures or emotional stress).

The cuticle is thick, hard, cracked, painful, and it bleeds occasionally. The nail becomes gradually narrower towards the apex and displays ridges and grooves; at worst it can lead to necrosis and destruction of the lunula.

Complications
Onychomadesis, onchyomycosis.

Treatment
Carefully sand off all sharp edges to prevent nail parts from getting caught on socks or blankets. Apply cuticle softener, such as Prontoman spray, to the cuticle, gently push the cuticle back with an excavator and remove it with cuticle nippers or scissors. This must be done very carefully so not to cause bleeding. The thick cuticle can also safely be removed with a rosehead bur without the application of a softening spray.

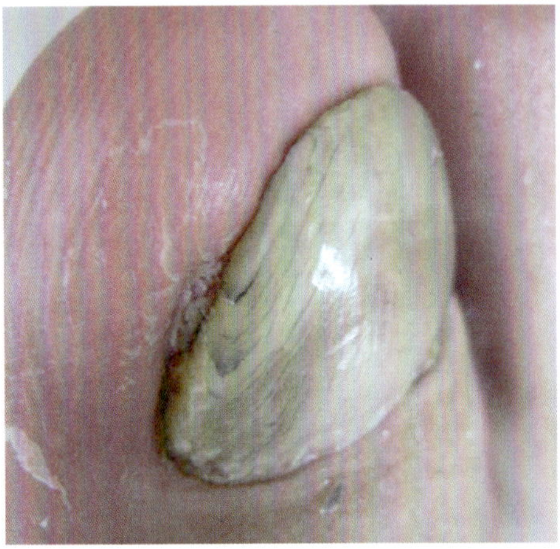

Image 3.259

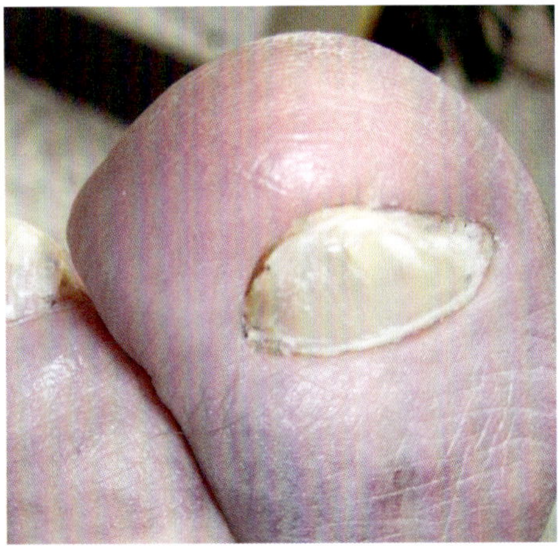

Image 3.260

Prophylaxis
None.

3.32 Tumors in the nail area

Definition

A tumor is a localized enlargement of tissue volume, a growth. The growth can also be an edema (fluid accumulation), warts, small periungual fibromas, exostoses, pigment naevi, glomus tumors, pseudo cysts, a malign melanoma, carcinoma or basalioma. Strictly speaking, the term tumor is used for the uncontrolled growth of the body's own cells; a tumor can be either benign or malign (images 3.261 to 3.263).

Causes

Tumors have various causes and affect the nail's growth and appearance.

Pathogenesis

Tumors in the nail fold area and on the matrix are easily recognizable. Subungual tumors are often just a blot resembling a subungual hematoma. The diagnosis or classification is not conclusive.

Differential diagnosis

The clinical diagnosis and differential diagnosis is done by a physician.

Treatment

The patient must be referred to a physician. However, it is helpful if the podiatrist draws a line below the dark discolouration with a fissure grinding bur and verifies at the next visit if the blot has changed in size (see 3.22 subungual hematoma). Documenting the changes of the growth and adding images is helpful for the physician (image 3.264).

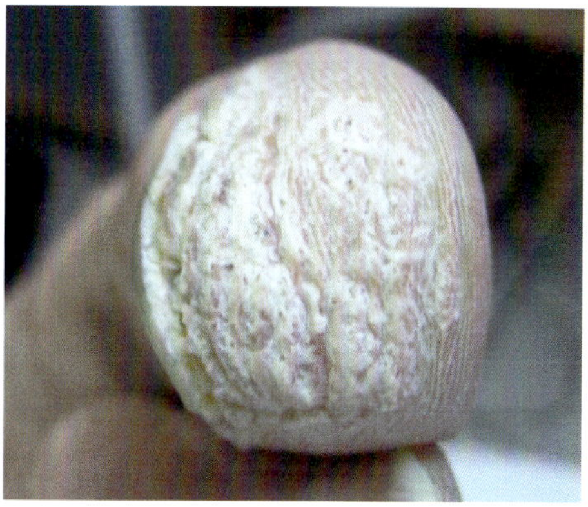

Image 3.261 Warts under and around the nail

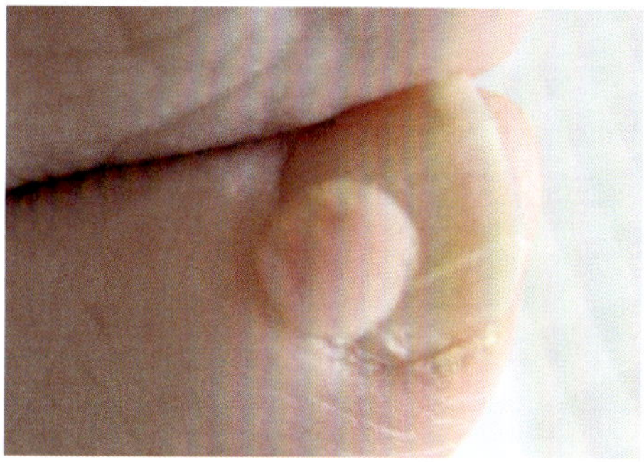

Image 3.262

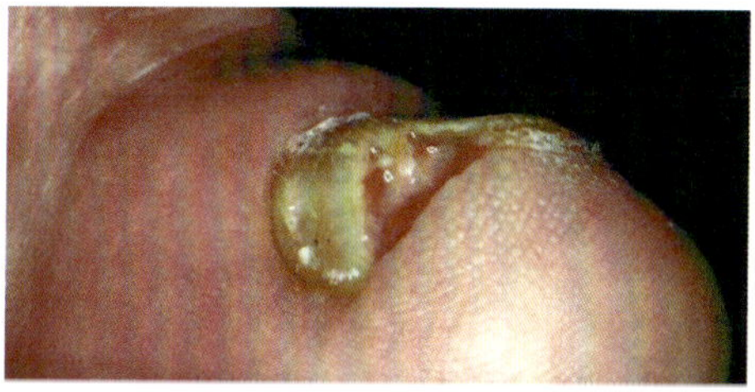

Image 3.263 Squamous cell carcinoma in the nail bed area

Source: Klaus Grünewald, Theorie der medizinischen Fußbehandlung, tome 2, 3rd edition 2016, Verlag Neuer Merkur

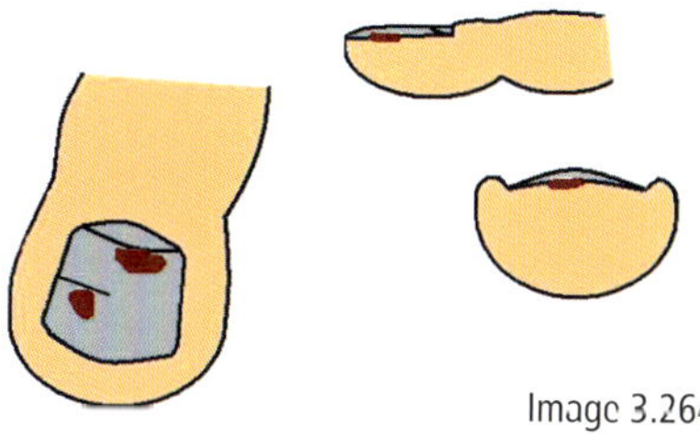

Image 3.264

3.33 Scleronychia
(Greek: sklēros = hard)

Definition
Permanently impaired nail growth up to complete arrest of growth (images 3.265 to 3.267).

Causes/symptoms/appearance
The nail is thick with a yellowish-grey discolouration. Often the cuticle is missing and the lunula is invisible. The nail is transversally curved. The connection between nail and nail bed is loose up to complete detachment. The cause is unknown, however, the disease is more often seen in women. Fifty per cent of the patients also suffer from respiratory diseases such as sinusitis, bronchitis, bronchiectasis, pleurisy and pulmonary fibrosis. The disease is often hereditary.

Complications
Onychomadesis, onychomycosis.

Treatment
Carefully smooth the nail's edges to prevent the nail from getting caught on socks or blankets. Medication prescribed by a physician can help in some cases. In rare cases, spontaneous healing occurs.

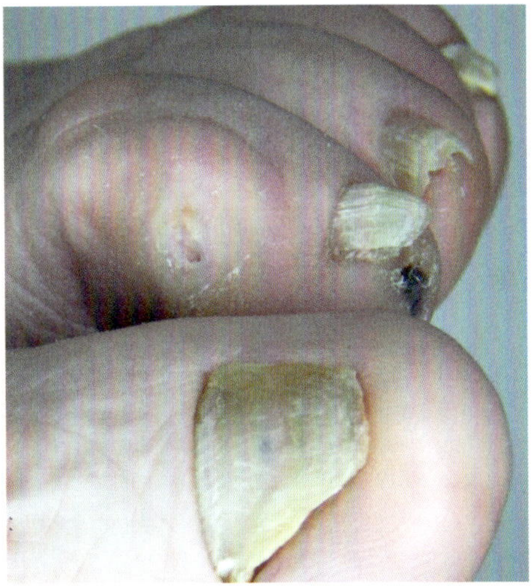

Image 3.266 Source: Liesel Sayferth

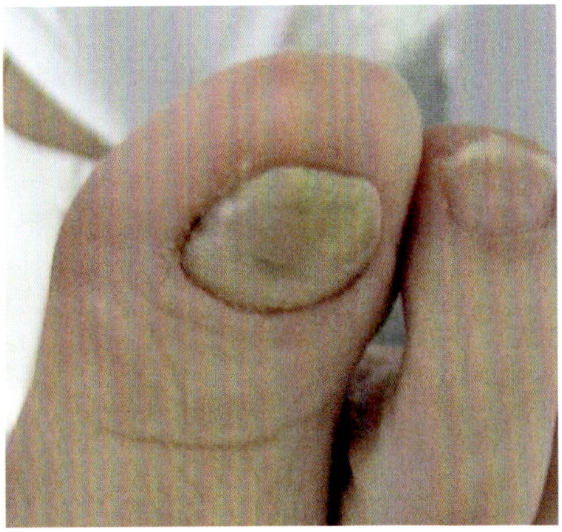

Image 3.267

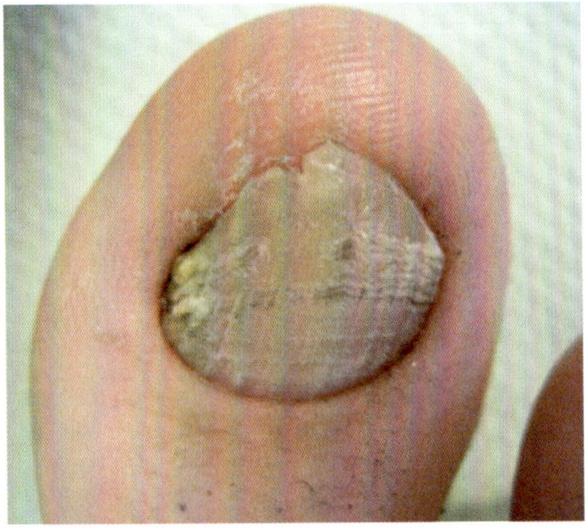

Image 3.265

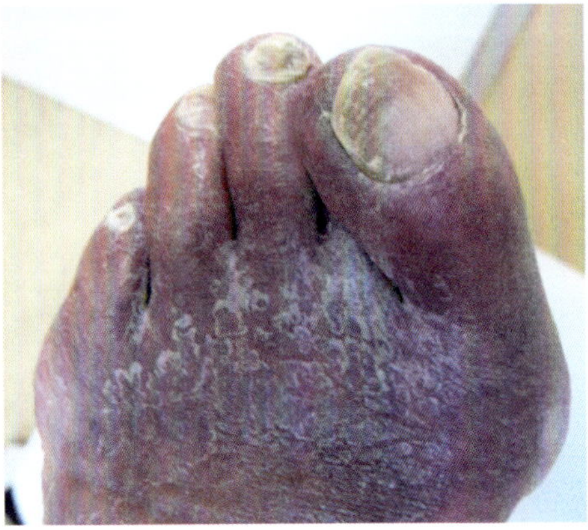

Image 3.268 Poor blood circulation

3.34 Dyschromia
(Lat.: dys = faulty, Greek: chrõma = colour)

Definition

Discolouration of the nail without changes to the shape or surface texture of the nail (images 3.268 to 3.271).

Causes

Discolouration of an otherwise healthy nail can be caused by a variety of exogenous factors, such as pigmentation deposits, colouring agents, medication, toxins, callus skin, hollow pockets under the nail, inflammation, tumors, foreign particles and hematoma.

Differential diagnosis

- white discolouration of the nail (leukonychia)
- dark discolouration of the nail: blue, blue-red, brown, yellow, green, red or black

A precise differential diagnosis must be performed by a physician who can determine if it is a harmless hematoma or a malign tumor. Discolouration of the nail is often a sign of various internal diseases, such as hepatopathy, haemochromatosis, kidney insufficiency, liver disease or heart disease. Therefore, a specialist for internal medicine should be consulted.

Treatment

From a podiatrist's viewpoint, there are no therapeutic treatment options available.

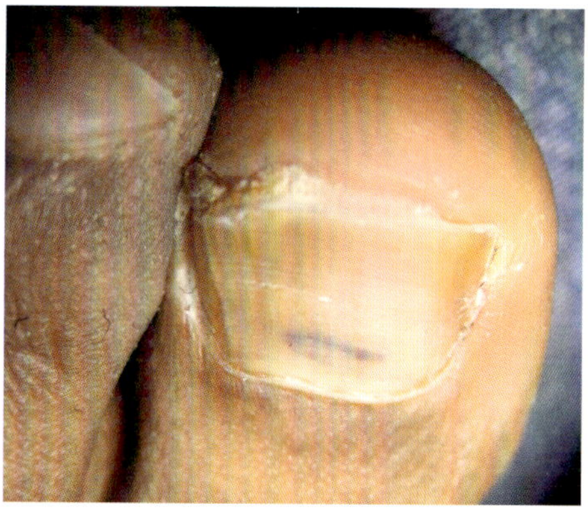

Image 3.269

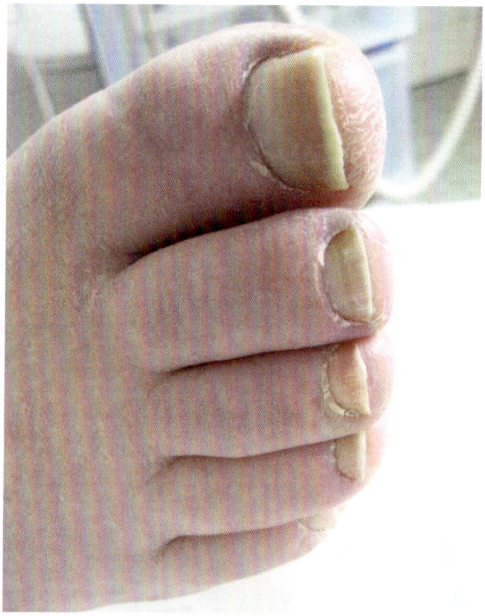

Image 3.270 Poor blood circulation

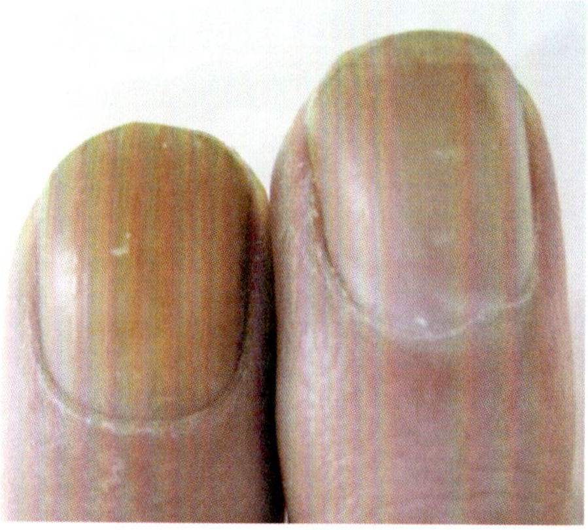

Image 3.271 Nicotine stains

4

Types of dressings

Every injury, even the smallest, is a reason for concern and must be taken seriously. Skin injuries in the foot area are prone to bacterial infections. The warm and moist environment in the foot region provides an excellent breeding ground for bacteria and spores, especially in the area between the toes and around the nails. For deep and large injuries, the follow-up treatment must, therefore, be performed after 24 to a maximum of 48 hours.

The dressings should fulfil the following requirements:

- **protection against the invasion of microorganisms** (bacteria, fungi, viruses and foreign particles) and act as a protective barrier against environmental factors, such as excessive heat, extreme dryness, unusual cold or wet conditions and UV rays
- **protection against mechanical stress**, such as shock and pressure and movements that cause the wound to reopen, resulting in the tearing of newly formed tissue
- **fixation of medicinal products**, such as ointments or medicine-impregnated gauze directly on the wound
- **compression dressing** to prevent swelling and scarring, as in thrombosis prophylaxis or in conjunction with manual lymphatic drainage
- **haemostasis**
- **secretion absorption** prevents tissue softening and removes denaturated protein, a healing resistant substance found in burn wounds and pus

A properly applied toe dressing should cover the wound completely without adding extra pressure on the wound that might suppress blood circulation. It is important to choose and prepare the dressing according to the patient's skin condition! For example, plasters should not be used on patients with thin parchment-like skin since it would damage the skin.

The presence of a hammer toe can cause pressure issues and requires additional pressure relief measures.

Choosing the correct dressing materials

The dressing material must be chosen according to the existing wound condition and should fulfil the following requirements:

- remove excessive wound secretion
- keep an adequate moisture level in the wound area
- ensure proper gas exchange
- protect the wound from heat and cold exposure
- must be impermeable to microorganisms
- The material must be lint- and impurity-free and able to be removed without causing trauma to the skin.

Changing the dressing

- A dressing must always be changed under sterile conditions.
- The "no-touch technique" must always be used during dressing changes, so that the wound and the dressing are never touched with bare hands.
- In case several wounds need to be treated, the following procedure must be followed: Aseptic wounds are treated first, then semi-aseptic wounds and lastly septic wounds.

Additional requirements for wound dressings

- It should promote wound healing.
- It should not stick to the wound.
- The dressing change process must be easy, quick and painless for the patient.
- The material ideally should also be versatile and cost-efficient.

Adhesive plasters

Adhesive plasters hold dressings, cannulas and tubes in place and have no direct skin contact.

They contain:

- caoutchouc
  - high adhesive strength
  - painful when removed from the skin
  - detoriates at high temperatures
  - e.g., Leucoplast
- polyacrylate
  - fully synthetic adhesive compound
  - excellent skin compatibility
  - rarely causes allergic reaction
  - ageing-resistant, porous, air and water permeable
  - e.g., Leukosilk

Emergency bandage

An emergency bandage is a plaster with a soft wound dressing pad in the center. The pad is a combination of sterile gauze, a layer of gauze-cotton compression material, nonwoven or synthetic material. The emergency bandage is used for the urgent treatment of small- to medium-sized wounds.

Different plaster shapes and sizes

The following must be considered when applying plaster in the toe area:

Different toe lengths or deformities require individually fitted plasters! The dorsal area of a toe is longer than the plantar area.

The plaster must completely cover the area to be protected and should not fray nor detach when the patient puts on or takes off his/her socks. If necessary, additional fixation tape must be applied!

Cutting the correct plaster size as shown in the images is important. The gauze dressing pad must be larger than the wound and must never be touched with bare hands. After cutting the correct size, remove the protective foil and place the wound dressing pad directly on the wound. The adhesive part of the plaster ideally should adhere smoothly and wrinkle-free to the skin (images 4.1 to 4.17). For applying a tubular bandage on a wound dressing, start by cutting a piece of tubular bandage that is double the length of the toe you want to dress and place it gently over the entire length of the toe. An applicator is helpful as it allows you to apply the bandage without putting pressure on the wound. Twist the bandage tube several times above the top of the toe, pull the remaining tube again over the entire length of the toe and gently secure the end piece with a plaster or, depending on the length of the material, tie it around the ankle of the foot without constricting the skin (images 4.18 to 4.22).

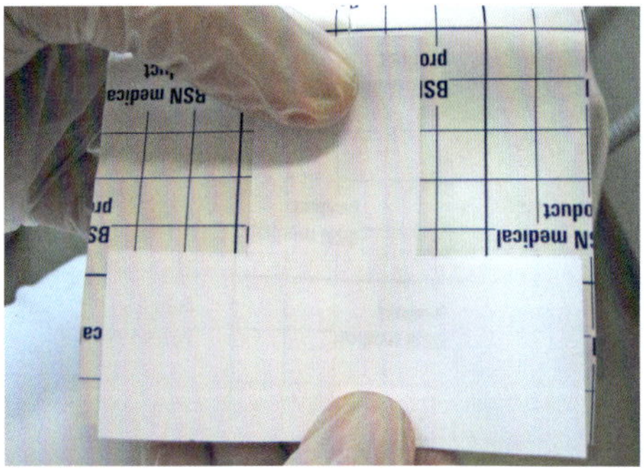

Image 4.1

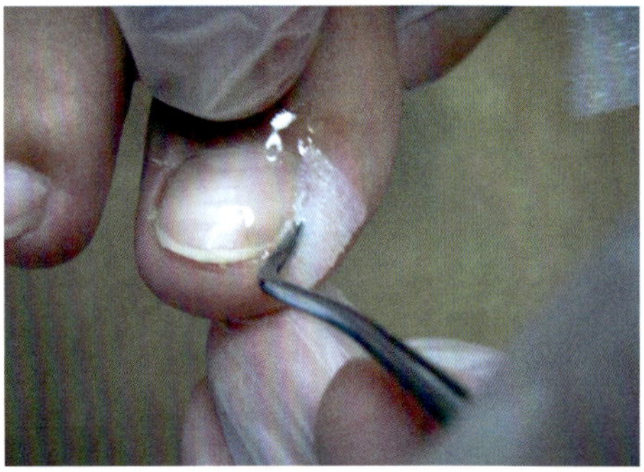

Image 4.2

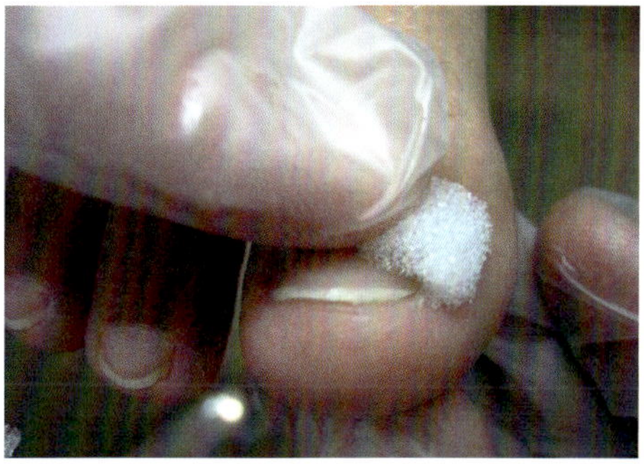

Image 4.3

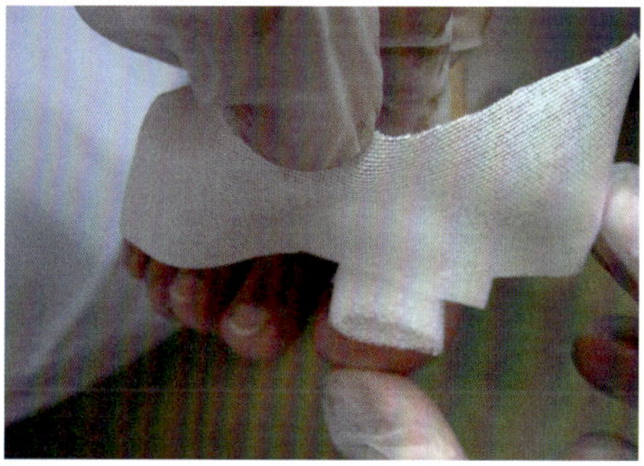

Image 4.4

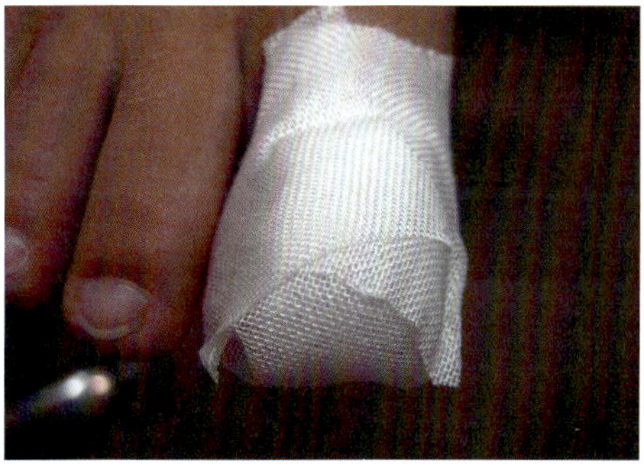

Image 4.5

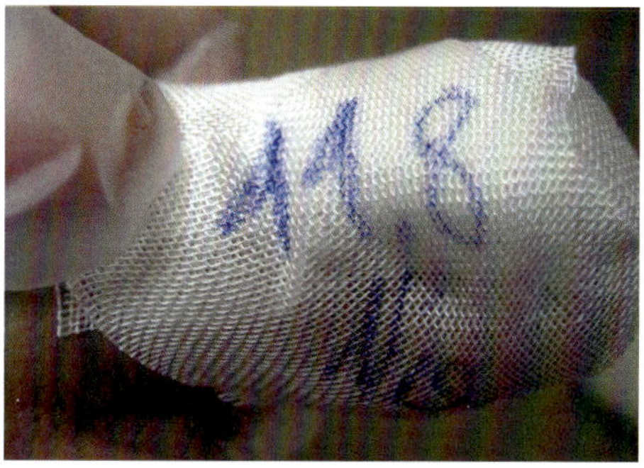

Image 4.6

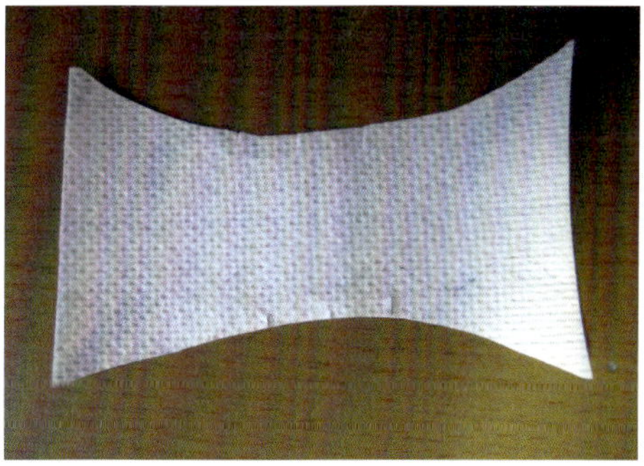

Image 4.7

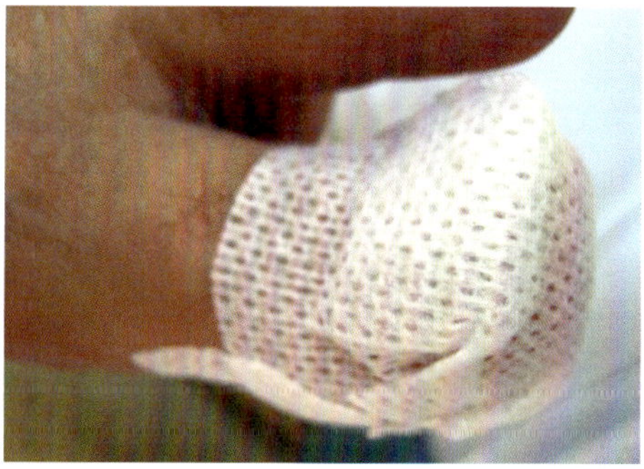

Image 4.8

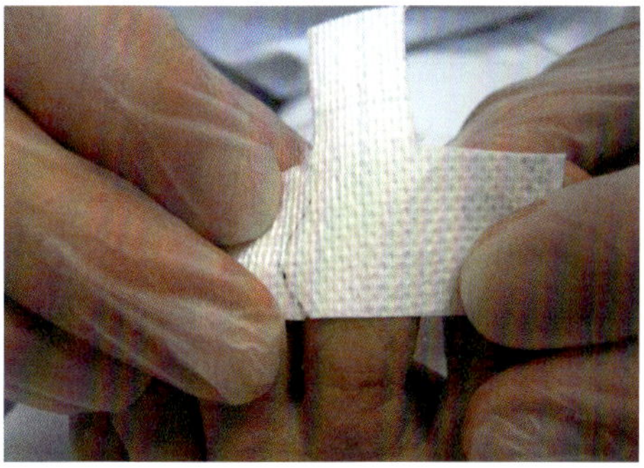

Image 4.9

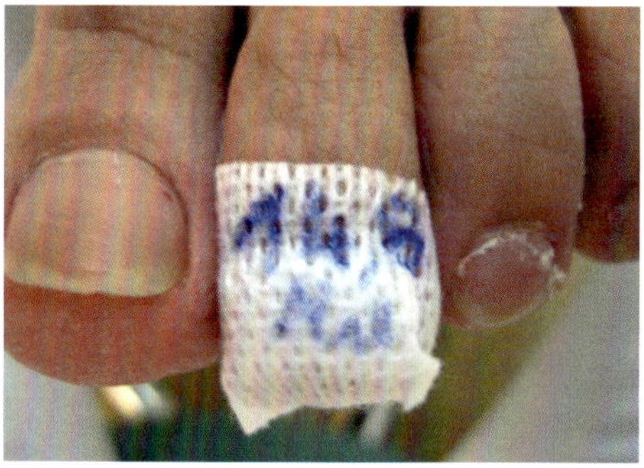

Image 4.10

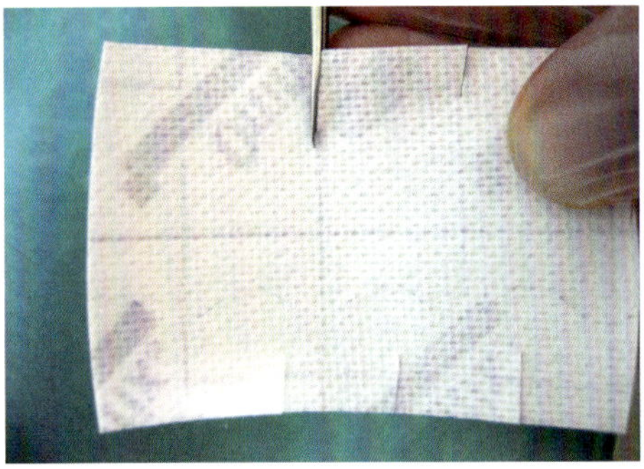
Image 4.11

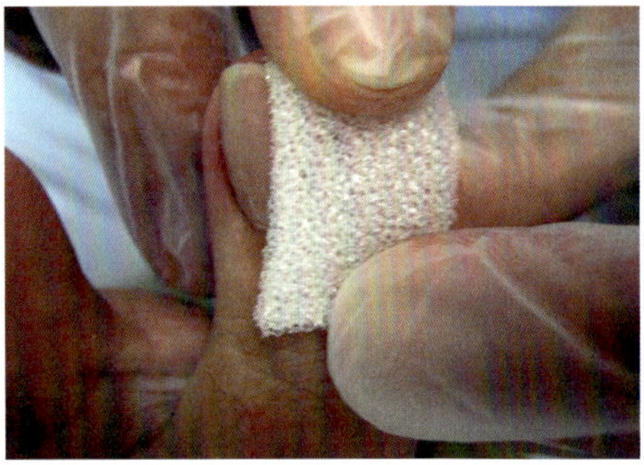
Image 4.12

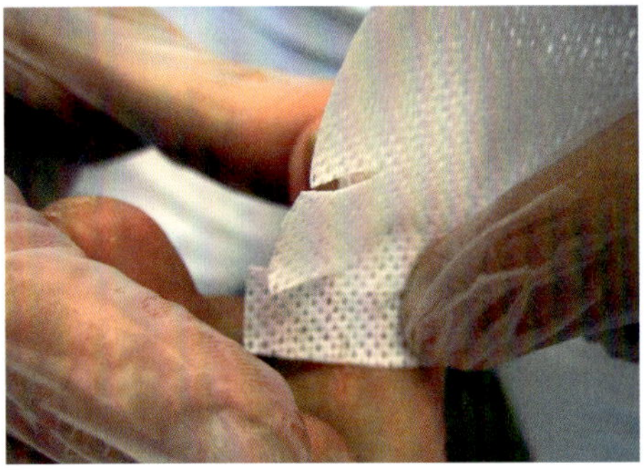
Image 4.13

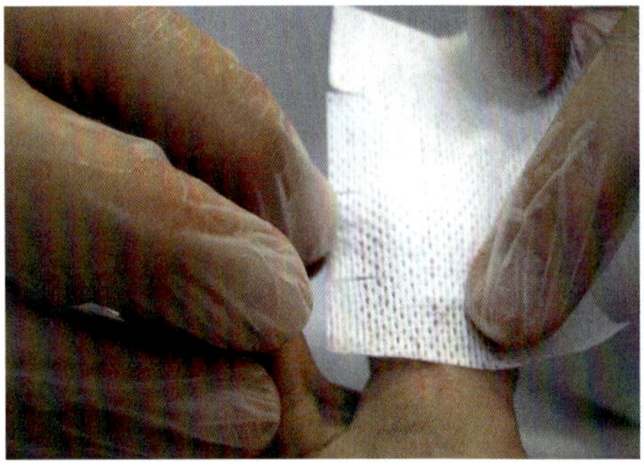
Image 4.14

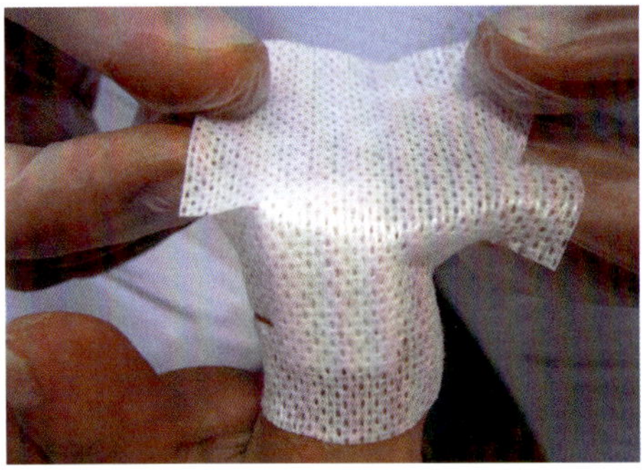
Image 4.15

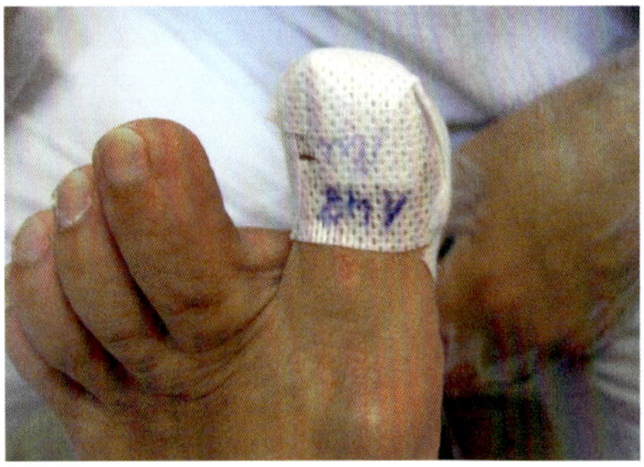
Image 4.16

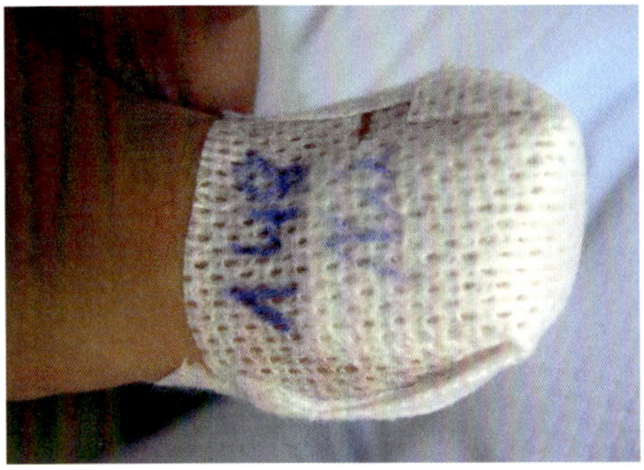
Image 4.17

Preparation and standard procedures for changing a dressing

- Prepare the work area (image 4.23).
- Close the windows and make sure the working space is well lit.
- Ensure that the patient is comfortable.
- Adjust the bed or chair to the desired working height.
- Clean and disinfect the hands.
- Inform the patient about the treatment procedure.
- Use disposable gloves.

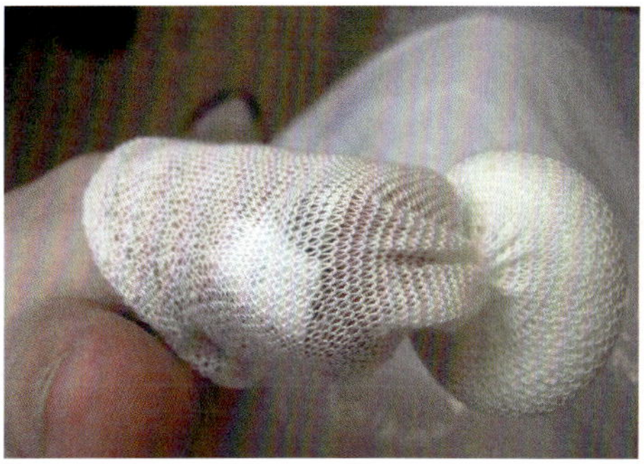

Image 4.18

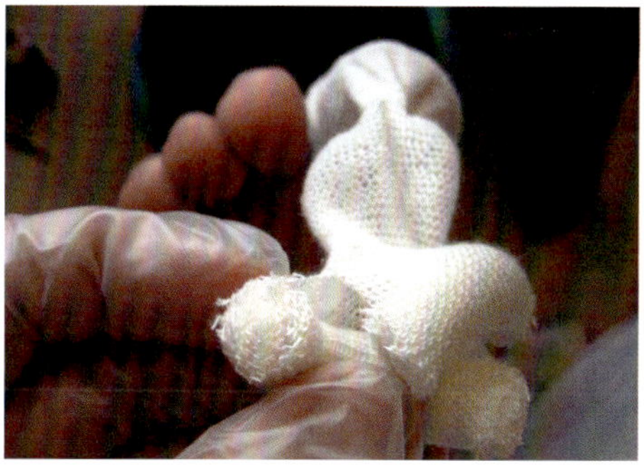

Image 4.19

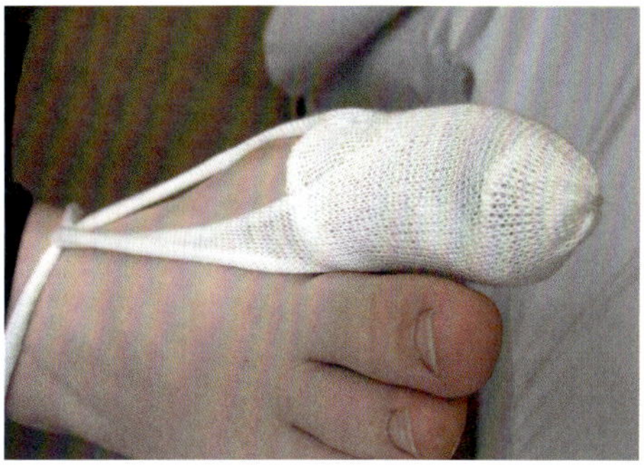

Image 4.20

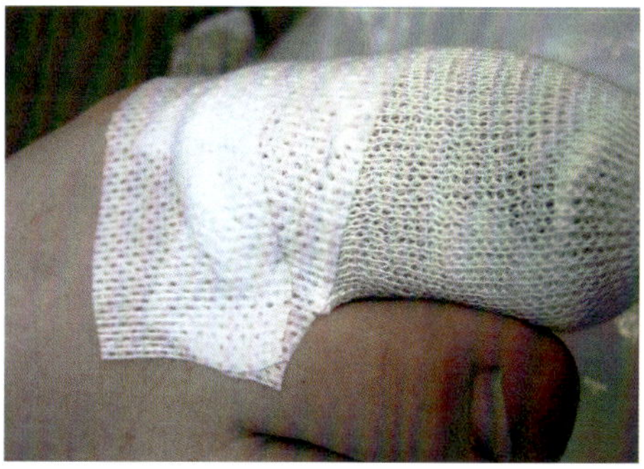

Image 4.21

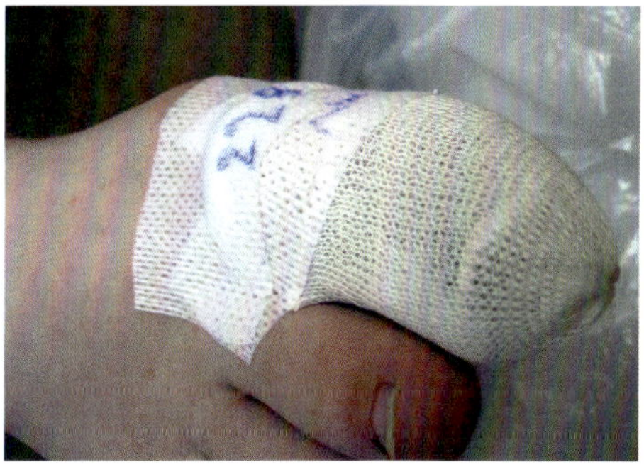

Image 4.22

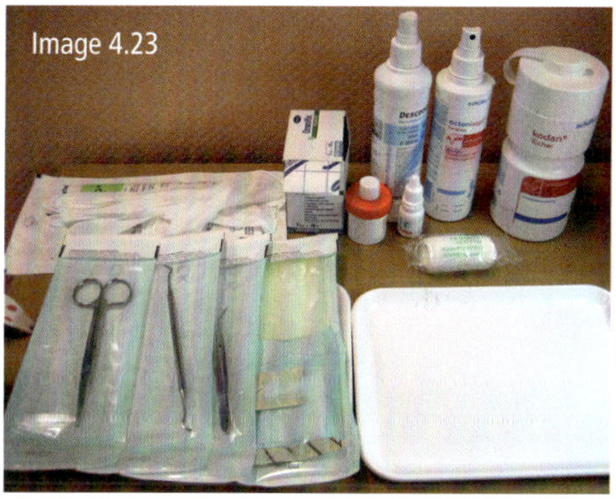

Image 4.23

- Remove old dressing and dispose of it, then inspect the wound carefully.
- Disinfect the hands again and wear a new pair of disposable gloves.
- Treat the wound (possibly as instructed by the physician, if the patient has been transferred)
- Apply the dressing.
- Disinfect the hands again.
- Document the wound care procedure.
- NGLProperly clean, disinfect and sterilize the instruments.
- Dispose of all used materials.
- Disinfect the work area.

5

Orthonyxia

5.1 The history of orthonyxia

The term orthonyxia was created in 1960 by the Scottish podiatrist Ross Fraser. It is a combination of the Greek words onyx (nail) and orthos (correct, straight) and means straightening of the nail.

Orthonyxia is an excellent alternative to surgical procedures, such as partial resection or complete removal of the nail, and provides instant pain relief for the patient. The method has been proven to generate successful treatment results for many patients.

Compared to a surgical procedure, orthonyxia offers the following advantages:

- the nail and the tip of the toe are preserved
- no scarring
- less pain
- covers a large application range

The most significant milestones in the field of nail correction techniques are listed below in chronological order:

1873	First wire brace patented by E. Stedman in 1873
1938	Rosenstein, two holes, one surgical thread
1946	Scholl, steel wire. Standard size, two centre loops; today Duplex
1960	Gifford, three parts with two end loops and centre spring
1961	Fraser 1, unilateral half-brace
1962	Fraser 2, bilateral brace, two end loops
1964	Waldmann, two parts; plastic brace for stabilization
1970	Kitzka, pre-assembled Fraser brace, 11–25 mm
1977	Gorkiewicz, flat spring brace without centre loop
1980	French version of the Fraser brace
1982	Erki-Technik, plastic hooks and rubber
1982	Link-method, regulatory instruments
1983	Full nail prosthesis by Erkodent, artificial nail, further development of the Greppmayr plate prosthetics
1986	Rading, universal tier pliers; preparation of the Fraser brace on the nail
1987	BS brace (Stolz), plastic platelets
1988	VHO brace (Osthold), three parts
1988	Glor, Swiss brace made of pure gold, soft gold wire, half adhesive brace with a large adhesive surface
1990	Gold brace or Goldstadt brace (Ruck)
1992	3TO brace, three-part brace
2006	Ora brace (Brigitte Rathenow), two-part brace
2007	Podofix active adhesive brace (3TO)
2010	Corectio Titan, Japanese brace, available in Germany since 2012
2010	SSO4U brace, three-part spring brace sold by the company Gerlach as GTO-brace (Gerlach-Technik-Orthonyxie)
2011	COMBIped, combination of a spring wire with an adhesive brace
2012	BS brace with magnetic applicator (adhesive brace)
2016	3TO PLUS I brace

5.2 Recommendations for the correct use of nail braces

Taping the nail fold supports the correction process. Place the base of the tape on the side of the nail wall, then pull the tape hard in plantar direction on the ball of the toe and secure the end piece of the tape. Rubbing the tape down ensures a strong adhesion. The tape must never be applied on wounds. The patient should not take a foot bath prior to taping and the foot must be warm.

Here is another useful tip for everybody who has difficulties measuring the brackets of wire braces:

Place a plaster over one half of the nail, mark the lateral nail margin and the highest point where the omega or the centre loop of the three-part brace will be positioned, then stick this plaster on an index card. It is now easy to determine the correct length of the brace brackets. Do not forget to include the length of the hooks.

To practice bending the brackets, draw different shapes on a piece of paper (see image below) and try to copy the shapes. Start at the omega or the hooks but be careful not to bend the long side pieces.

Podiatrist and patient protection

When applying nail correction braces, always wear safety glasses, disposable gloves and a face mask and also ask the patient to wear safety glasses to protect him/her from wire pieces while cutting the brace wire.

Safety information

The braces are intended to provide relief for patients who suffer from ingrown toe nails, with the focus on restoring the natural growth process of the nail.

Children must never be allowed to handle the wires since the ends are extremely sharp and can cause serious injury. Always store the wires in a childproof container.

Use the sterile brace explicitly for the intended treatment purpose following specified instructions and avoid any misapplications.

Contraindications of brace application

- onychomycosis (the nail plate is soft, and the static will be impaired)
- onycholysis/subungual hematoma (the braces force the already loose nail to detach even further)
- onychogryposis/onychauxis (it can cause the nail edges to loosen with an abnormally thick nail and may trigger onycholysis)
- onychorrhexis (static problems)
- onychoschizia (static problems)
- onychodystrophy, e.g., psoriatic nail dystrophy (static problems)
- inadequate patient compliance

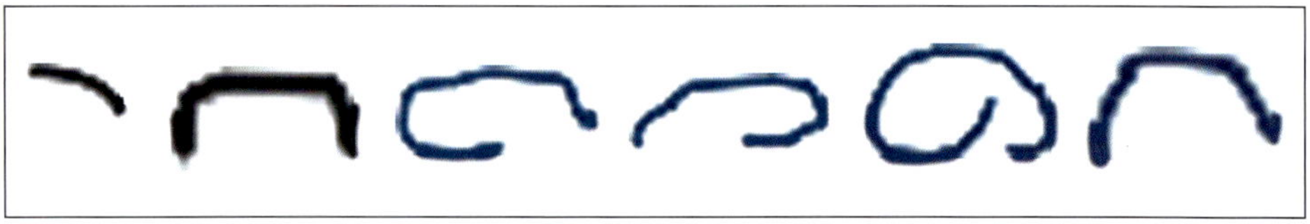

5.3 Fraser nail bracing system with omega loop

The Fraser brace is considered the classic nail correction brace.

1946 First mention of a brace made of sterling silver in the book "The Human Foot" by Dr. W. M. Scholl. Published by Foot Specialist Publishing Co., Chicago, USA.

1960 Advanced development of the technique by Ross Fraser, Dundee, Scotland.

1964 Introduction of the technique in Germany by the podiatrist Josef Greppmayr, Munich.

Material

The brace is made from a round 0.4 to 0.6 mm thick stainless steel wire.

Work materials (image 5.1)

- rounded pliers
- flat pliers
- edge cutter
- fixation pliers
- hammer
- anvil with rounded-off edges

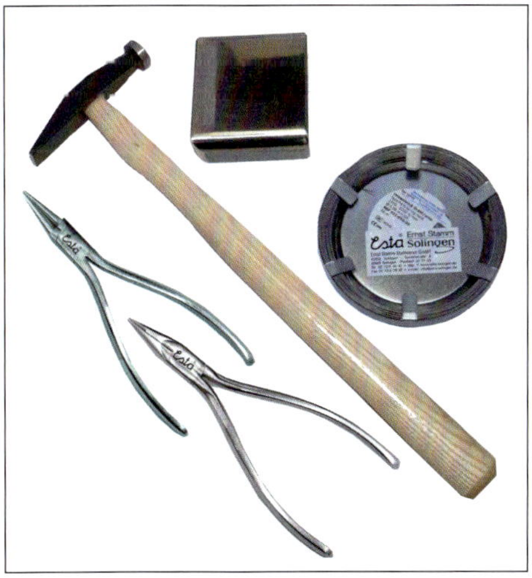

Image 5.1

- corundum grinder
- springwire 0.4 mm or 0.5 mm depending on the thickness of the nail (thick nails: 0.5 mm, thin to normal nails: 0.4 mm)
- dappen dish
- spatula
- impression material
- resin material
- mixing pad
- tamponade

Effectiveness

This is a bilateral nail correction brace (images 5.2 and 5.3).

It affects both or only one lateral nail margin. This brace offers optimal results. It

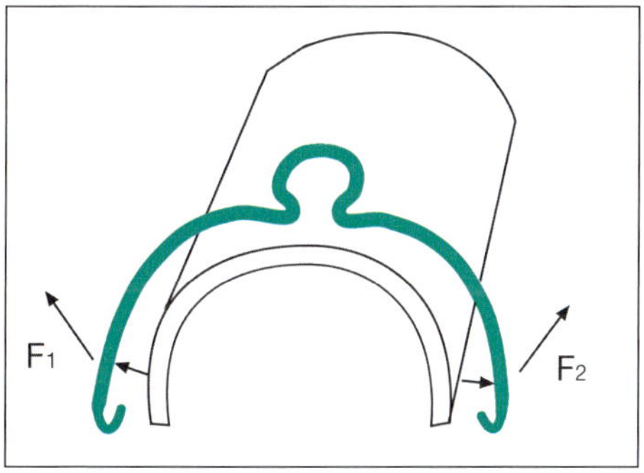

Image 5.2 Tensile force caused by elasticity

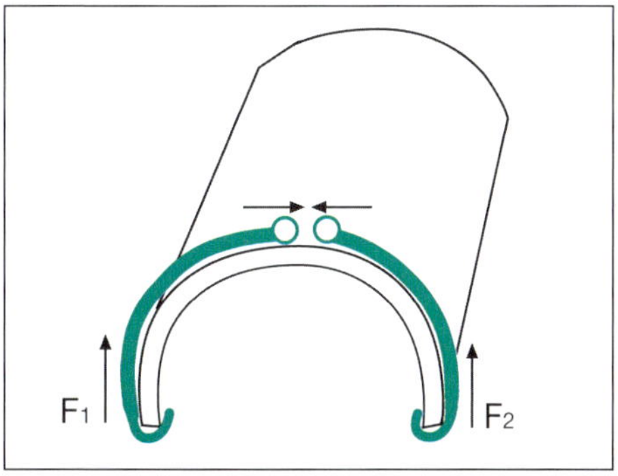

Image 5.3 Tensile force on the width of the nail

Images 5.2 and 5.3 Source: Klaus Grünewald, Theorie der medizinischen Fußbehandlung, tome 2, 3rd edition 2016, Verlag Neuer Merkur allows individual adjustment of the spring's tension on each side of the brace. The tensioned wire gently lifts the edges of the nail away from the skin, reducing and correcting its curvature. The nail bed adjusts to the growing nail, therefore achieving a permanent correction. This prevents secondary disorders, such as onycholysis. The spring tension can be adjusted with the omega.

Indications

- unguis incarnatus
- unguis convolutus
- callositas
- hyperkeratosis
- clavus in the sulcus area or under the nail plate

Additional contraindication

- paronychia (the brace application is painful)

Conditional contraindication

This involves diabetics or patients with a neuropathic disorder. These patients cannot feel if the tension of the brace is too strong, which can impair proper wound healing.

Preparation

If the nail fold is infected, the infection must be treated first. Once the infection has completely healed, carefully and thoroughly remove existing hyperkeratosis, callositas or clavi with an excavator or another adequate instrument. Applying an adhesive brace to the nail provides relief and promotes faster healing.

Fabrication

The negative impression
A condensation-cured silicone is commonly used for the impression. Blend the appropriate amount of silicone material with the hardener (according to the manufacturer's specifications) on a mixing pad.

Mix the silicone and the hardener swiftly, respecting the curing time. Then press the impression material into the nail fold with a spatula and cover the nail completely with the material. Once the material has cured, carefully start at the proximal end and lift the impression of the nail.

The positive impression (images 5.4 to 5.14)
Use a resin compound or plaster (breaks easily) for the positive impression.

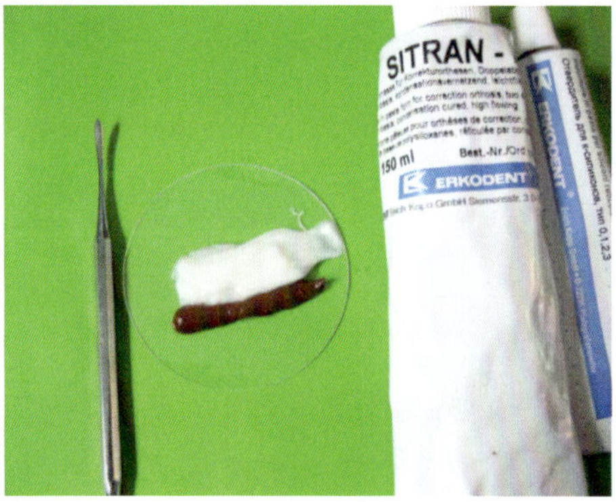

Image 5.4

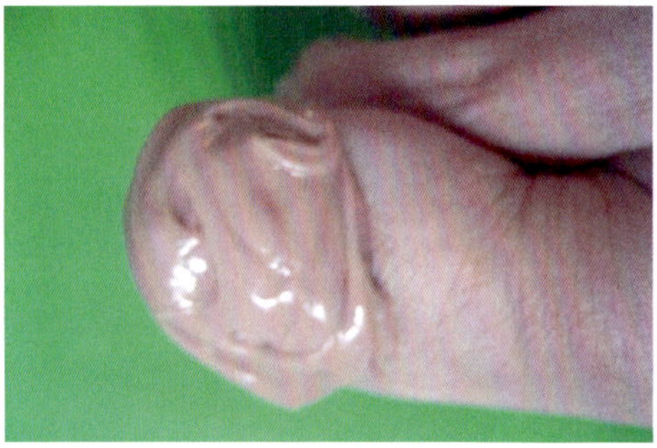

Image 5.5 Preparation of a negative impression

Image 5.6

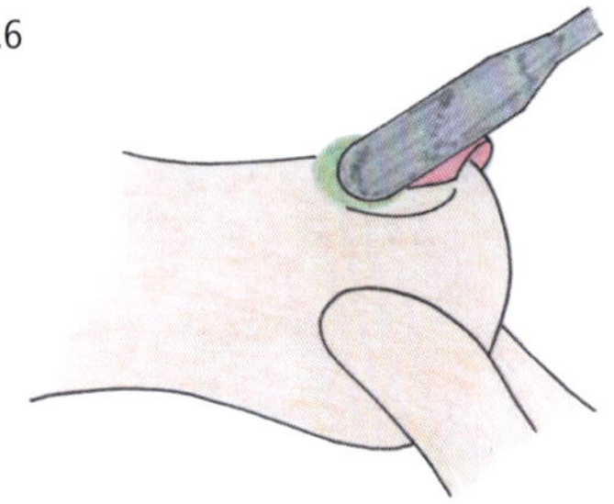

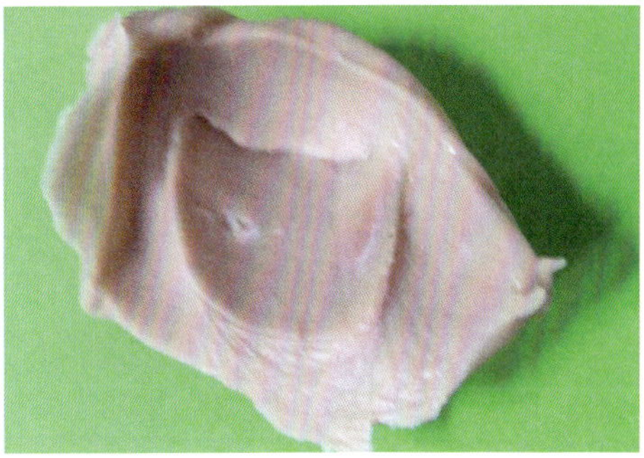

Image 5.7

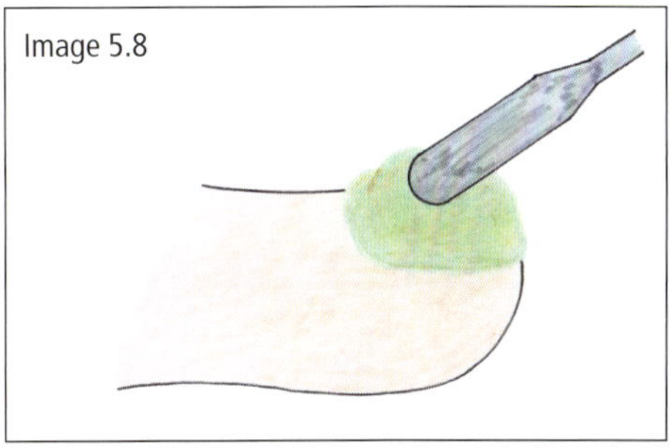

Image 5.8

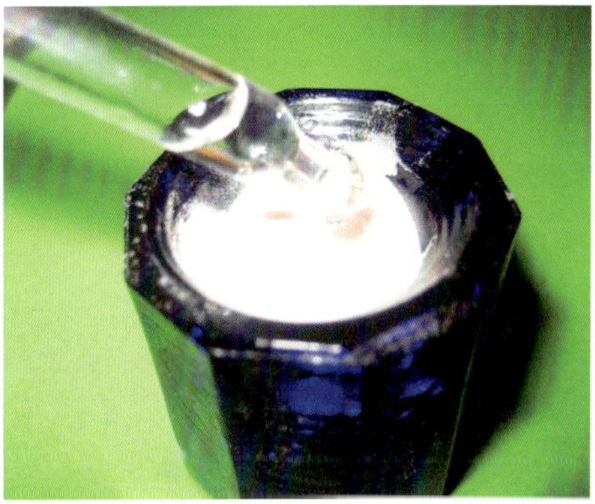

Image 5.9

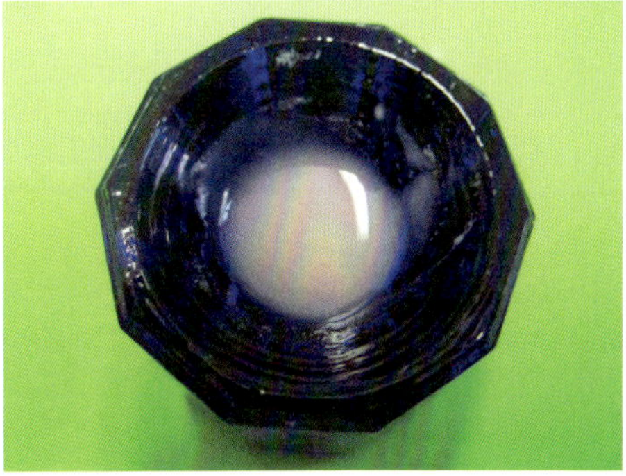

Image 5.10

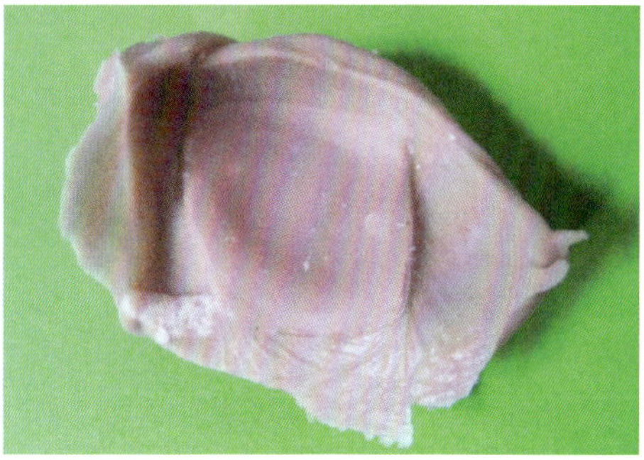

Image 5.11

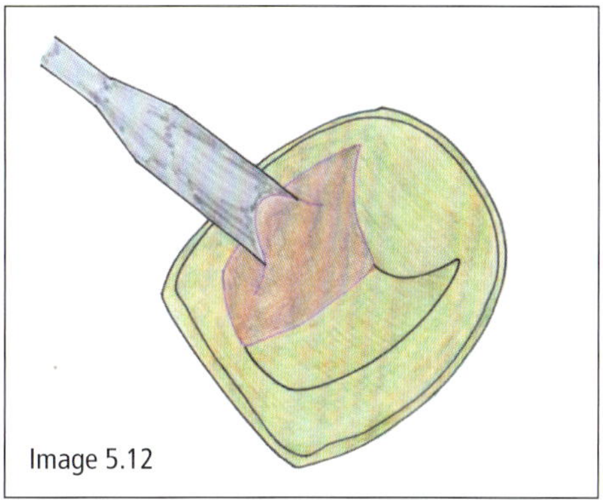

Image 5.12

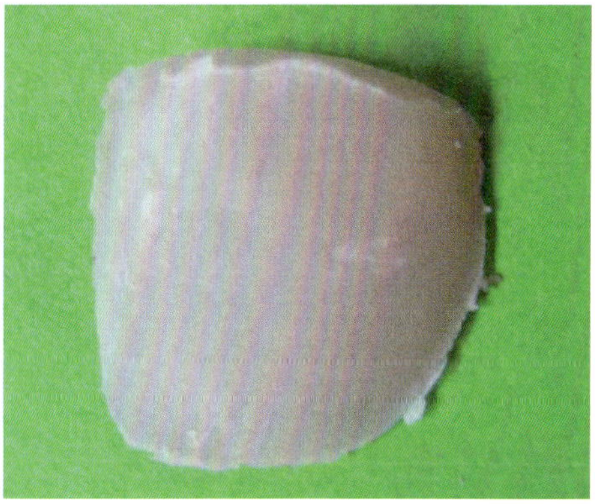

Image 5.13

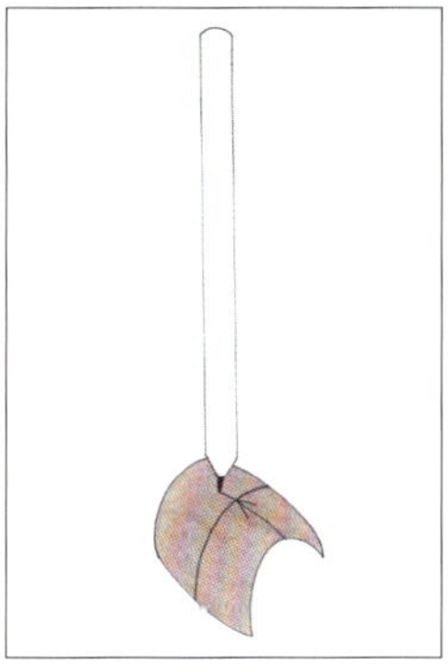

Image 5.14

Fabrication of the artificial nail with resin material

Mix the resin material in a dappen dish. It should have a consistency similar to honey. Pour the material into the negative impression and distribute it evenly with a spatula.

Ensure that the artificial nail is neither too thick nor too thin. The thickness of the artificial nail must have the same thickness as the natural nail.

In order to prevent distortion, the resin must have completely hardened before the nail can be removed from the mould.

Manufacture of the brace

Cut an approximately 5 cm long piece from the 0.5 mm thick spring wire with a wire cutter.

Mark the highest point on the artificial nail with a dot and draw an arrow pointing to the matrix (proximal direction). This procedure is helpful in determining the correct positioning of the omega (image 5.15).

To create the omega:

1. Grab the wire centre with rounded pliers and bend both sides of the wire down (images 5.16 to 5.19).

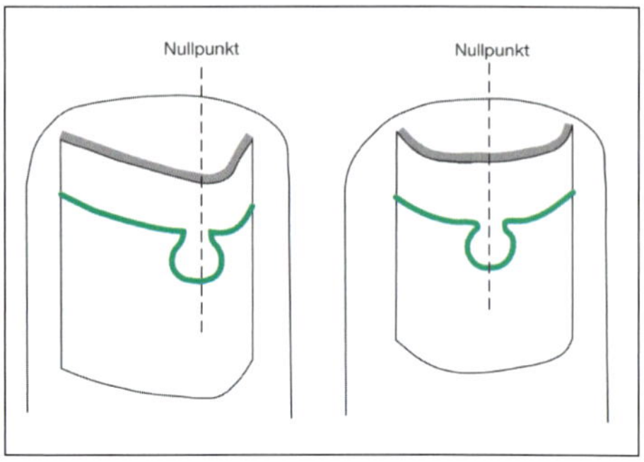

Image 5.15 Examples of the position of the nail's natural point

Source: Klaus Grünewald, Theorie der medizinischen Fußbehandlung, tome 2, 3rd edition 2016, Verlag Neuer Merkur

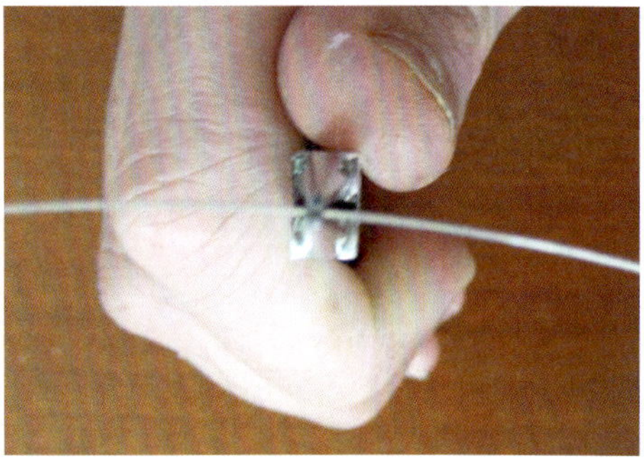

Image 5.16

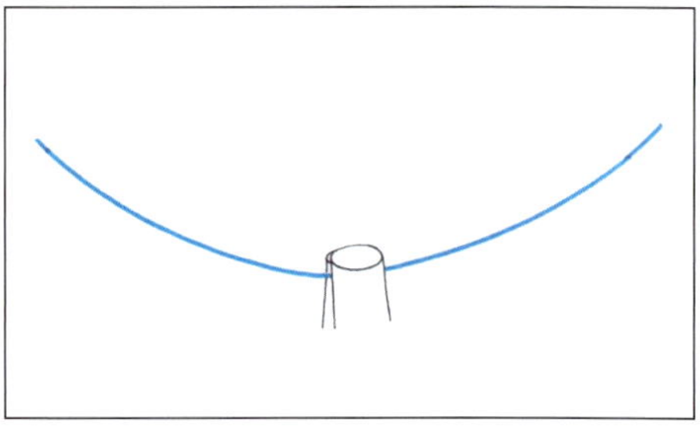

Image 5.17

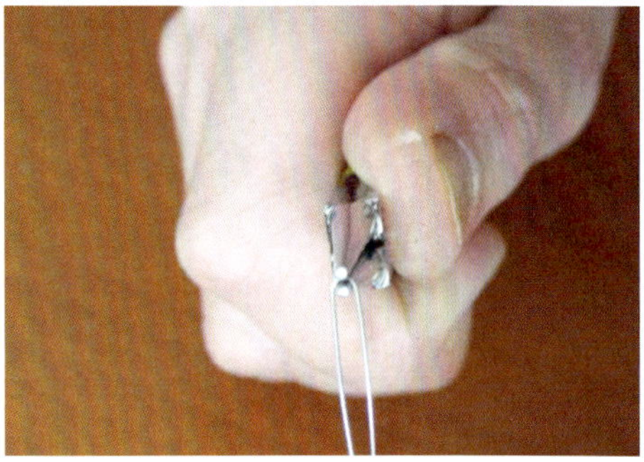

Image 5.18

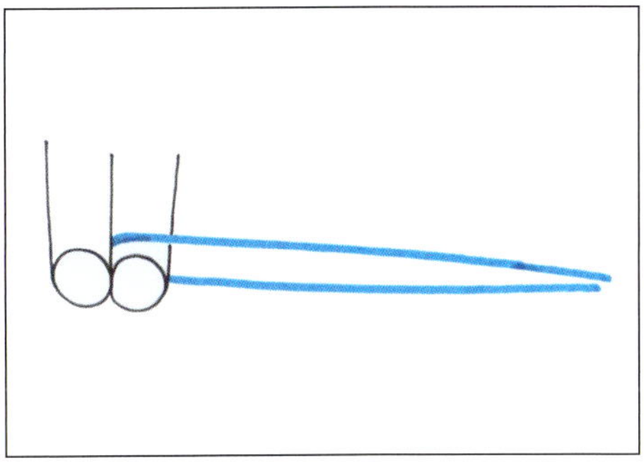

Image 5.19

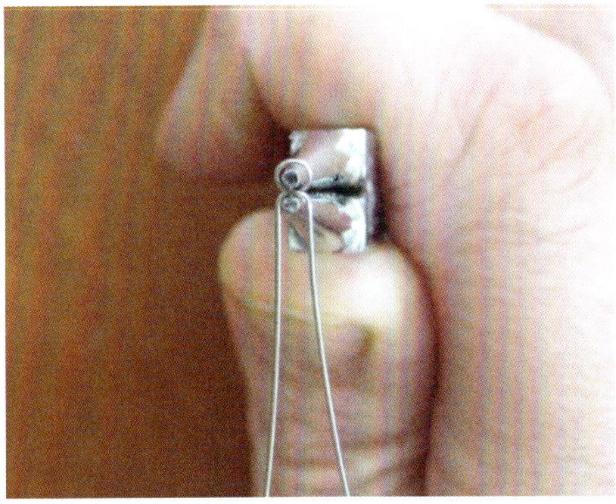

Image 5.20

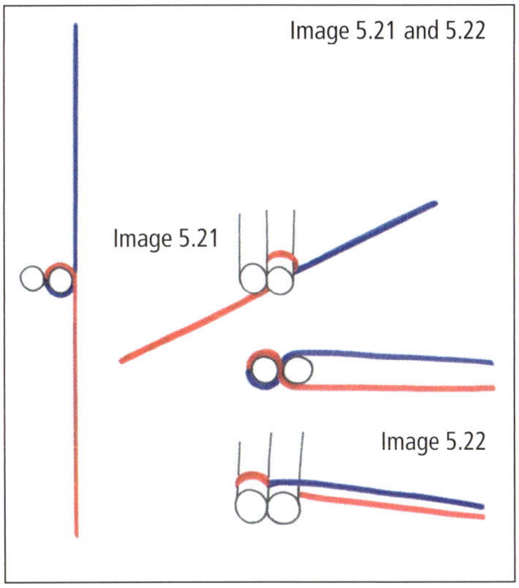

2. Cross the two long parts of the wire close to the tip of the pliers thereby creating a small loop (image 5.20).
3. Slip the wire loop onto the upper jaw of the pliers (images 5.23 and 5.24).
4. Bend both long wire pieces downwards, then cross them close to the pliers. Ensure that the front piece stays in front and the back piece stays behind, allowing the omega to be pulled apart (image 5.25).

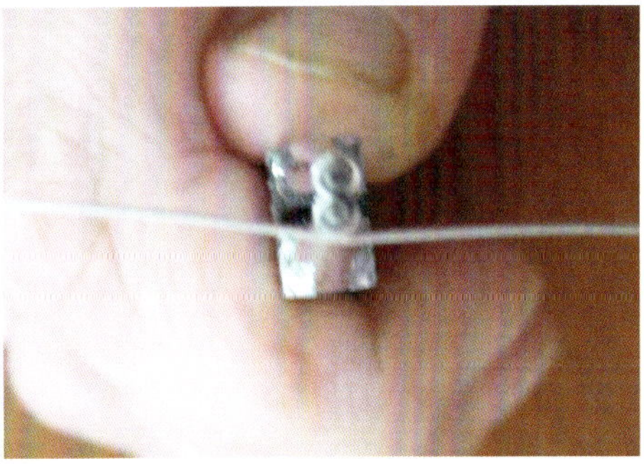

Image 5.23

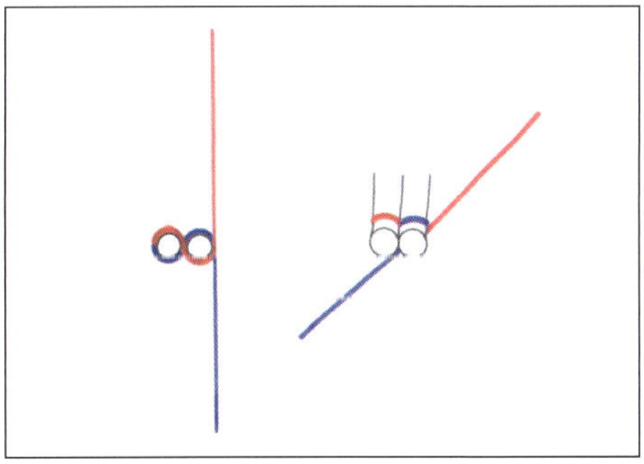

Image 5.24

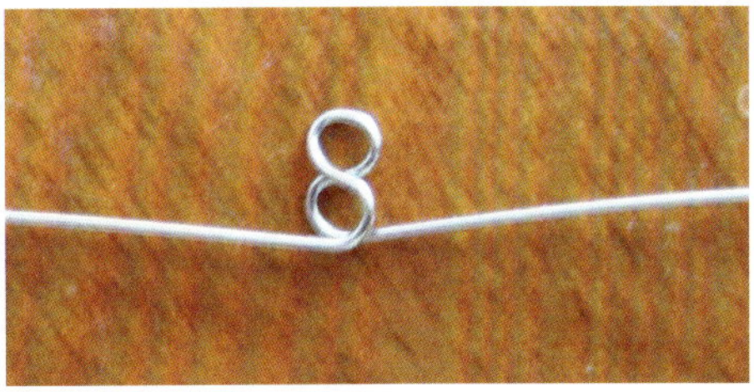

Image 5.25

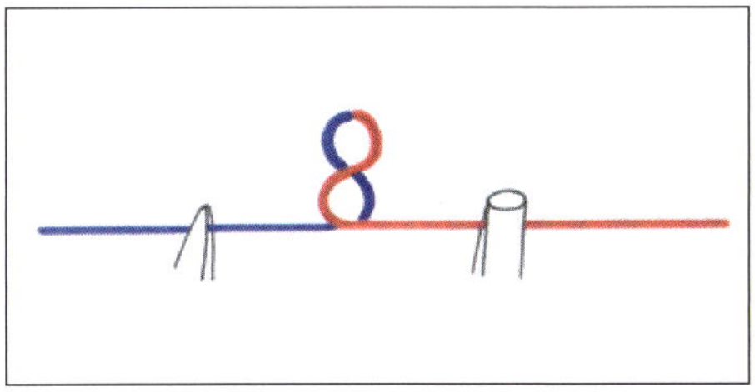

Image 5.26

5. Pull the omega apart with two pliers until there is a space of at least one wire thickness between the two sides (images 5.27 to 5.30).

6. Now align the omega with flat pliers (images 5.31 to 5.36).

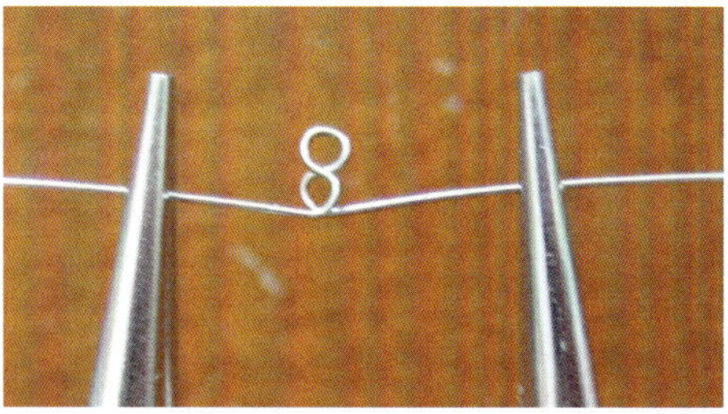
Image 5.27

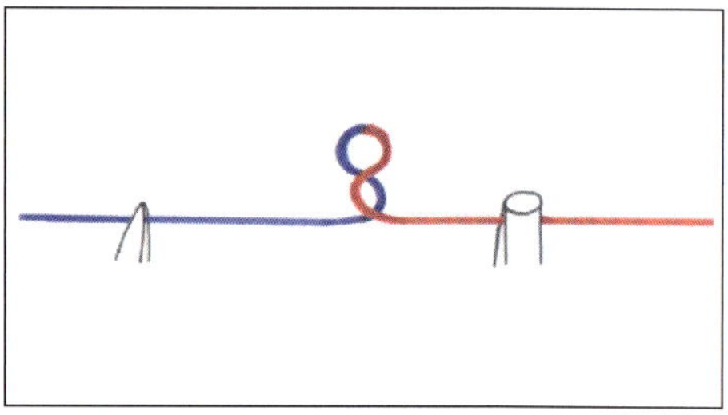
Image 5.28

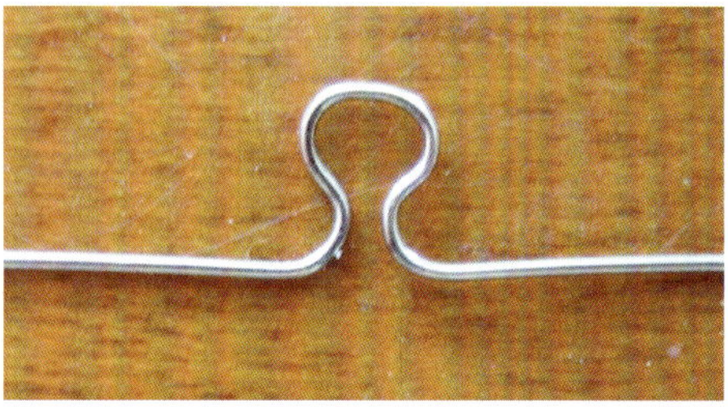
Image 5.29

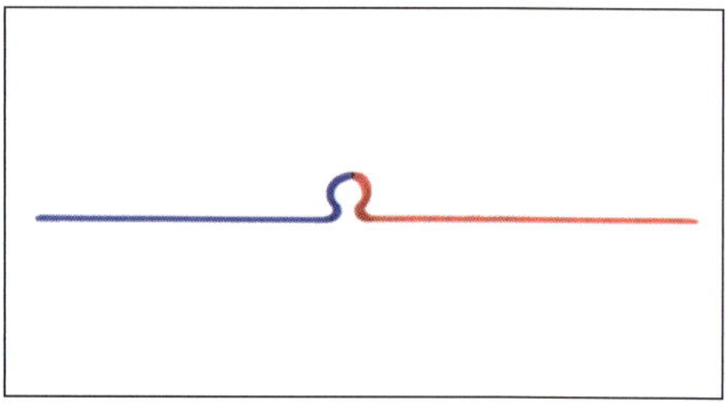
Image 5.30

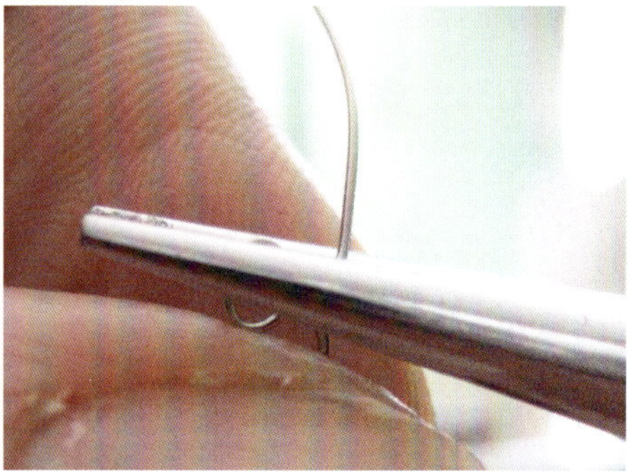
Image 5.31

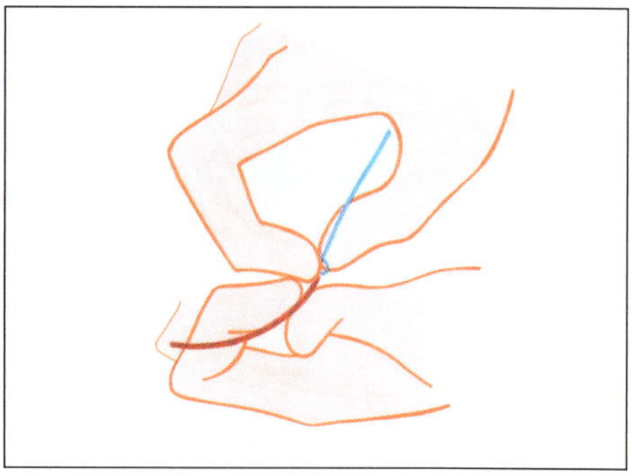
Image 5.32

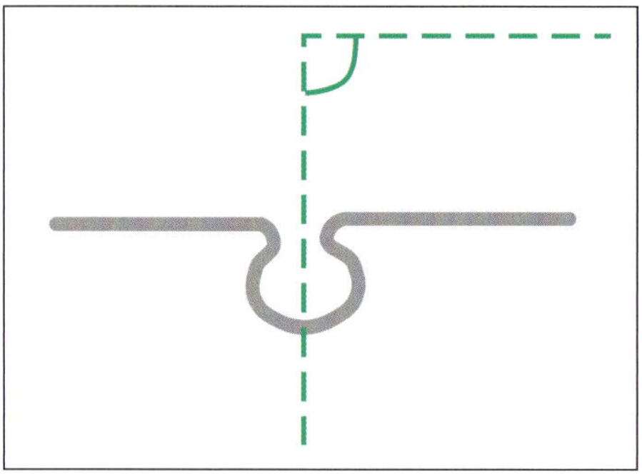
Image 5.33 The loop's centre line orthogonally aligning with the wire pieces

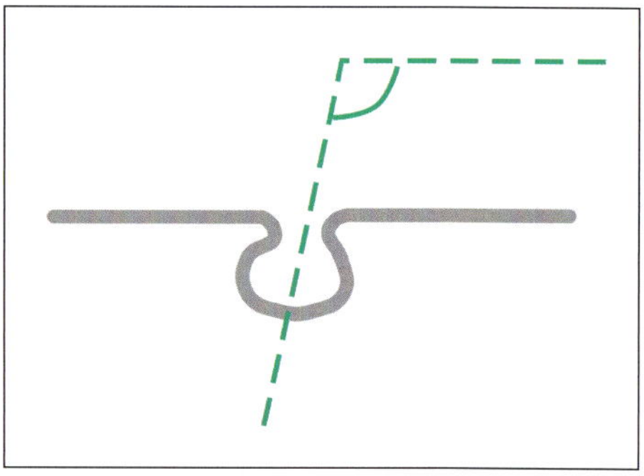
Image 5.34 The loop's centre line not orthogonally aligned with the wire pieces

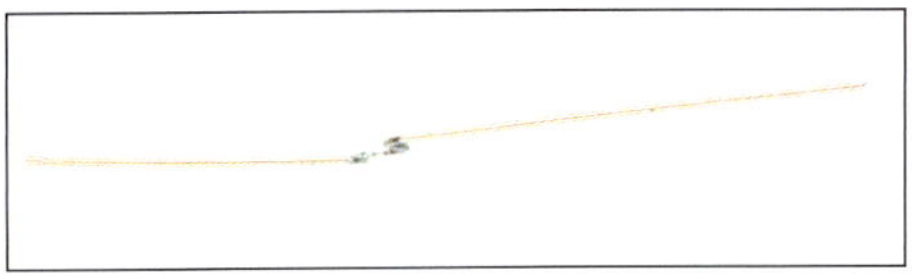

Image 5.35 Misaligned loop

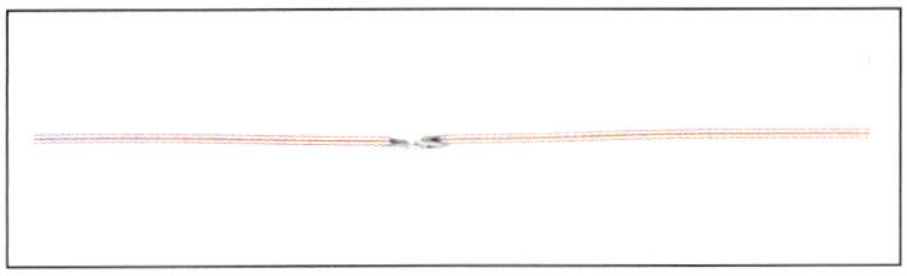

Image 5.36 Correctly aligned loop

Image 5.36 Source: Klaus Grünewald, Theorie der medizinischen Fußbehandlung, tome 2, 3rd edition 2016, Verlag Neuer Merkur

7. Place the brace on the artificial nail and cut the wire on each side to the desired length (images 5.39 and 5.40).

8. Cut approximately 2 mm below the artificial nail edges (images 5.41 and 5.42).

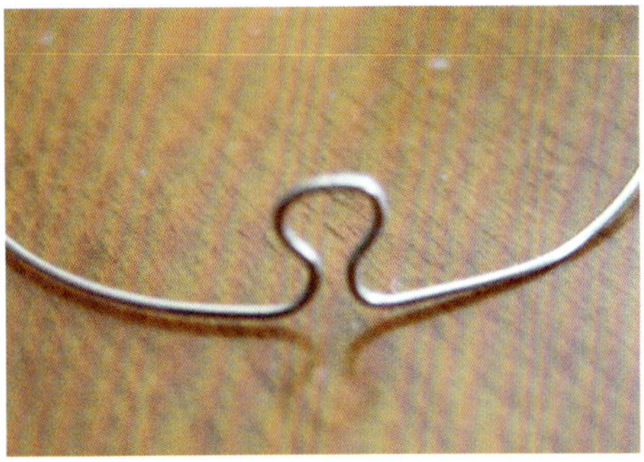

Image 5.37

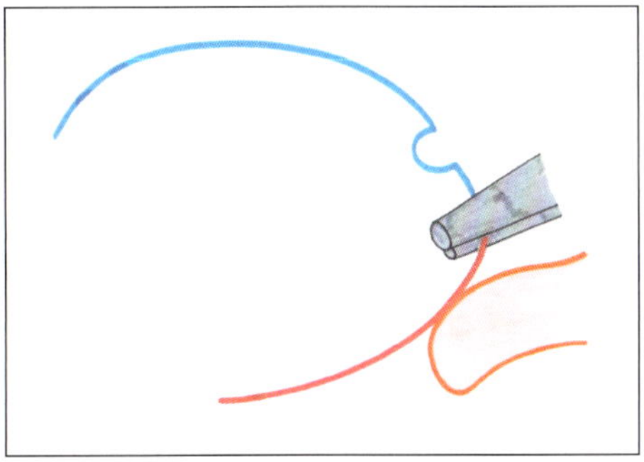

Image 5.38

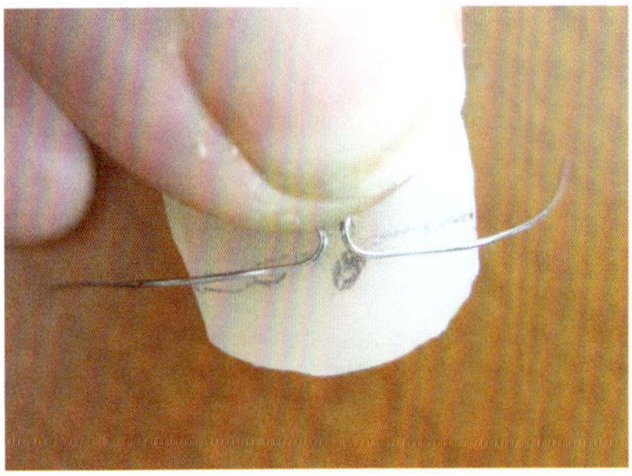

Image 5.39

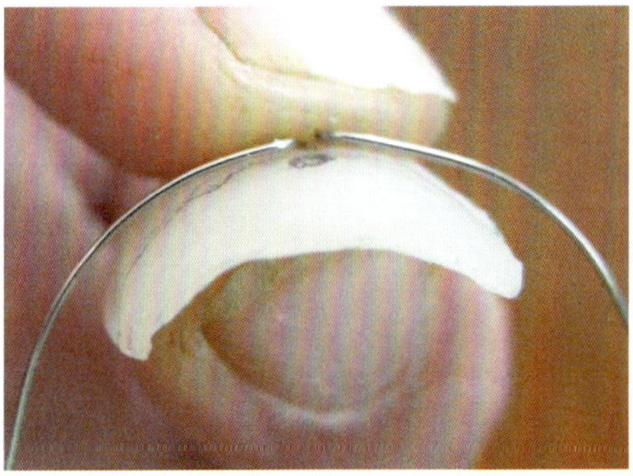

Image 5.40

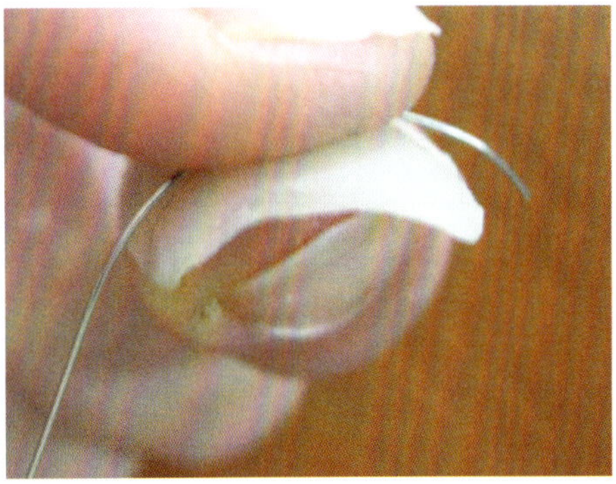

Image 5.41

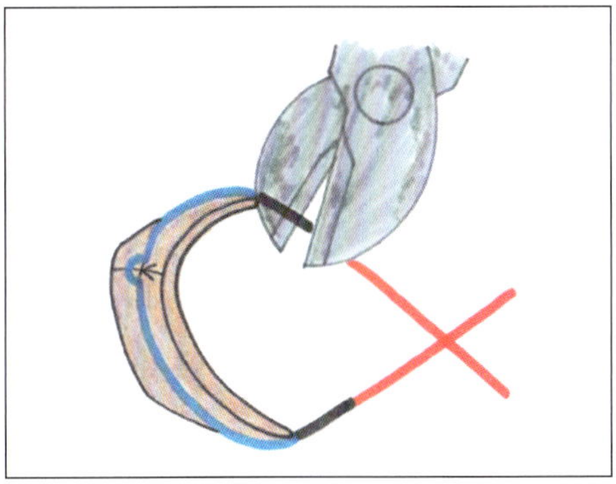

Image 5.42

9. Grab the omega with fixation pliers and hammer the ends of the wire flat to prevent nail fold irritation (images 5.43 and 5.44).

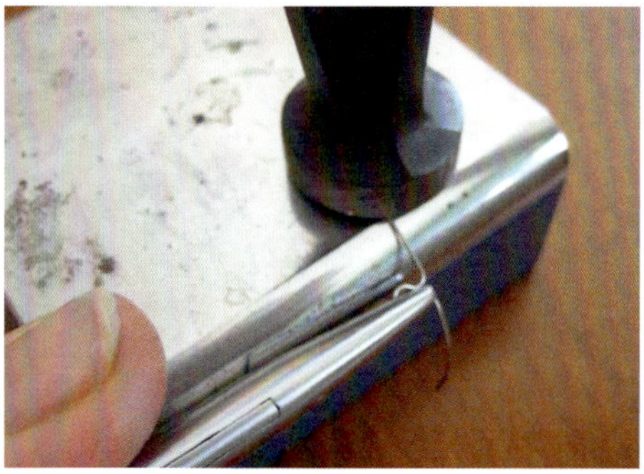

Image 5.43

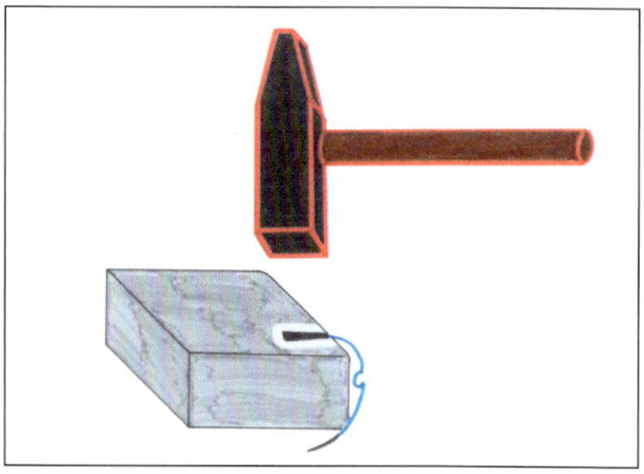

Image 5.44

10. Bend the wire pieces with round pliers until they fit tightly and tension-free on the artificial nail (images 5.45 and 5.46).

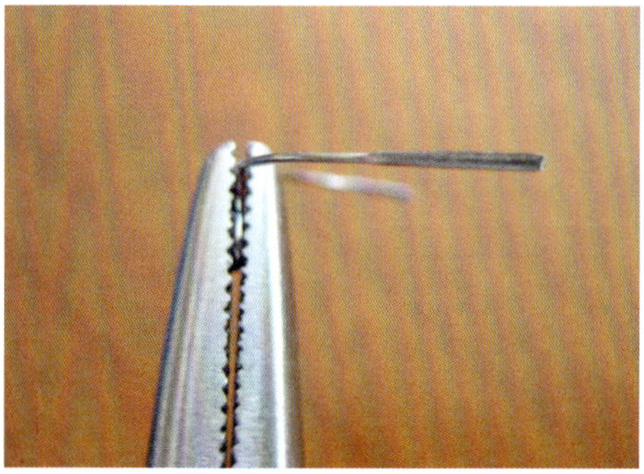

Image 5.45

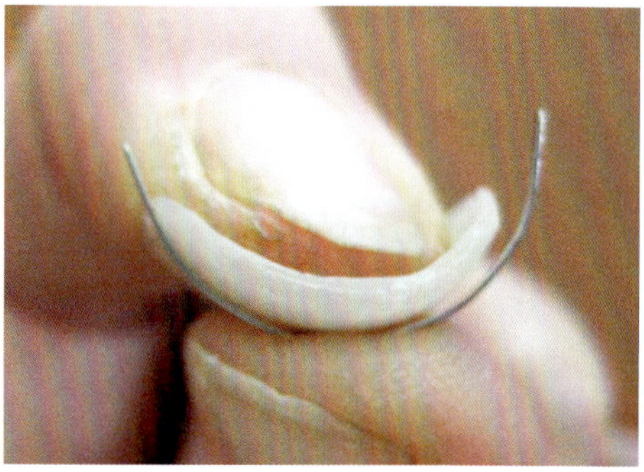

Image 5.46

11. Create small hooks with rounded pliers. Ensure that the hooks are parallel and evenly aligned (images 5.47 to 5.50).

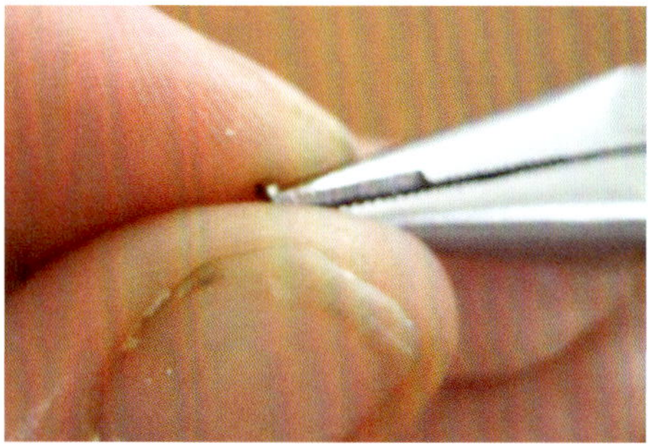

Image 5.47

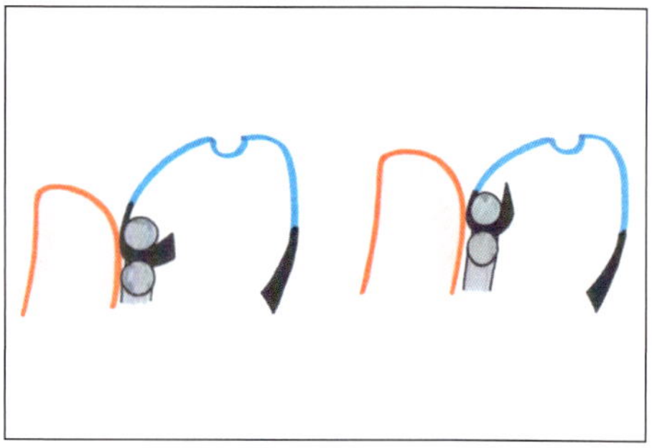

Image 5.48

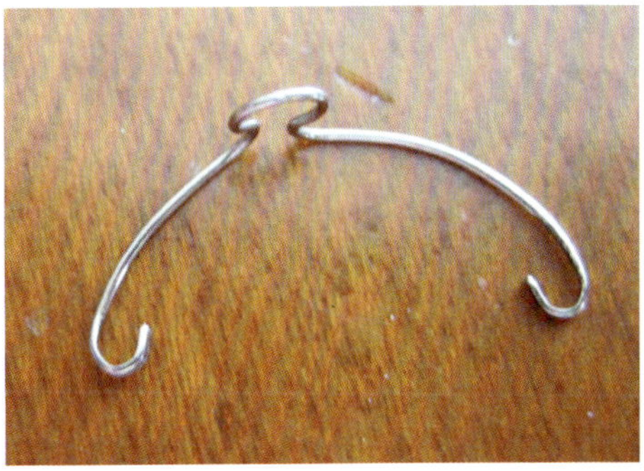

Image 5.49

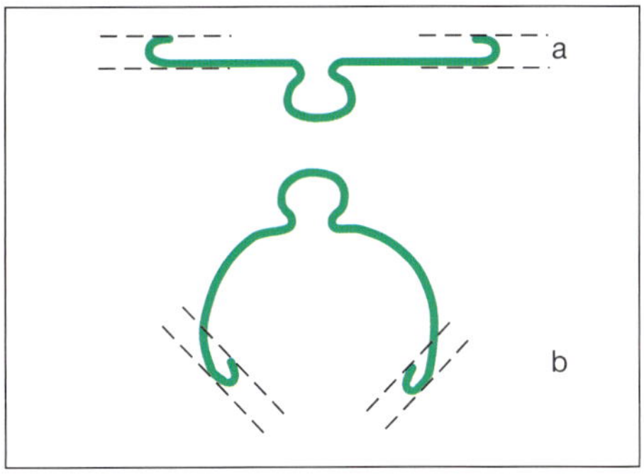

Image 5.50 Parallel alignment of the hooks
Source: Klaus Grünewald, Theorie der medizinischen Fußbehandlung, tome 2, 3rd edition 2016, Verlag Neuer Merkur

12. Place the brace without pressure on the artificial nail (images 5.51 to 5.55).

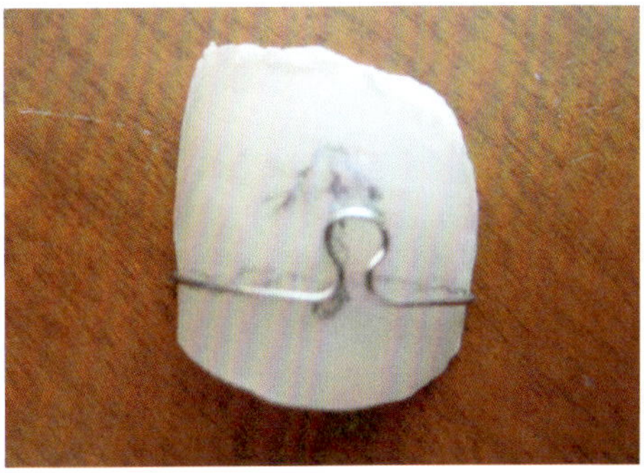

Image 5.51

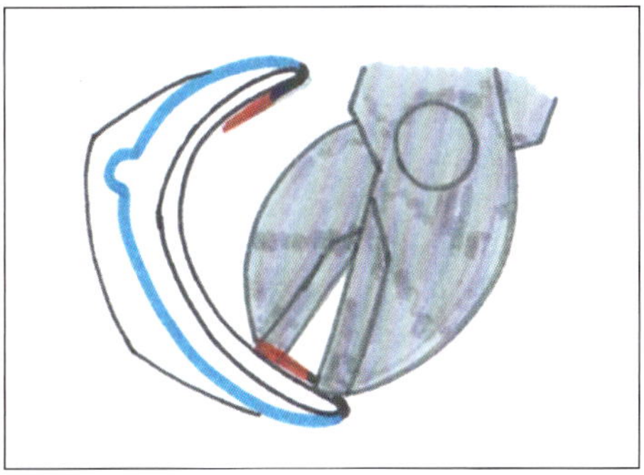

Image 5.52

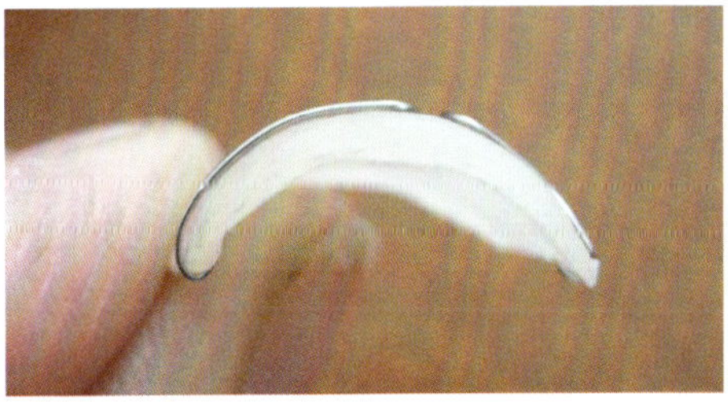

Image 5.53

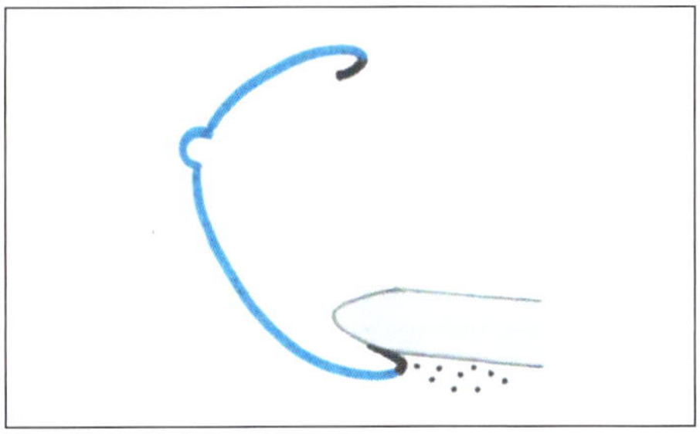

Image 5.54

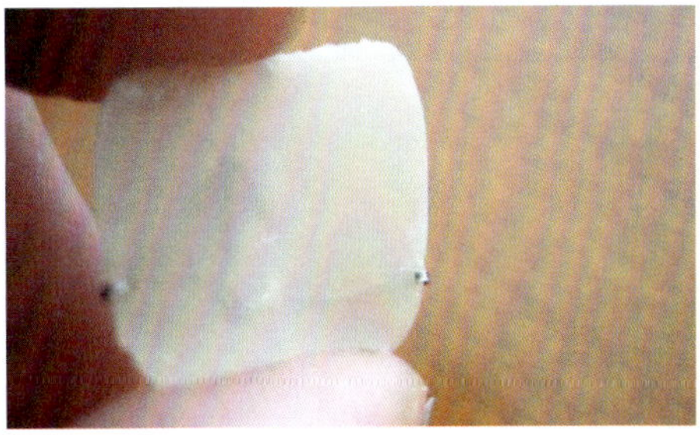

Image 5.55

Special loop-forming pliers or a tier plier (Rading) can also be used to shape the omega loop (image 5.56).

Positioning and fixation

Ensure that the nail fold is free of sharp edges and hyperkeratosis (image 5.58). Do not trim the nail's edges nor sand the surface of the nail since this will interfere with the nail's static.

Disinfect the brace and place it on the natural nail to verify the fit. Then remove the brace and activate each side with flat pliers. Place the pliers below the curve of the wire and press the jaws of the pliers together. The curvature will be slightly reduced (image 5.59). A simple technique to activate the sides of the brace is to hold the brace with needle pliers, then lift one side of the wire carefully with your finger, but no more than the width of a hook (image 5.60). The activation must be done in accordance with the nail's thickness so not to risk nail damage (koilonychia, lysis). Position one hook on one side, check the wire tension and repeat (image 5.61) for the other side.

Carefully glide the activated and disinfected brace from distal towards proximal direction onto the nail. The brace must be positioned in the front third of the nail plate (image 5.62).

Verify that the brace does not apply pressure or tension on the nail and that the hooks do not penetrate the skin.

Insert tamponades into the nail fold to prevent irritation and remove any oily substances from the nail plate with acetone.

Secure the omega with an acrylic bonding agent, cyanoacrylate or gel adhesive. Do not cover the entire brace with adhesive since this will impair its functionality.

Repositioning

The brace must be repositioned and reactivated after four to six weeks. For the removal of the brace, the following two methods are recommended:

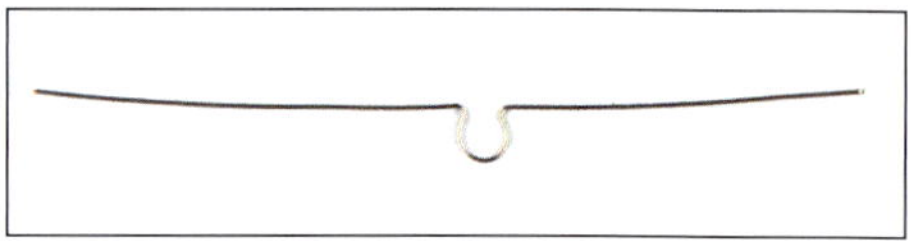

Image 5.56 Omega loop created with loop-forming pliers

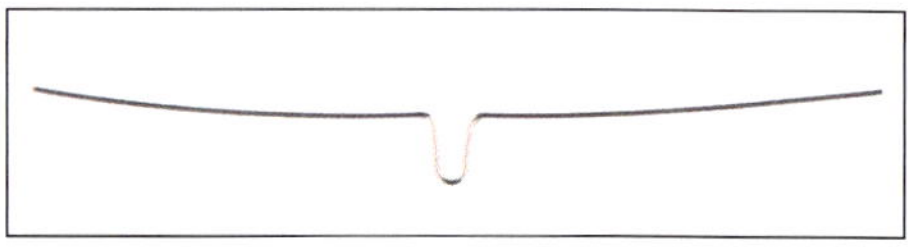

Image 5.57 Loop created with tier pliers (Rading).

Images 5.56 and 5.57 Source: Klaus Grünewald, Theorie der medizinischen Fußbehandlung, tome 2, 3rd edition 2016, Verlag Neuer Merkur

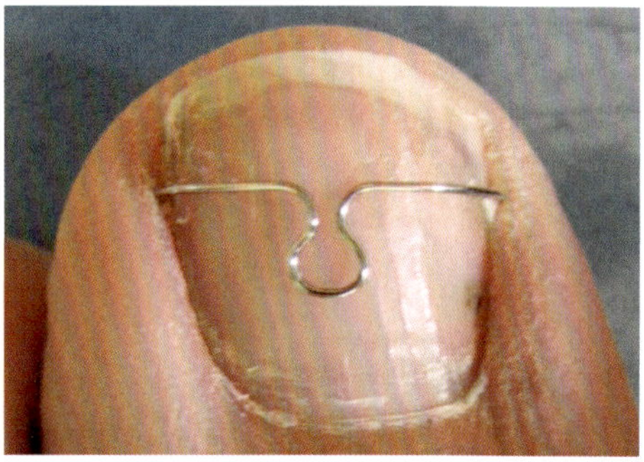

Image 5.58

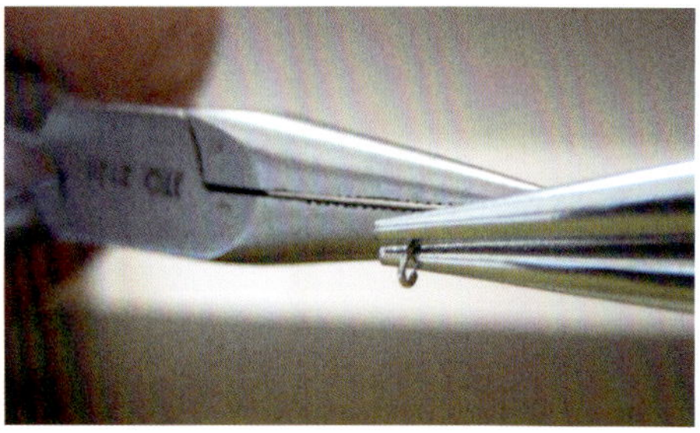

Image 5.59

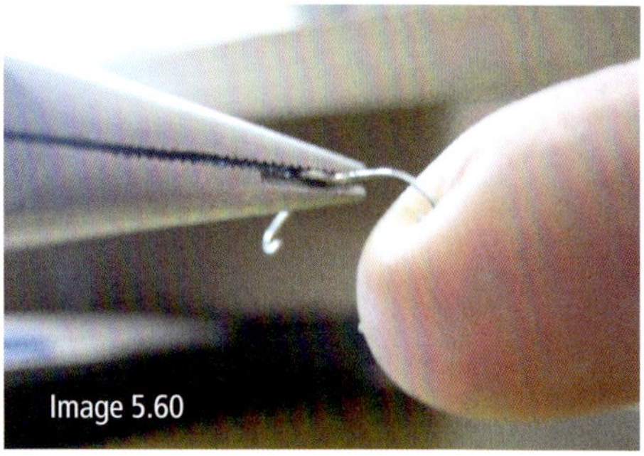

Image 5.60

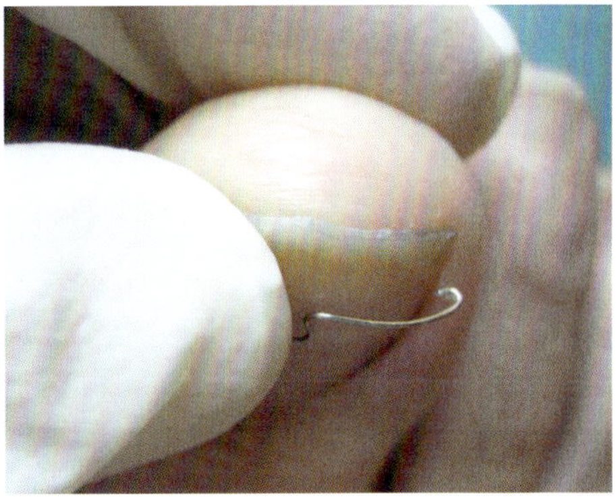

Image 5.61

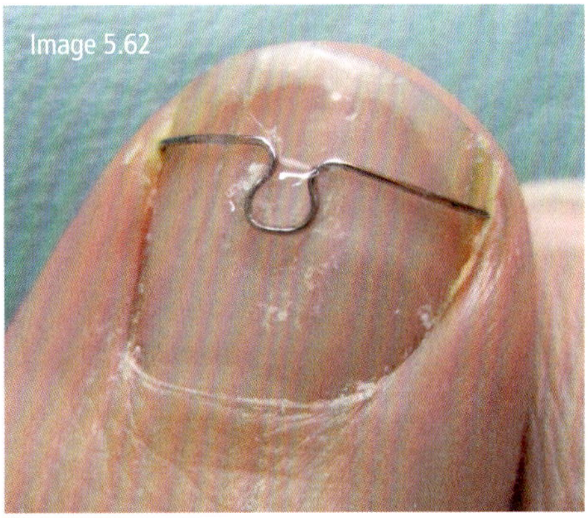

Image 5.62

- Carefully sand off the adhesive without damaging the wire and loosen the brace with a nail knife.
- Carefully cut into the adhesive with side-cutting nippers and remove the brace.

Remove the remaining adhesive, realign, reactivate and disinfect the brace and proceed with regular nail care. Afterwards, reposition the brace and apply tamponades.

Treatment period

Nine to 14 months. During this period, the brace must be readjusted every four to eight weeks.

Important information for the patient

Inform the patient about the procedure by supplying him/her with an information leaflet.

5.4 The physical strength of all three-part brace systems

The effectiveness of three-part braces is based on physical forces such as leverage, tensile-, loop- and spring force.

Tensile force

The small inserted hooks ensure that tensile force is distributed over the entire nail plate. At a 90 degree angle, the tensile force is fully transmitted, however the tensile force decreases if the angle between the wires and the nail plate's longitudinal axis changes.

Leverage

Leverage causes the lifting of the lateral nail plate edges whereby the pivot point on the nail surface determines the tensile force via a long lever.

Loop force

The centre loop must be positioned exactly in the centre of the two wires. This creates accurate tensile force after twisting the wire.

Spring force

Sealing the centre loop with adhesive creates a "button" through which the top of the shoe applies pressure on the brace while walking. The elasticity of the brace and the resetting force activate the spring force.

5.5 3TO brace system

The 3TO brace consists of three parts and is made of thin stainless steel wire. The two sides of the wire are attached individually to the lateral edges of the nail with small hooks. The long ends of the wires are then pulled through a centre loop and tightened, depending on the treatment.

The purchase and application of this brace requires attendance at an introduction course on its use.

Material

Thin preformed spring wire of various diameters (image 5.63).

Work materials

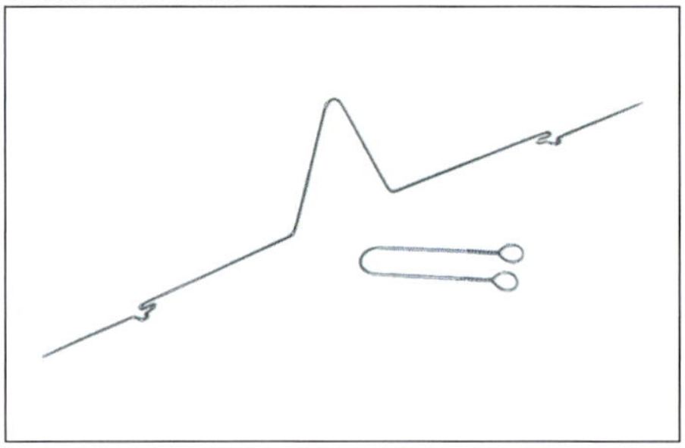

Image 5.63 Source: 3TO

- preformed brace
- centre wire = 3TO-loop
- combination pliers
- side-cutting pliers
- needle holder
- winding hook
- for sealing: gel technique, nail compound, Onycholit or Unguisan

Effectiveness

It is the perfect brace to be applied to nails that need immediate attention, PLUS+ its placement is almost pain-free.

The three-part design allows the individual positioning of each piece. The brace is activated via the connection loop. The activation is done in direct agreement with the patient.

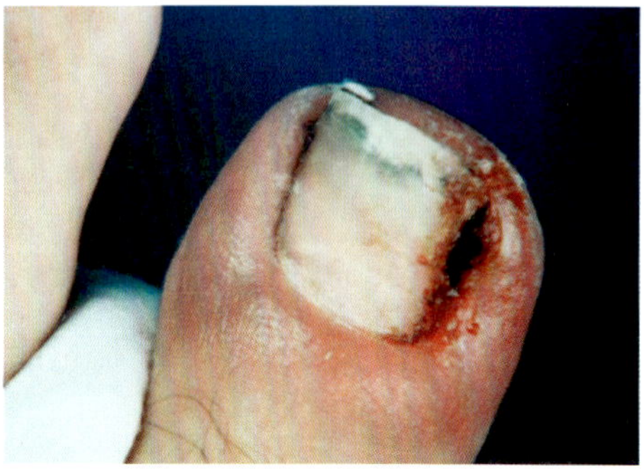

Image 5.64 Prior to the treatment

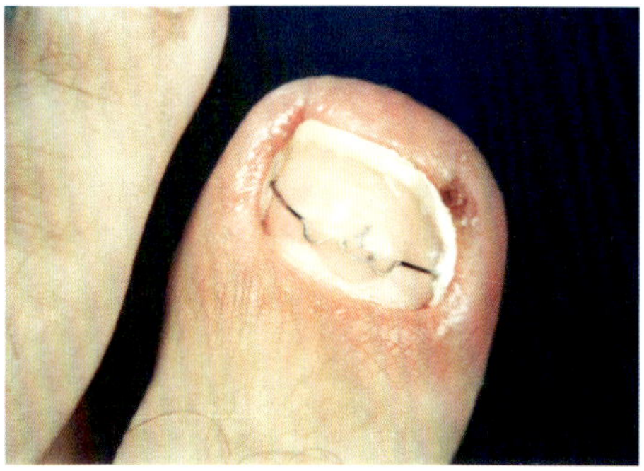

Image 5.65 10 days post treatment

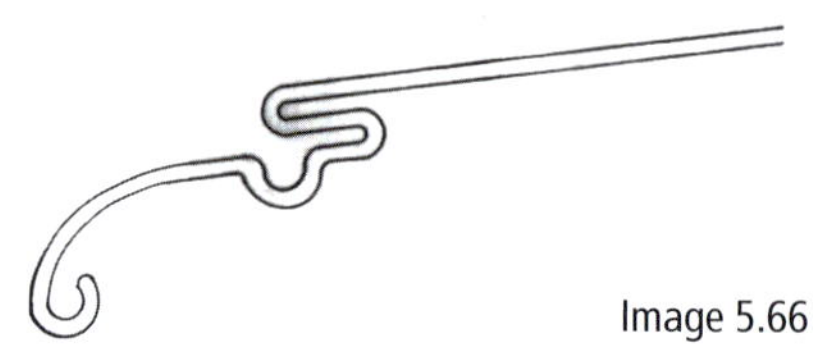

Image 5.66

The 3TO brace relieves pain immediately, provided the nail fold has been well prepared prior to application.

Very deep ingrown nail parts can often be removed only once the brace has lifted the nail. This brace system is very well received by patients and physicians alike (images 5.64 and 5.65).

Indications

- unguis convolutus
- unguis incarnatus
- clavi in the sulcus
- onychophosis
- paronychia
- granulation tissue

Preparation

Prior to placing the brace, disinfect the nail fold and clean it with a probe. The brace can be placed even if the nail shows signs of infection or if granulation tissue is present. However, if there are signs of suppuration or granulation tissue in the nail fold, an appropriate treatment must be performed in accordance with a physician. A plaster model is not required.

Brace preparation

The brace is assembled from two preformed elements made of 0.4 mm thick steel spring wire, which can be adjusted to fit the individual shape of any nail. Create small hooks by bending the wire ends and place the hooks under the lateral nail edge (image 5.66).

Positioning and fixation (images 5.67 to 5.69)

Hook the individual brace pieces carefully onto the lateral nail edges. Connect both pieces with a centre loop and tighten the loop by twisting it with a winding hook. The strength of the tension can be controlled for each side individually by twisting the loop. Adjust the brace's tension until the patient notices pressure and pain relief in the nailfold.

Cut the protruding wire pieces, cover them with artificial nail material and sand the hardened material to make it less noticeable.

Finally, apply an anti inflammatory ointment on the nail fold prior to inserting the tamponade.

Complications

It is important that the tension adjustment is not too strong to avoid tearing the nail's edges or detaching the nail plate.

Existing infections must be checked frequently to prevent them from spreading.

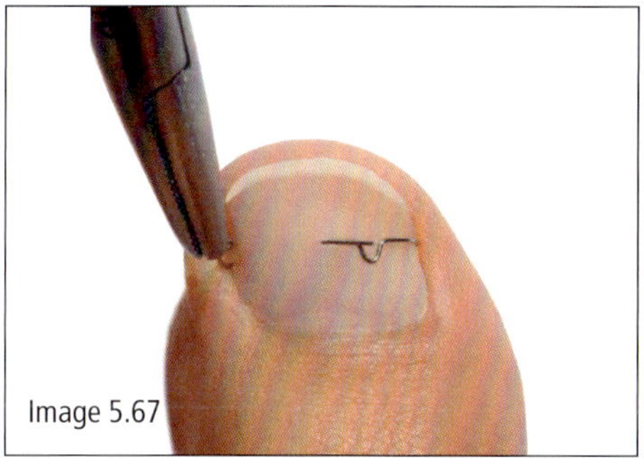

Image 5.67

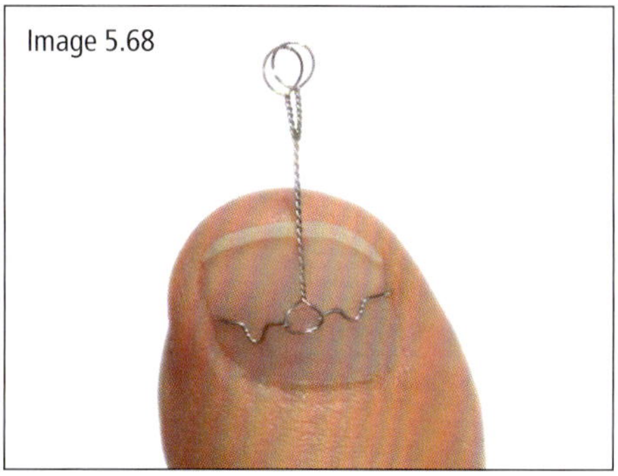

Image 5.68

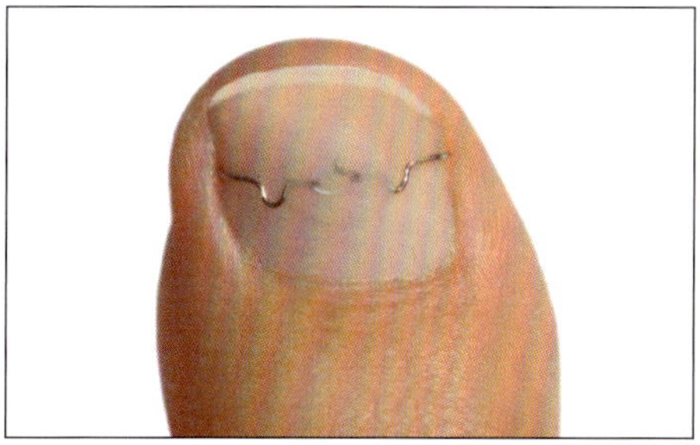

Image 5.69

Images 5.64 to 5.69 Source: 3TO

Important information for the patient

- The brace must be checked every night.
- In the event that the nail becomes painful, the brace loosens or for any other problems that might occur, visit the podiatrist.
- See the podiatrist for a follow-up visit within one to three days.
- Schedule a visit within four to six weeks with the podiatrist to reposition and align the brace.

5.6 Ortogrip brace

(Manufacturer: Ruck GmbH)

Material

A thin prefabricated spring wire. Available in different daimeters.

Work materials (image 5.70)

- preformed brace
- centre wire
- round tier pliers
- needle-nosed pliers
- side-cutting pliers
- hook spatula
- double-ended nail lifter
- silicone mixing bowl
- sealant material: nail compound, Onycholit, Unguisan or gel technique

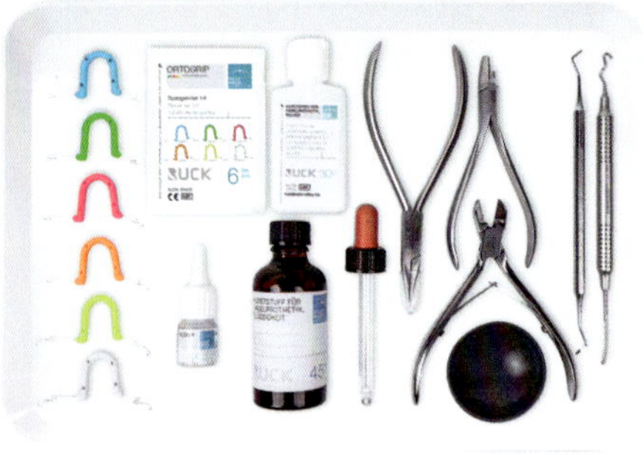

Image 5.70

Effectiveness

It is the perfect brace to apply to nails that need immediate attention, PLUS+ its placement is almost pain-free.

The three-part design allows individual positioning of each piece. The brace is activated via the connection loop.

Very deep ingrown nail parts can often be removed only once the brace has lifted the nail. This brace system is very well received by patients and physicians alike.

Indications

- Unguis convolutus
- unguis incarnatus
- clavi in the sulcus
- onychophosis
- paronychia
- granulation tissue

Preparation (image 5.71)

Clean the nail folds with a gauge blade or nail lifter and remove ingrown nail particles. For better adhesion, roughen the nail surface and clean it with an anti-grease solution.

Tamponade application (image 5.72)

To expand the nail folds, insert Copoline or Ligasano white tamponades and apply peclavus pre-treatment (application time: 5–8 minutes) to prevent irritation in the nail fold.

Brace preparation (image 5.73)

Measure and determine the correct brace size; the important selection criteria are the length of the action part (roof length) and the diameter of the wire. The following rule applies: The longer the roof length, the wider the nail; the thicker the wire, the more force can be applied.

Hook preparation (image 5.74)

Trim the end hooks with rounded tier pliers, if necessary, and deburr the ends with a diamond file. Remove the tamponades.

Positioning and fixation (image 5.75)

Start by inserting one side of the brace in the nail fold; the roof of the brace (V-stamp) must always face the patient. Fixate the brace end with a tamponade and secure the roof of the brace with an adhesive. Cut off the brace wire at the plastic holder with a side-cutting plier (hold the wire down with your thumb). Repeat on the other side. In this instance, the application of an adhesive is not necessary. Do not yet cut the wire on this side.

Loop application (image 5.76)

Adjust the space between the two side pieces of the brace with a needle-nosed plier. Hook the loop into the curved end pieces (the wire ends must face upwards). Place the winding hook in both loops and turn clockwise causing the side pieces of the brace to connect. This will ensure that the tension is distributed evenly.

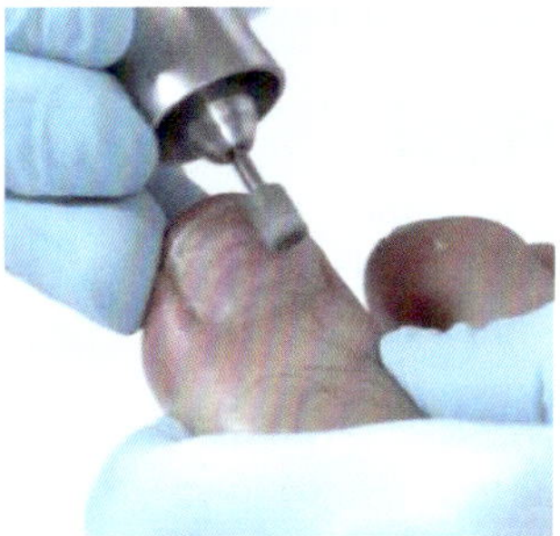
Image 5.71

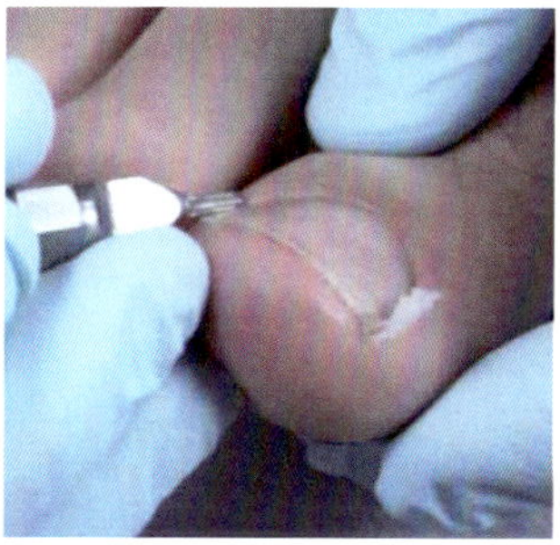
Image 5.72

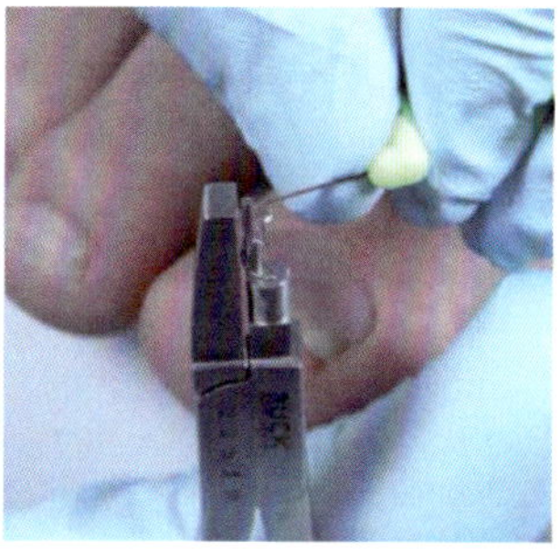
Image 5.73

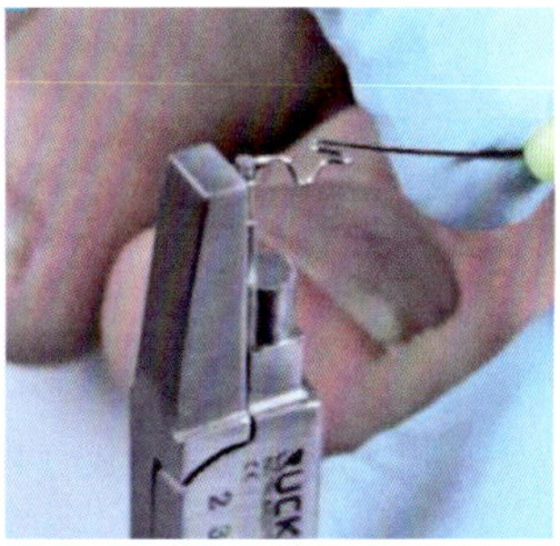
Image 5.74

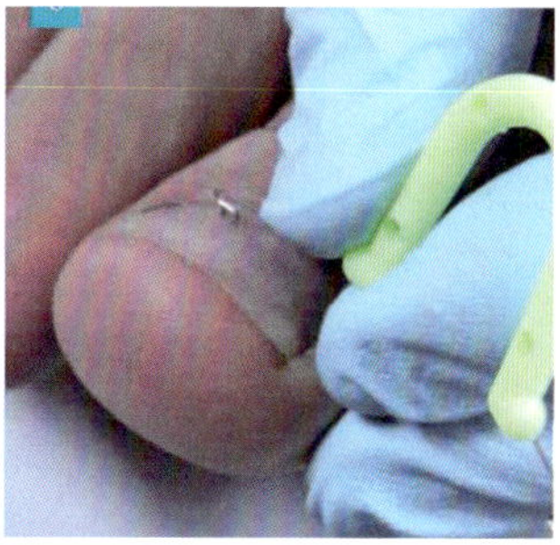
Image 5.75

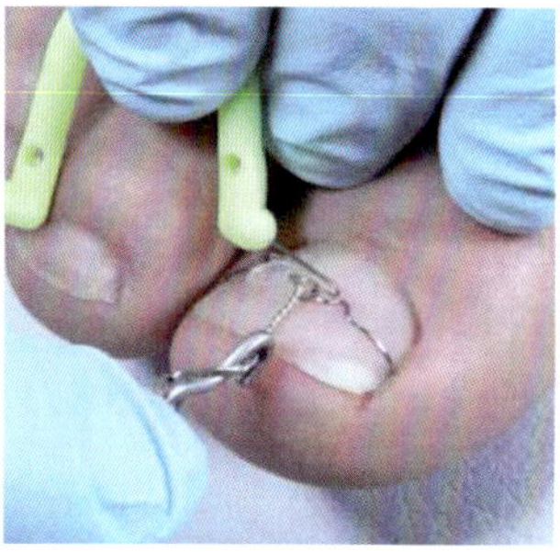
Image 5.76

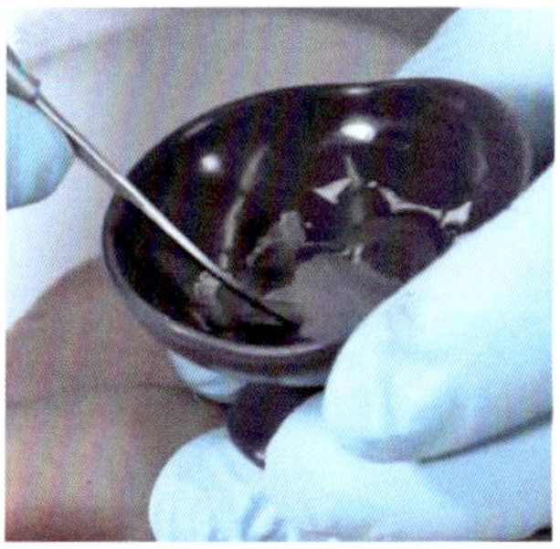
Image 5.77

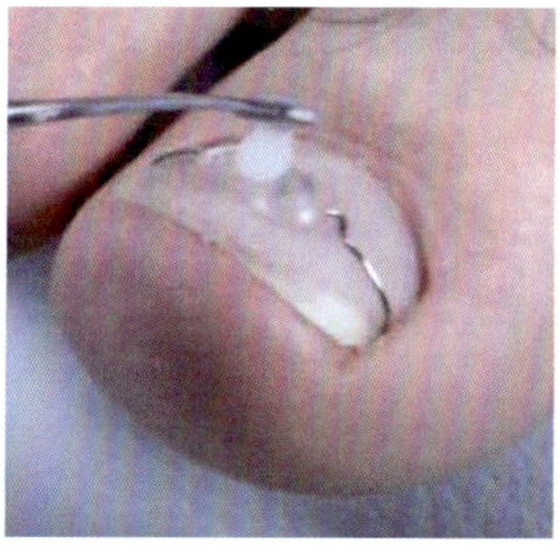
Image 5.78

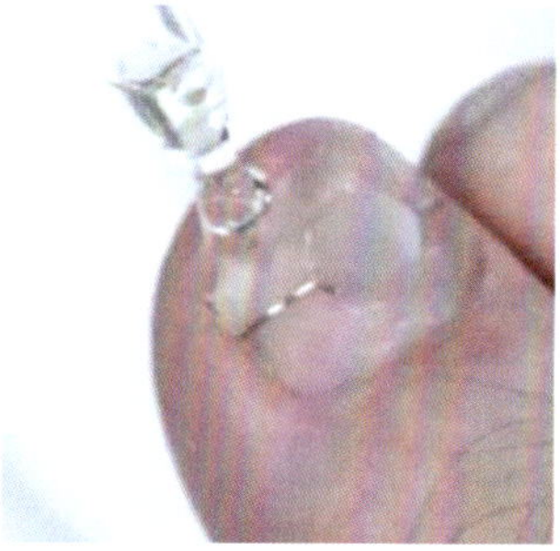
Image 5.79

Images 5.71 to 5.79 Source: Ortogrip-Anwendungsbroschüre der Fa. Ruck

Cut the twisted wire loop above two to three turn threads.

Covering (image 5.77)
Cut all protruding wire pieces as short as possible. Blend acrylic powder and hardener liquid (lukewarm) in a mixing bowl until it has a creamy consistency. Apply the mixture on the wire ends with a spatula until a "button" has formed which covers the wire ends completely. Apply a little bit more hardener, if needed, to shape the button. Clean the mixing bowl and spatula immediately after use.

Rework (images 5.78 and 5.79)
Replace a soiled tamponade with one that has been impregnated with peclavus post-treatment which has a pain-relieving and soothing effect.

Tamponade application in three steps
The application of Copoline tamponades is important to ensure treatment success. It expands the nail fold, protects it from irritating adhesive material residue and, if impregnated with peclavus pre-and post-treatment, has a pain-relieving and soothing effect.

For nail brace applications, it is categorized in three phases:

1. **Pre-tamponade application**
   Expands the nail fold and impregnation with peclavus pre-treatment relieves pain and soothes.
2. **Interim-tamponade application**
   Protects the nail fold from adhesive material residue and serves as a fixation aid.
3. **Post-tamponade application**
   Serves as a fixation aid to secure the brace's end pieces, protects the nail fold and impregnation with peclavus post-treatment or AntiMYX silver promotes healing.

Two tamponade functions (image 5.80)

1. The classic variant protects and is used for the application of tinctures and ointments.
2. The filler tamponade increases the leverage effect of braces.

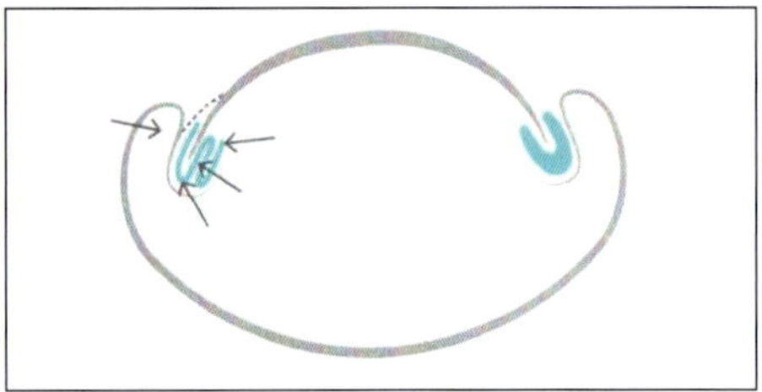

Image 5.80

Complications

It is important that the tension is not adjusted too tightly to avoid tearing the nail's edges or detaching the nail plate. Existing infections must be checked frequently to prevent them from spreading.

Important information for the patient

- The brace must be checked every night.
- In the event that the nail becomes painful, the brace loosens or for any other problems that might occur, visit the podiatrist.
- See the podiatrist for a follow-up visit within one to three days.
- Schedule a visit within four to six weeks with the podiatrist to reposition and align the brace.

Documentation is obligatory.

5.7 SSO4U brace

(Manufacturer: MCI medical care instruments UG)

The SSO brace is used on ingrown toe nails (unguis incarnatus) to straighten the growing nail. It temporarily relieves or eliminates painful impairments and injuries so that painful surgical procedures on the nail or nail bed can be avoided.

Contrary to the case of a surgical intervention, the use of this brace does not require the patient to take sick leave. This brace is non-sterile and is intended for a one-time temporary application.

It is made of a thin spring steel wire. The small fixation hooks on the end of the side wires are individually hooked to each lateral nail edge and then tightened, according to the required tension force, via a centre loop.

The purchase and application of this brace requires attendance at an introduction course on its use.

Material

Thin preformed wire with a centre loop available in different thicknesses.

Work materials

- brace
- U-loop
- holding pliers
- bending pliers
- file
- side-cutting pliers
- winding hook
- gloves and two pairs of safety glasses

Indications

- unguis convolutus
- unguis incarnatus
- clavi in the sulcus
- onychophosis
- paronychia
- granulation tissue

Preparation

Ensure that you and the patient wear safety glasses before nipping off wire ends!

Ensure that each side of the brace conforms to the nail shape. The highest point of the nail serves as a reference point and determines the length of each side of the brace. Leave a gap of approximately 5 mm between the wire ends to ensure that there is enough space for the loop.

The highest point of a nail is not always in its centre. This means that the sides of the brace have different lengths.

Tighten the loop until the patient feels a gentle tug and the brace is secured. The applied tension should not cause pain. Always check with your patient.

Brace preparation

Bend the wire ends 180 degrees with bending pliers. This step is in preparation for the small hooks that will be hooked under the nail.

Image 5.81 shows the bending of the wire.

Then cut off the unneeded wire pieces and ensure that there are no sharp pieces left on the hook (image 5.82).

Ensure that the wire adapts to the curvature of the nail surface. Press the wire with your thumb over the round handle of the conic MCI winding hook. This will create a nice curvature in the wire.

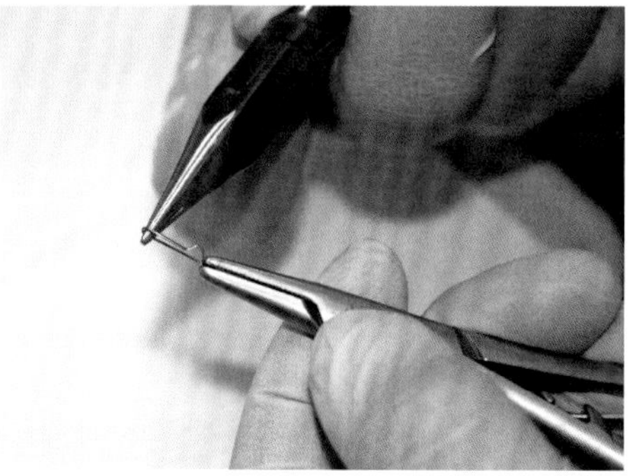

Image 5.81

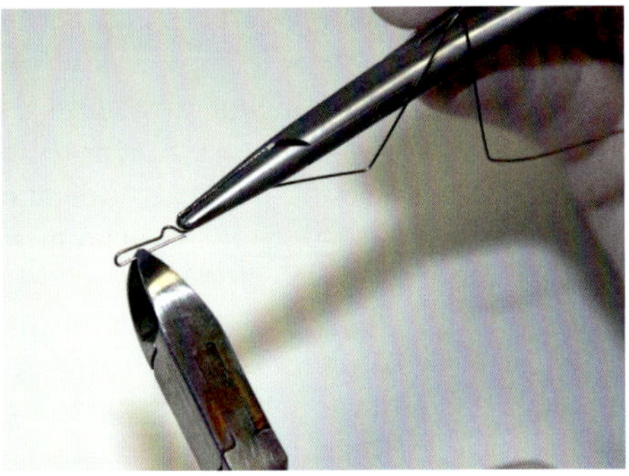

Image 5.82

Trim and smooth sharp wire pieces with a grinding bur or a metal file before inserting the hooks under the nail.

Positioning

Carefully hook one end of the prepared wire under the nail and align the remaining wire piece with the omega so that the small hook points forward and the omega points to the nail bed.

Cut off unneeded wire behind the S-curve with side-cutting pliers, leaving the rest of the wire.

Image 5.83 shows the result after the first piece of the brace has been placed. Repeat the previous steps with the second piece.

Both pieces should now be aligned with the omegas to the centre of the nail (reference point is the highest point of the nail) and there should be a 5 mm gap between them.

Connect the two wires with the U-loop by placing the loop in the S-curve of each wire.

Grab the loop with the winding hook.

Caution: Apply the correct tensile force. Do not pull too hard!

Press both S-curves together with your thumb and index finger. This already applies tension. With the other hand, twist the loop clockwise until the patient feels a tug without pain.

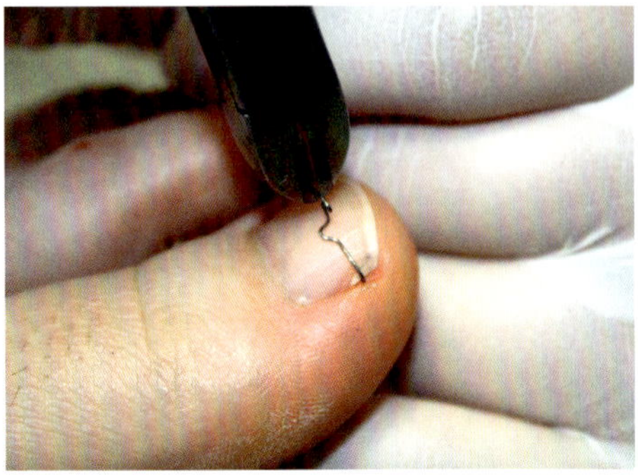

Image 5.83

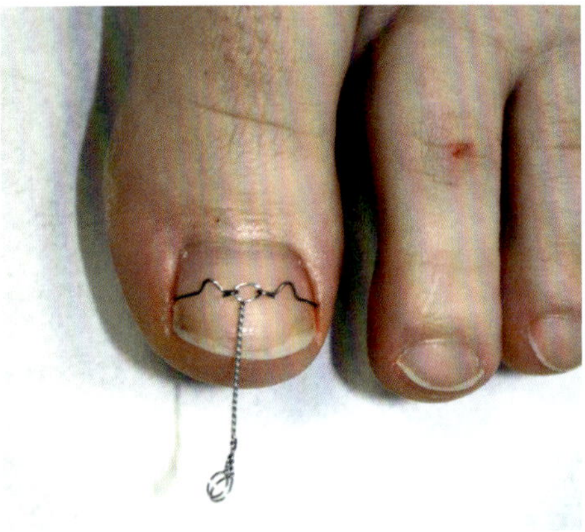

Image 5.84

Image 5.84 shows the result after the loop has been tightened.

Nip off the protruding S-curve pieces and the unneeded piece of the loop.

Image 5.85 shows the end result after all protruding wire pieces have been cut off.

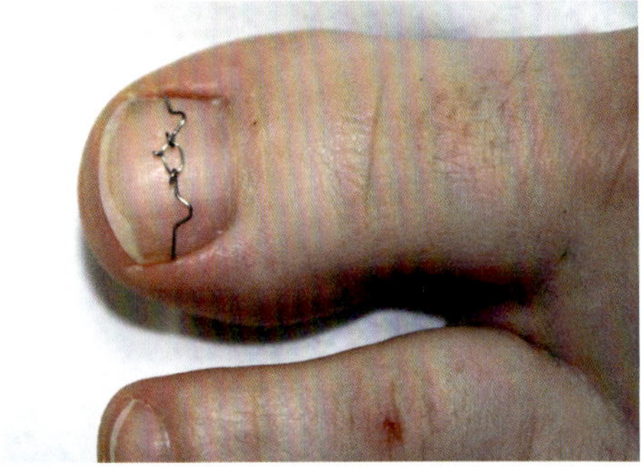

Image 5.85

Next seal the centre loop with light-curing Unguisan blue light gel and an LED light.

Finally, insert Ligasano or cotton gauze in both nail folds.

Important information for the patient

- The brace must be checked every night.
- In the event that the nail becomes painful, the brace loosens or for any other problems that might occur, visit the podiatrist.
- See the podiatrist for a follow-up visit within one to three days.
- Schedule a visit within four to six weeks with the podiatrist to reposition and align the brace.

Documentation is obligatory.

5.8 VHO-Osthold brace

The VHO (Virtuose Human Orthonyxie)-Osthold brace perfect was originally invented by Elvira Osthold under the name VHO-Osthold brace and patented in 1992. This nail correction brace already displayed the basic characteristics of the three-part brace technique. In the beginning, it was a simple brace wire that had to be shaped manually. This has been modified over the years and developed into a modular system which was patented in 2001 as VHO-Osthold brace perfect. The three pieces that make up the brace are made of thin spring steel wire. Each wire piece is individually hooked under the lateral nail plate and the other ends of the wire are connected via a centre loop that can be tightened until the correct tension has been achieved.

The purchase and application of this brace requires attendance at an introduction course on its use.

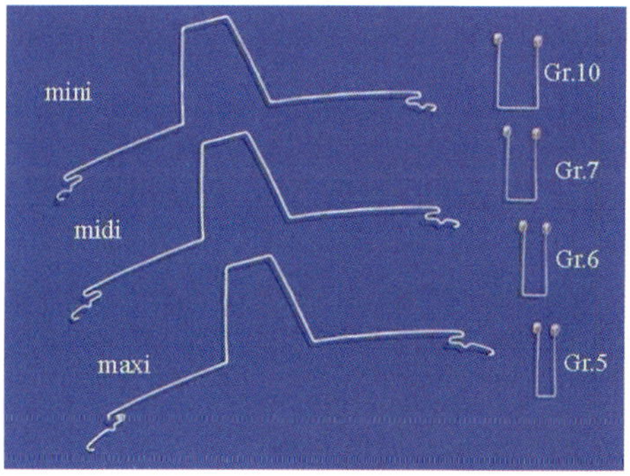

Image 5.86

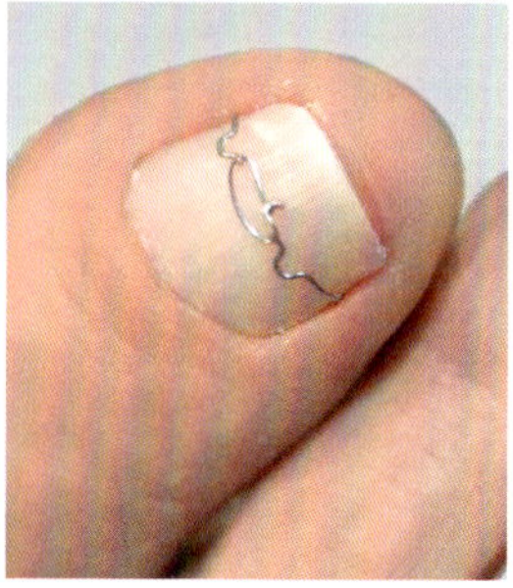

Image 5.87

Material

A thin preformed spring steel wire that comes in different diameters (images 5.86 and 5.87).

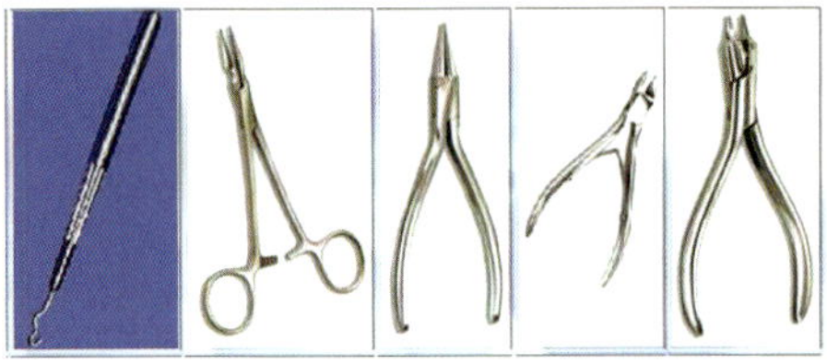

Image 5.88

Image 5.89 Functional principle

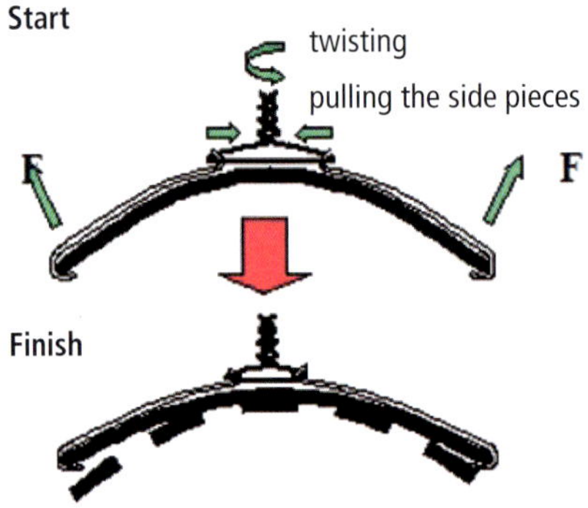

- Two hooked wire pieces are placed under the nail. This is a virtually painless procedure.
- The gap in the centre of the nail between the two side pieces is bridged with a preformed loop which is twisted with a winding hook until the desired tension has been achieved.
- The applied force lifts the edges of the nail of the inflamed tissue, providing immediate pain relief.

Work materials (image 5.88)
- preformed brace mezzo, mini, midi, maxi
- loops of different widths
- long nose pliers
- side-cutting pliers
- needle nose pliers, rounded pliers
- winding hook
- for sealing: gel technique, nail compound, Onycholit or Unguisan

Effectiveness and principle (image 5.89)

Indications
- unguis convolutus
- unguis incarnatus
- clavi in the sulcus
- onychophosis
- paronychia
- granulation tissue

Preparation
- Examine the nail fold with a probe to check where the brace should be placed.
- Disinfect the brace parts with an approved disinfectant.
- The brace can also be placed if inflammation or granulation tissue is present.
- If there are signs of suppuration in the nail fold, an appropriate treatment must be performed prior to placing the brace.
- A plaster model is not required.

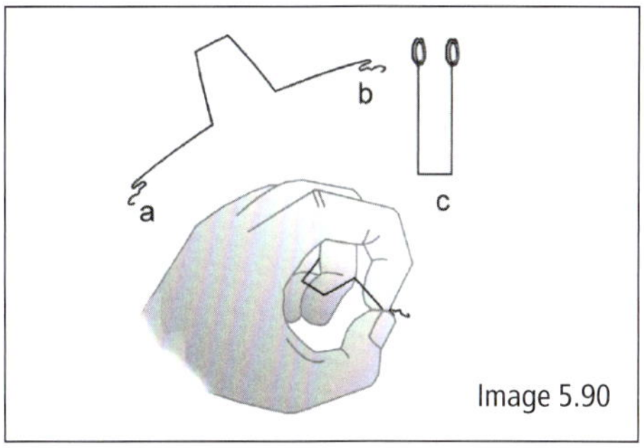

Image 5.90

Brace preparation

The brace system consists of the brace with its two mini levers (a and b) and a loop (part c).

The brace wire is made of high quality 0.3, 0.4 and 0.5 mm thick spring steel wire (image 5.90). The loop is made of a softer stainless steel wire (0.3 and 0.4 mm) (image 5.91).

Positioning and fixation

Position the first lever on the non- or less infected or damaged side of the nail and cut to the appropriate length (image 5.92). Repeat on the other side. The "handle" in the centre of the brace allows the podiatrist to proceed with great sensitivity so not to cause any pain for the patient.

Place the loop and twist it with a winding hook. The three parts of the VHO brace are now joined together. The resulting leverage force lifts the edge of the nail out of the inflamed area causing instant pressure and pain relief (images 5.93 and 5.94).

Cut off all protruding brace and loop wire pieces and cover the centre of the brace with an artificial nail compound to protect socks and blankets (image 5.95).

During the initial treatment of serious infections, do not seal the brace with artificial nail compound. Instead, apply a dressing and bandage the toe. This way the brace can easily be removed at the patient's next follow-up visit.

Complications

It is important that the tension is not adjusted too tightly to avoid tearing the nail's edges or detaching the nail plate. With existing infection, frequent control visits are crucial to check if the infection has spread.

Important information for the patient

- The brace must be checked every night.
- In the event that the nail becomes painful, the brace loosens or for any other problems that might occur, visit the podiatrist.
- See the podiatrist for a follow-up visit within one to two days in acute cases, otherwise in four to six weeks.
- Schedule a visit within four to six weeks with the podiatrist to reposition and align the brace.

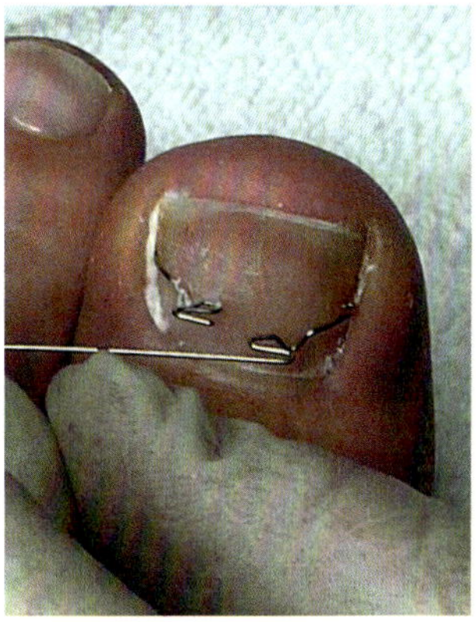
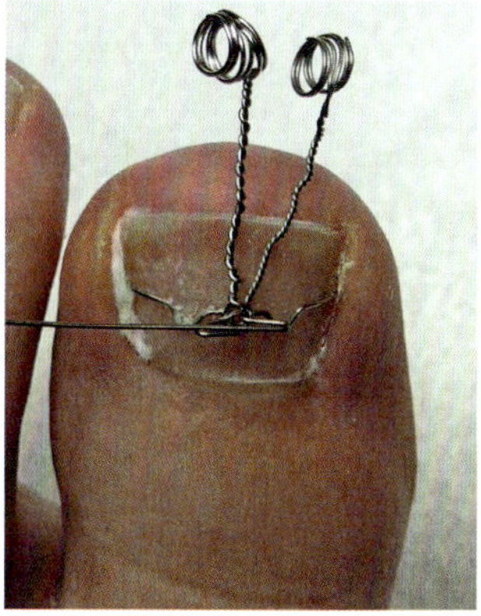
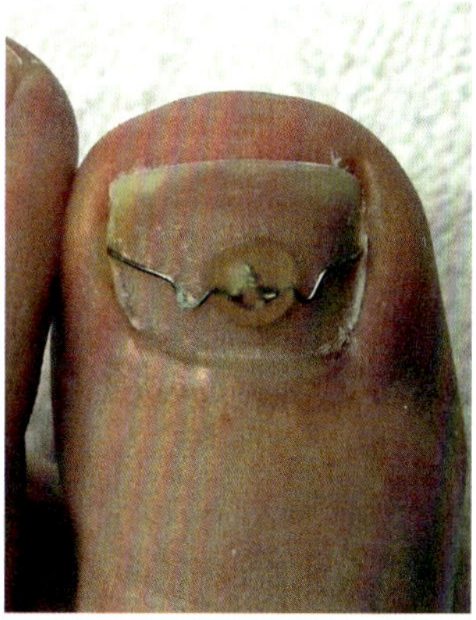

Image 5.91

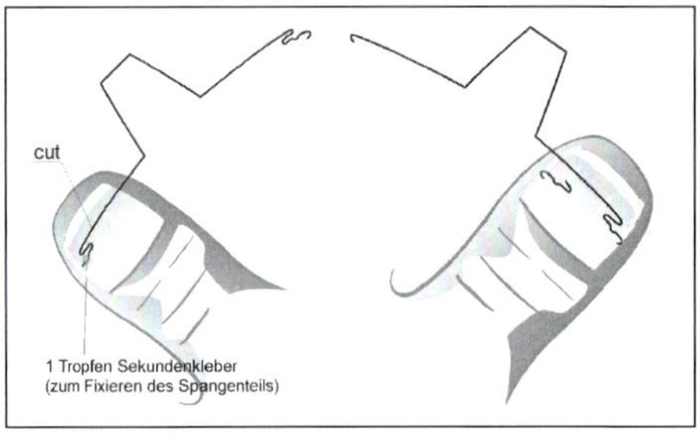

Image 5.92

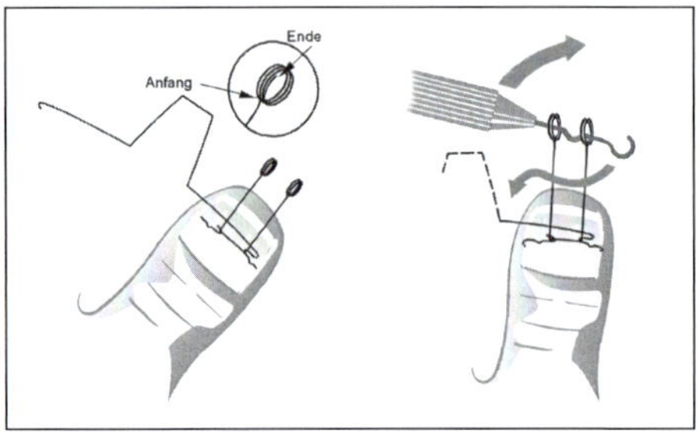

Image 5.93

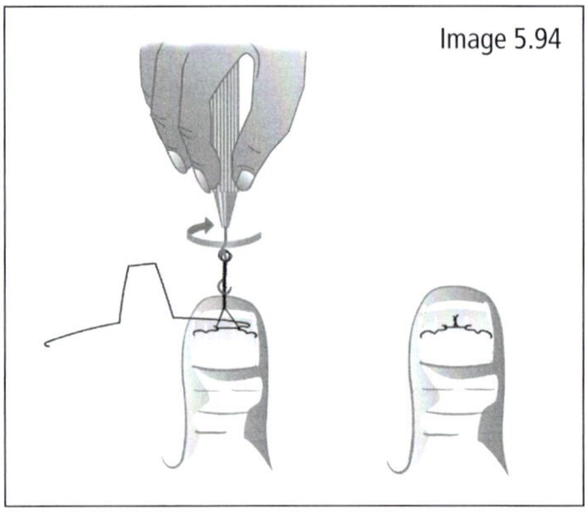

Image 5.94

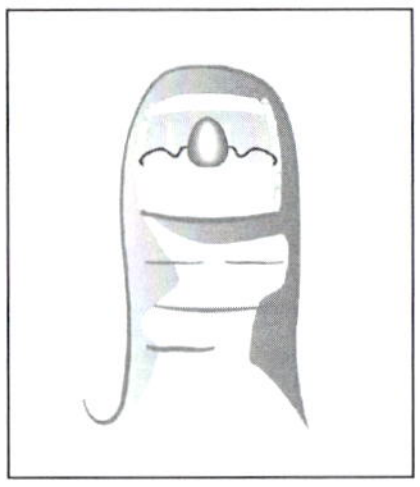

Image 5.95

Images 5.86 to 5.95
Source: VHO

5.9 ORa brace

All images in this chapter are courtesy of Brigitte Rathenow, inventor of the brace.

Material

Stainless steel spring wire. Left and right side 0.3 mm and 0.4 mm diameter (images 5.96 and 5.97).

Work materials (images 5.98 and 5.99)

- flat-nosed pliers, with holes
- round pliers and round bending pliers
- needle holder
- side-cutting pliers
- brace hooks left/right

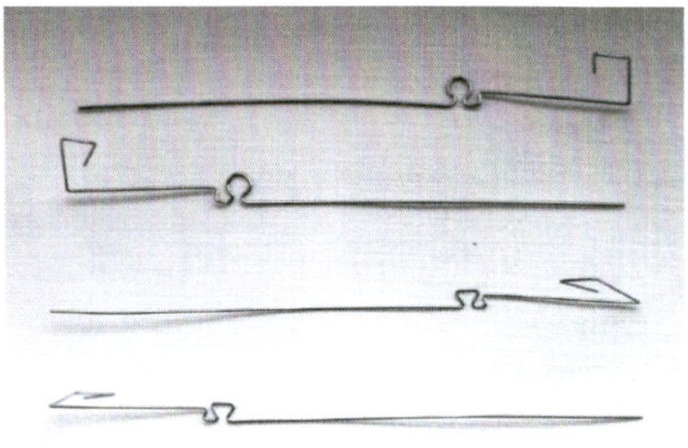

Image 5.96 Braces

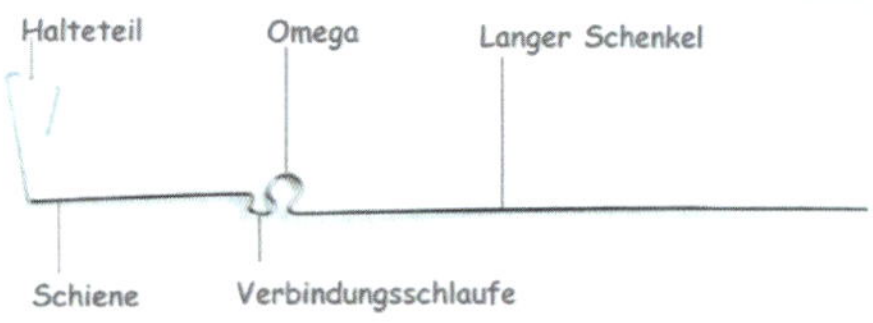

Image 5.97 The different parts of the brace

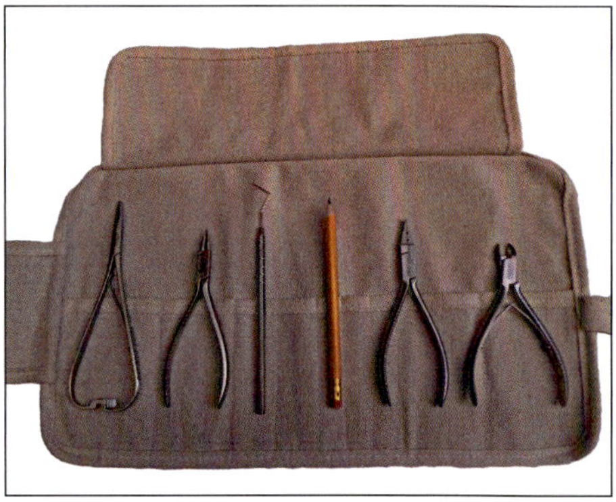

Image 5.98 Professional instrument set

Effectiveness

- **Unguis convolutus on both sides**

Start by attaching the side of the brace either on the left or right side of the nail. After adjusting the length of the wires on each side, activate the brace using single to triple nail thickness as a guideline. Increase the tension for healthy and flexible nails by shortening both side wires of the brace, if necessary.

The difference in length must not exceed single to maximal triple wire diameter (1.2 mm) (images 5.103 to 5.108).

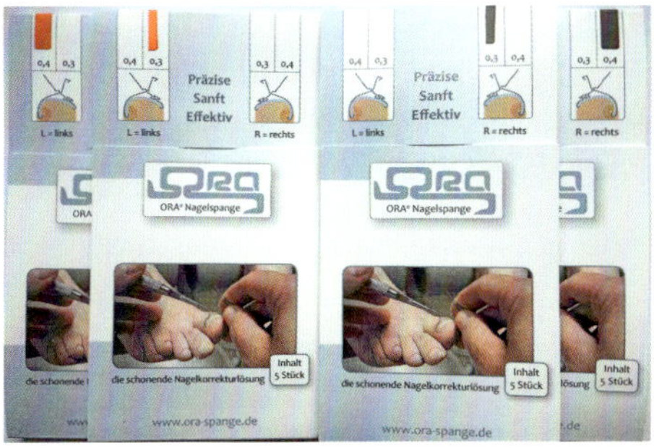

Image 5.99 Different brace designs

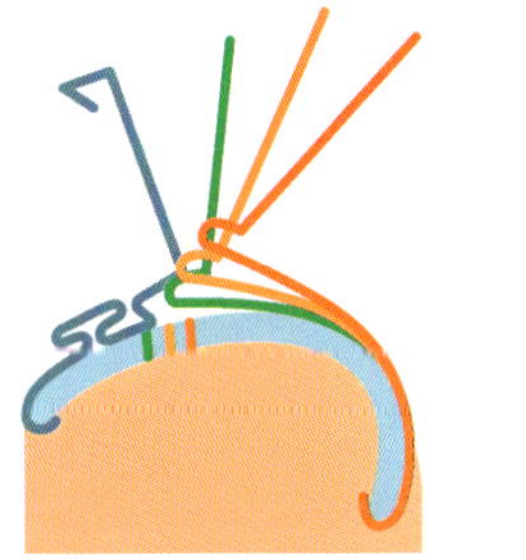

Image 5.100 Customized nail correction

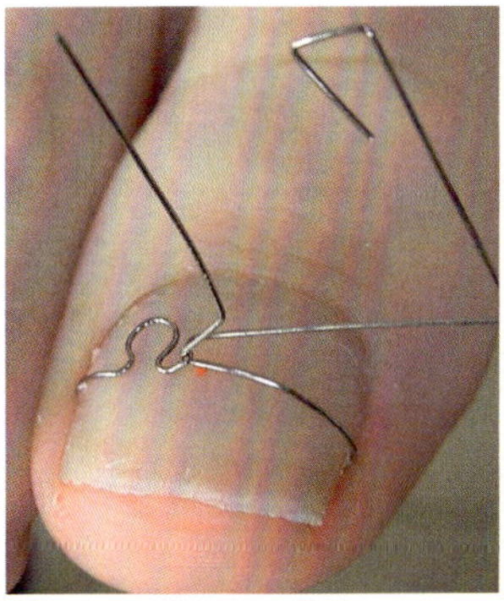

Image 5.101 Hooking the two sides together

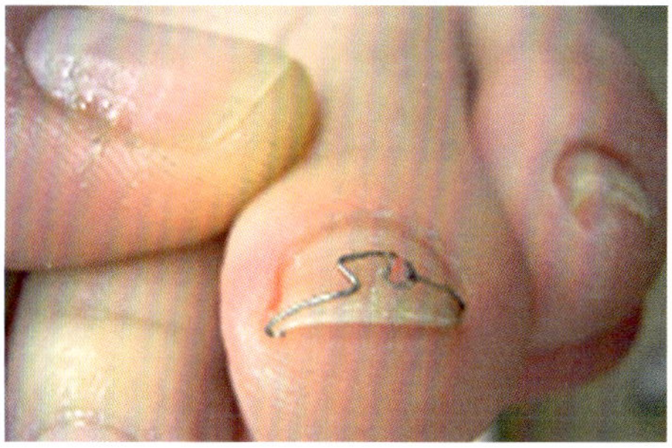

Image 5.102 0.3 mm brace suitable for small toes

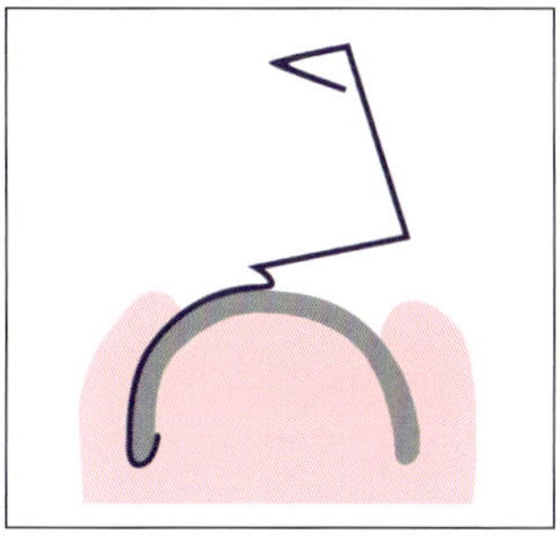

Image 5.103

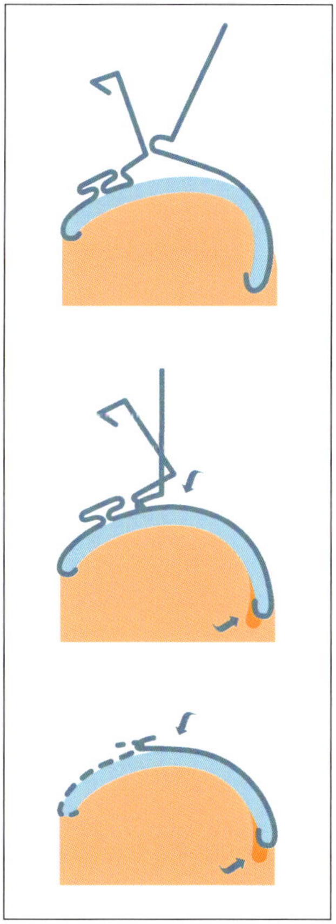

Image 5.104 Ora brace, single-sided

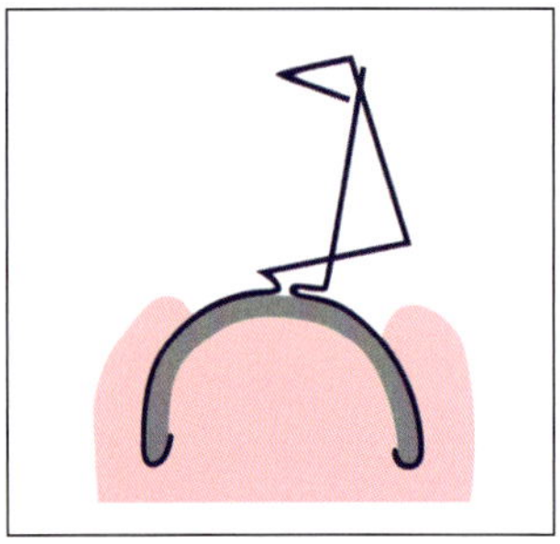

Image 5.105

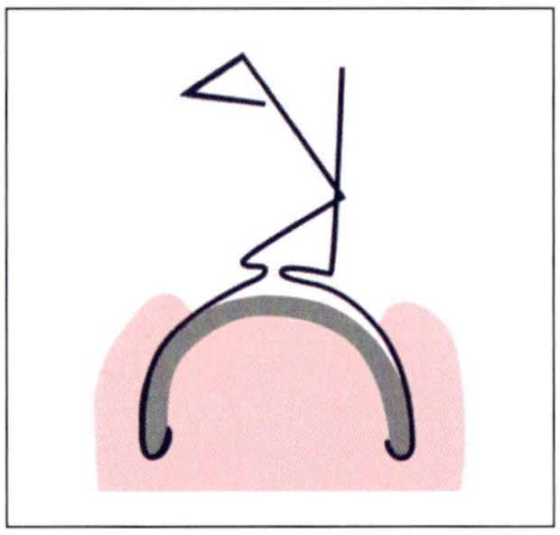

Image 5.106

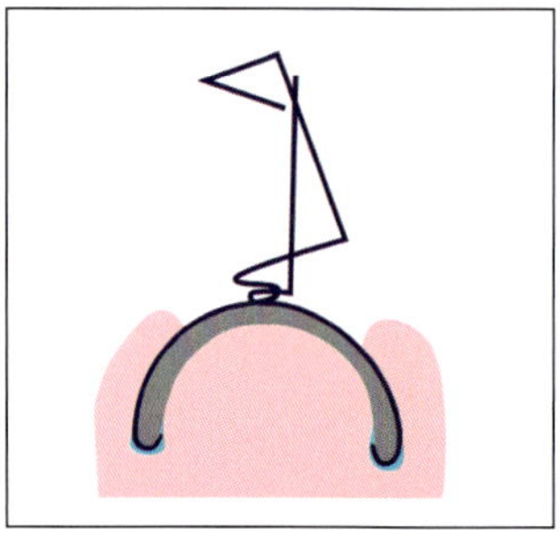

Image 5.107

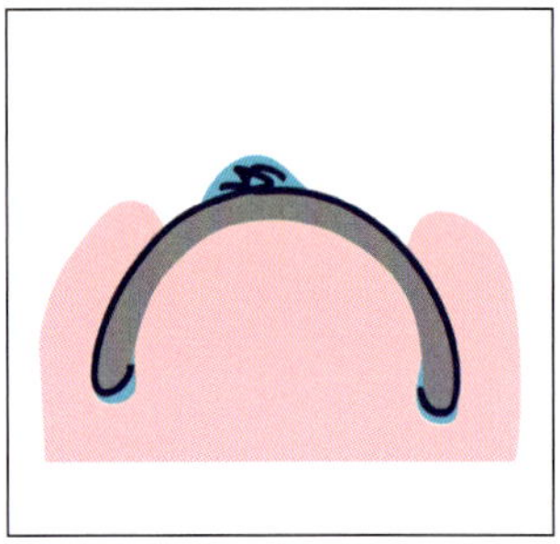

Image 5.108

• Unguis incarnatus one side

Insert one side of the brace first in the healthy nail edge. Keep it as short as possible. The connection point–the point where the two sides of the brace are hooked together–is on the side of the nail that is not affected by unguis incarnatus. Custom fit the second wire and attach it to the edge of the ingrown nail. This wire is responsible for the nail correction process via activation of the brace. The longer the second wire, the larger the nail area over which the correcting forces are distributed (images 5.109 to 5.114).

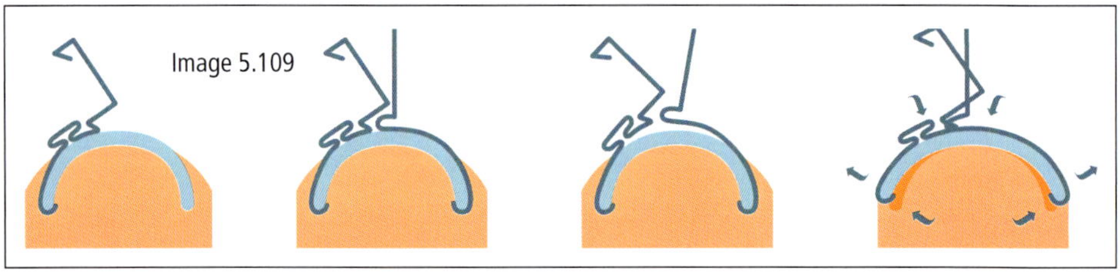

Image 5.109

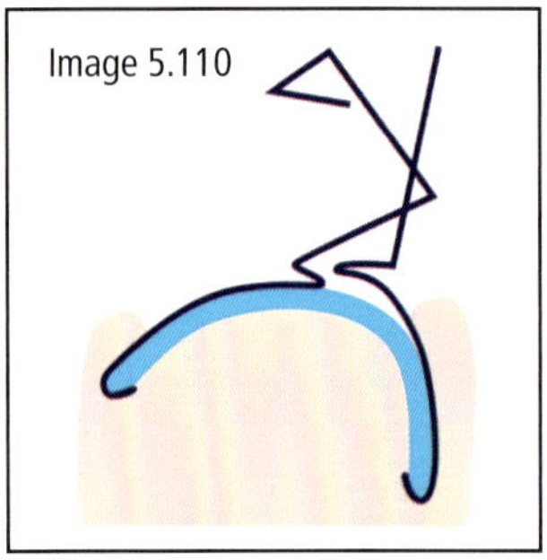

Image 5.110

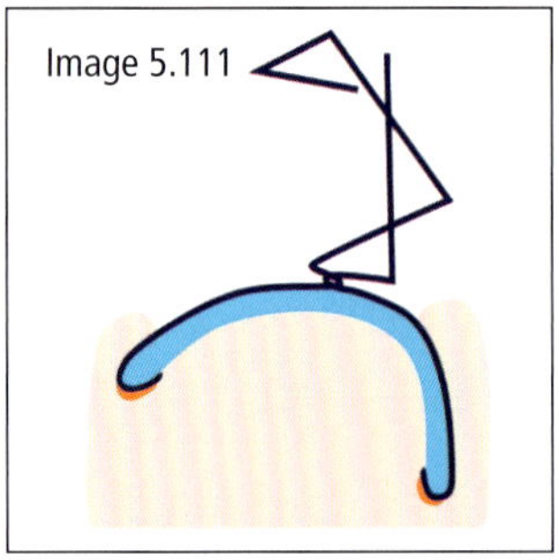

Image 5.111

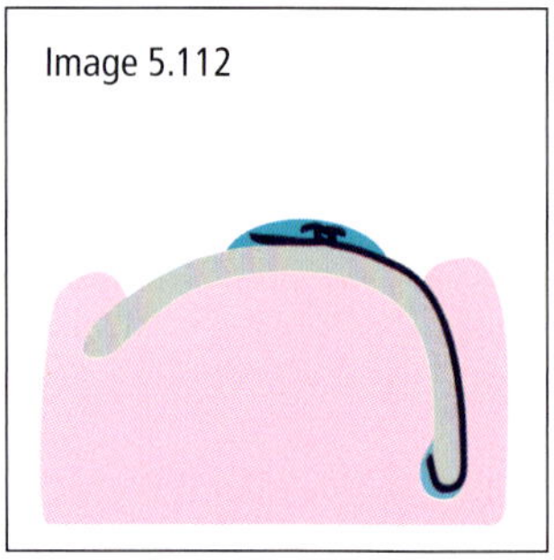

Image 5.112

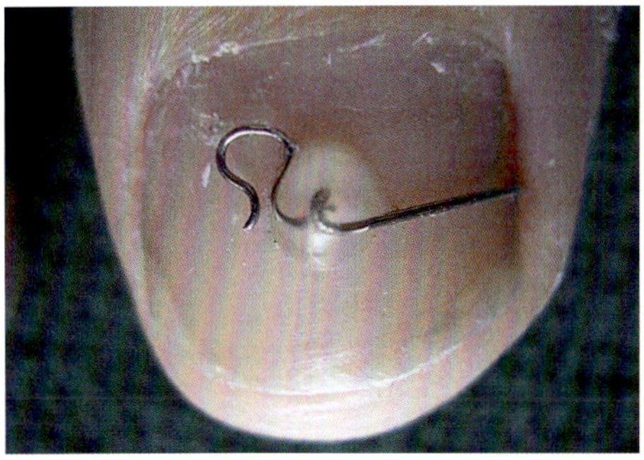

Image 5.113 Single-sided Ora bracee

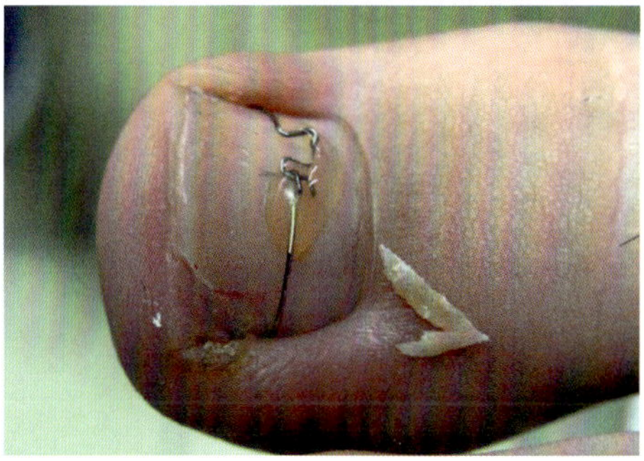

Image 5.114 The applied brace with a section of the nail cut off

Acute brace

This brace is optimal for application on acutely painful nails because it can be applied pressure-free. The open two-part design offers a precise application in the problematic area of the nail and its activation can be easily controlled. It offers immediate pain relief, provided the nail fold has been properly prepared. Deeply impacted nail parts can often be removed only once the nail has been lifted by a brace.

Due to its effectiveness and its pain-free application, the ORa brace is well accepted by physicians and patients alike (image 5.114).

Indications

- unguis convolutus
- unguis incarnatus
- clavi in the sulcus
- onychophosis
- paronychia
- granulation tissue

Limited indication

- onychogryposis/onychauxis (the extreme thickness of the nail causes the brace sides to loosen and can trigger onycholysis)
- onychorrhexis (static issues)
- onychoschizia (static issues)
- onychodystrophy, psoriatic nail

Podiatric treatment prior to applying the ORa brace is imperative.

Preparation

- Disinfect, clean and dry the nail.
- Check for hornification and/or ingrown nail particles.
- Remove hornification with cuticle nippers, a grinding bur or apply propolis tincture and carefully scrape with a probe.
- Dry the granulation tissue and moisten the nail plate by applying tamponades.
- Expand the nail fold area by applying a tamponade.

Brace preparation

The images on the package facilitates choosing the correct brace design. For instance, if the left side of the nail is problematic, choose the left brace in the orange package. Place the side of the brace with the omega in the nail edge opposite the painful side of the nail, the right side.

Positioning and fixation

Positioning the first side of the brace: Fixate the brace with the omega in the needle holder. Pre-bend the long brace wire with your hand, cut with side-cutting pliers and shape a small end hook with flat-nosed pliers. Bend the short piece with round-nose pliers to fit the nail's shape. Hook the end hook into the lateral nail edge, turning it 45 degrees. The wire lies now flush on the nail surface. The tension can be adjusted, depending on the existing nail situation. For this, mark the nail with a small dot. The closer the dot is to the end of the first wire, the less difference in length there is and, therefore, the less necessary tensile force (images 5.115 to 5.117).

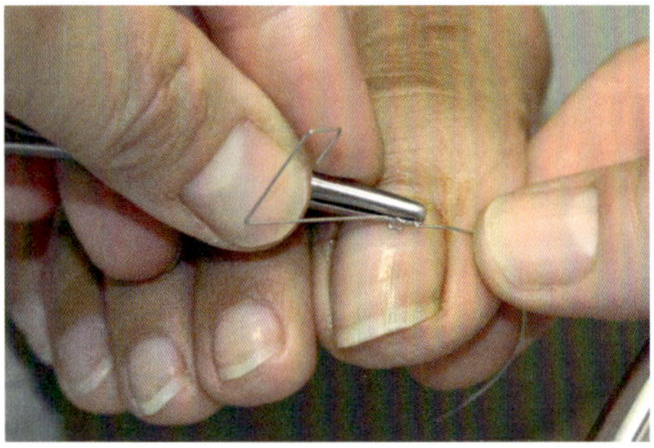

Image 5.115 Preparation

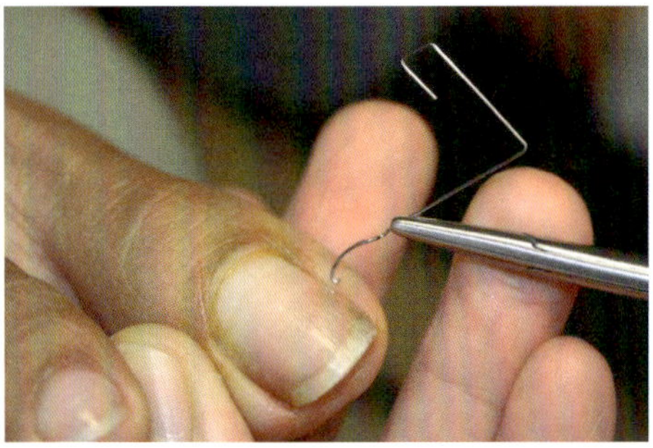

Image 5.116 Hooking the wire under the nail's edge

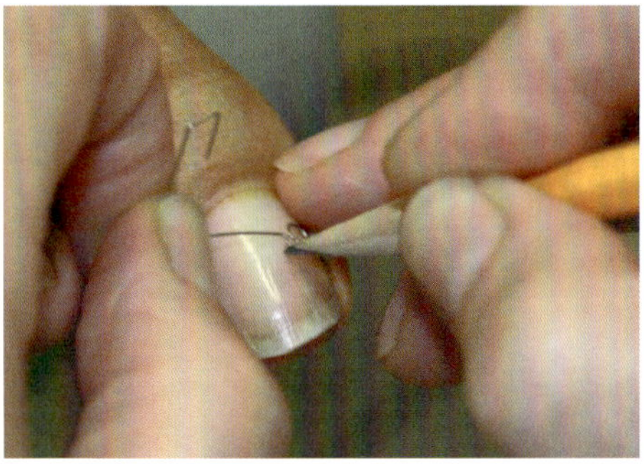

Image 5.117 Marking the nail

Positioning the second side of the brace: Use the cut-off leftover piece of the first wire for the other side of the brace. Prepare the wire and hook it under the problematic nail edge as proximal as possible. The straight long piece lies now over the mark. Bend the wire over the mark with flat-nosed pliers and create a tight connection loop.

Now activate the second piece by bending the wire a single to triple nail thickness away from the nail (images 5.118 and 5.119).

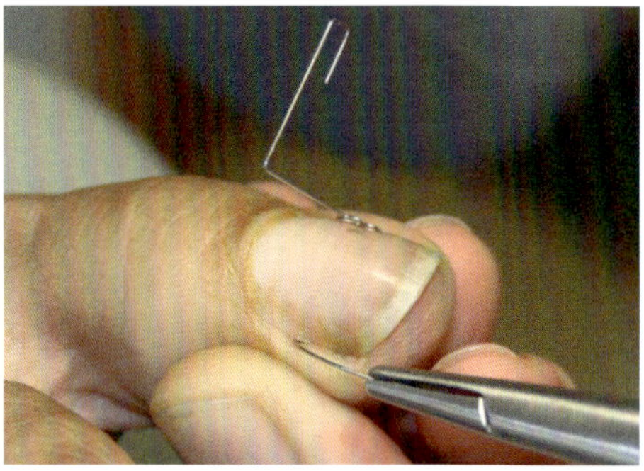

Image 5.118 Bending the wire

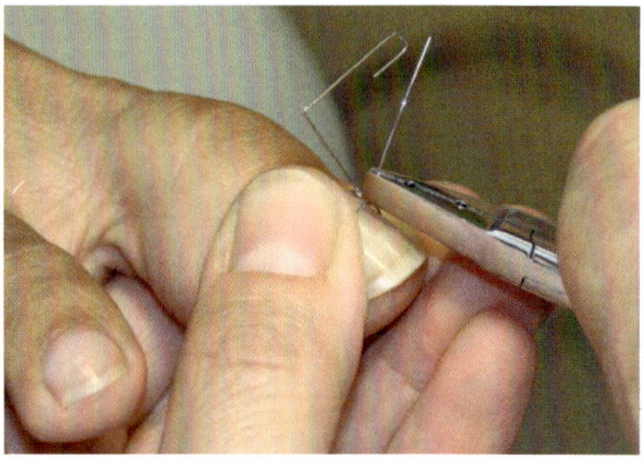

Image 5.119 Activation

Hook the two brace pieces together without pulling. Press the activated side onto the nail plate with your finger. Now pull the elastic omega from the front through the connection loop of the two wires. The brace has now been activated. Nip off protruding wire pieces and seal with resin. Once the resin has hardened, sand it down (image 5.120).

Insert a Ligasano tamponade into the nail fold (images 5.121 and 5.122).

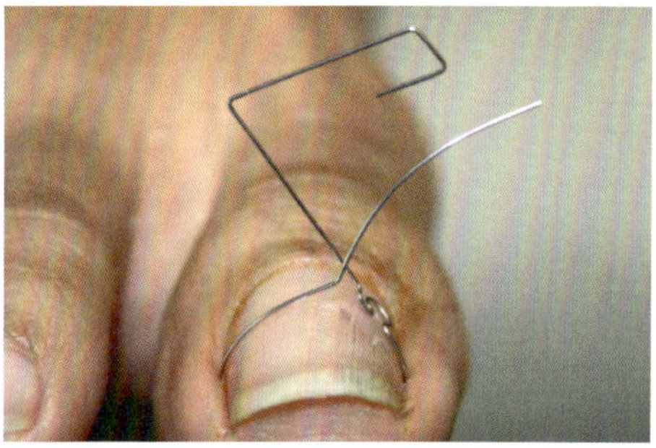

Image 5.120 Activation

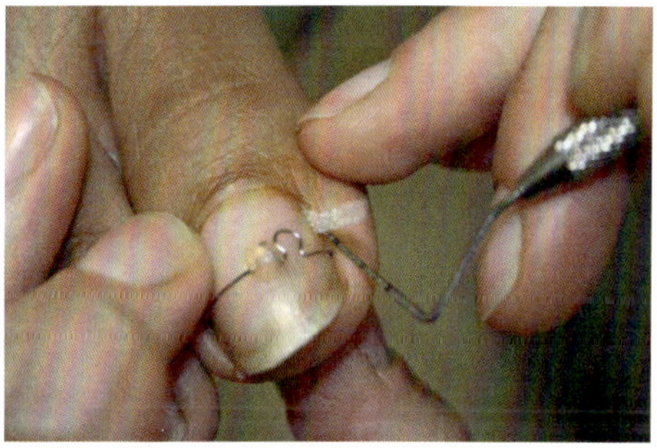

Image 5.121 Image 5.122 ▼

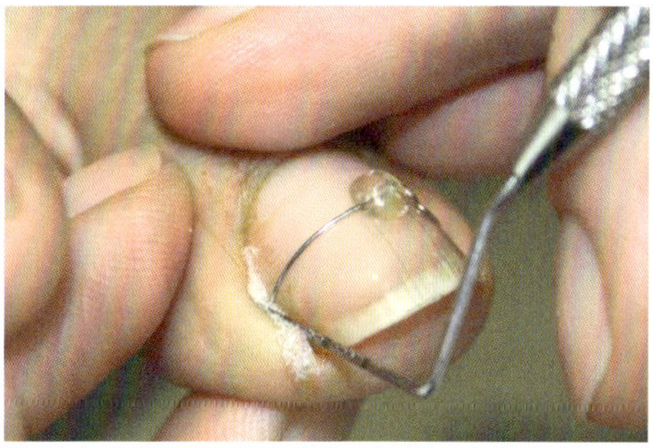

Important information for the patient

- The brace must be checked every night.
- In the event that the nail becomes painful, the brace loosens or for any other problems that might occur, visit the podiatrist.
- See the podiatrist for a follow-up visit within one to two days.
- The ORa brace stays on the nail approximately three to twelve weeks and grows with the nail. Once the brace wire reaches the distal nail margin, it must be removed and maybe replaced, depending on the nail situation.

5.10 Corectio titanium brace

This two-part wire brace was developed in Japan. It is easily applied since the hooks are already pre-shaped. Smoothing the tip of the wire is not necessary since it has been treated with a special surface finish. Its bowline knot is 100-per-cent secure. Another advantage to promote stability: the brace comes in one piece, as compared to other brace designs, which require two or three wires to be connected. The brace risks loosening only if it is pulled too hard (very rarely). High quality workmanship and the special welding process of soft and hard wires are valuable features of this product made in Japan.

The specially processed wire prevents injury at the nail's edge. The titanium coating is not known to cause irritation. Titanium is usually used with invasive surgical procedures such as artificial joint surgery. Titanium is, therefore, suitable for patients suffering from allergies.

The brace is intended for one-time use.

Work materials (images 5.123 and 5.124)

Three designs are available:

- **Corectio titanium regular**: basic brace (0.3 mm wire in the top part of the brace)
- **Corectio titanium hard:** for hard nails (0.4 mm wire in the top part of the brace)
- **Corectio titanium wide:** for wide, thick and severely rolled nails (0.4 mm wire in the top part of the brace)
  "Hard" and "wide" can be combined on the same nail.
- holding pliers
- winding hook
- round nose pliers
- sealant: gel technique, Onycholit, Unguisan, nail compound

Effectiveness (image 5.125)

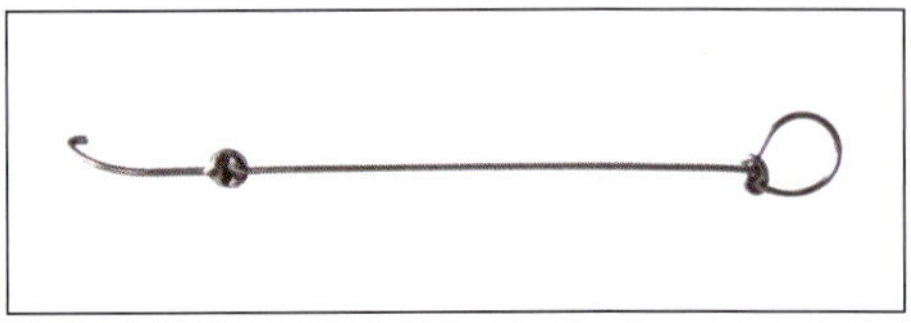

Image 5.123

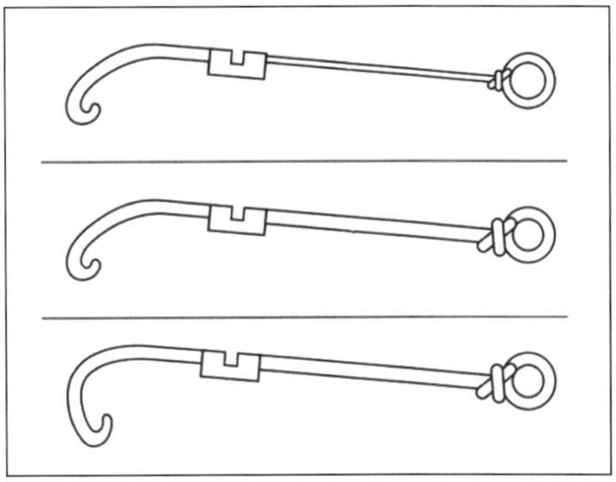

Image 5.124

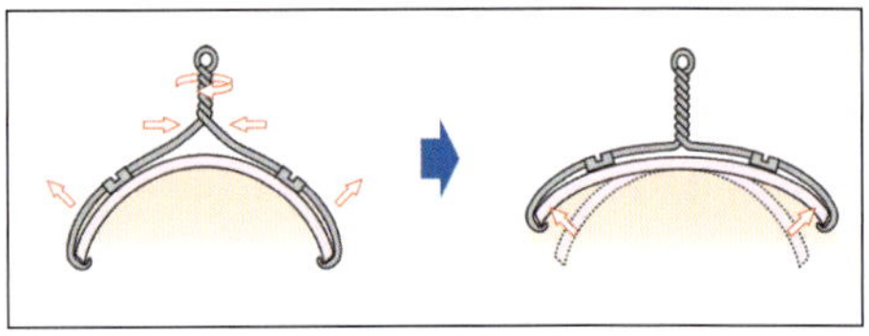

Image 5.125 Effect mechanism

Indications

- unguis incarnatus
- unguis convolutus
- callositas
- hyperkeratosis
- clavi in the sulcus or beneath the nail plate

Contraindication

Paronychia (the application of the brace may be painful).

Conditional contraindication

This involves diabetics or patients with a neuropathic disorder. These patients cannot feel if the tension of the brace is too tight, and wound healing is impaired.

Preparation

If the nail fold is infected, the infection must be treated first in consultation with a physician. Once the infection has healed, probe the nail fold carefully with an excavator or another adequate instrument.

Thoroughly remove hyperkeratosis build-up or clavi without injuring the area.

Image 5.126 Numbers 1 to 8: positioning of the Corectio titanium brace

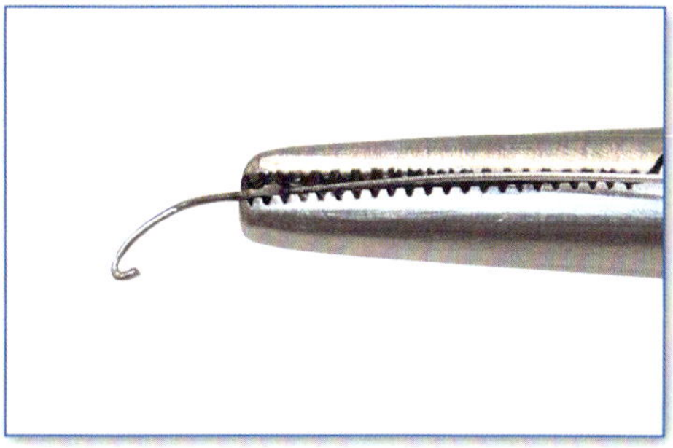

1

After properly preparing the nail, grab the brace plate with holding forceps so that the hook of the brace is pointing downwards. Ensure that you also grab some wire with the brace plate and support the wire with your finger.

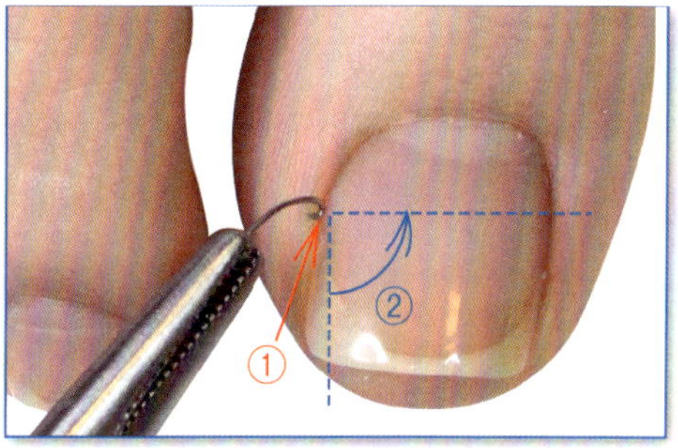

2

1. Check the hook's length and fit and, if necessary, adjust it with round-nosed pliers. The braces come pre-bent (image 5.127) but can be shaped if needed (image 5.127). For application on small nails (children's toenails) the tip must be cut and re-bent.
2. Hook the hook in the first third part of the nail at an angle in the lateral nail edge. Then twist the wire 90 degrees towards the centre of the nail.

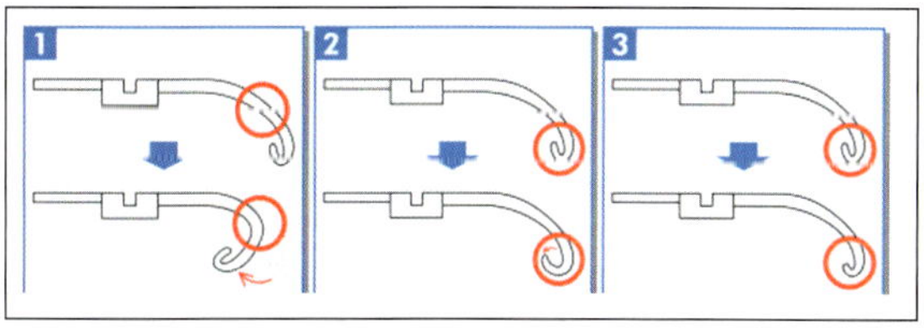

Image 5.127

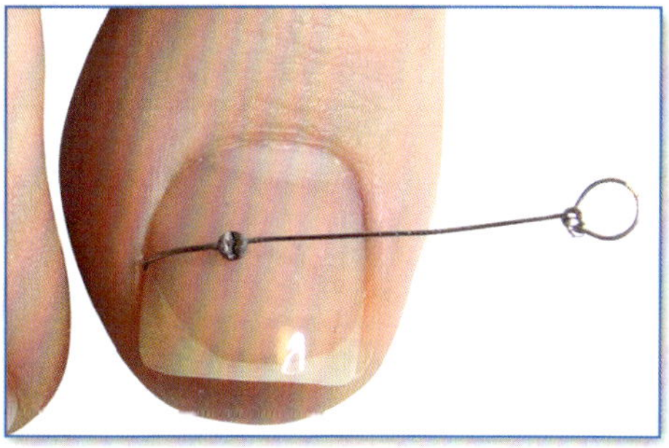

3

Put the pliers on the side and position the brace plate on the nail and press it down with your finger simultaneously bending the wire vertically upwards.

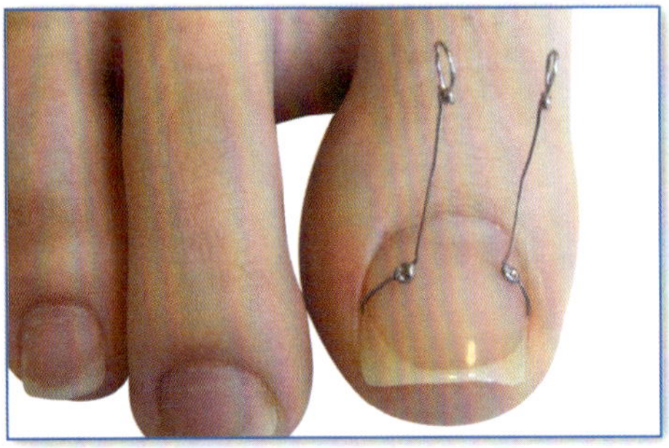

4

Repeat steps 1 to 3 with the second brace element on the other side of the nail (image 5.128).

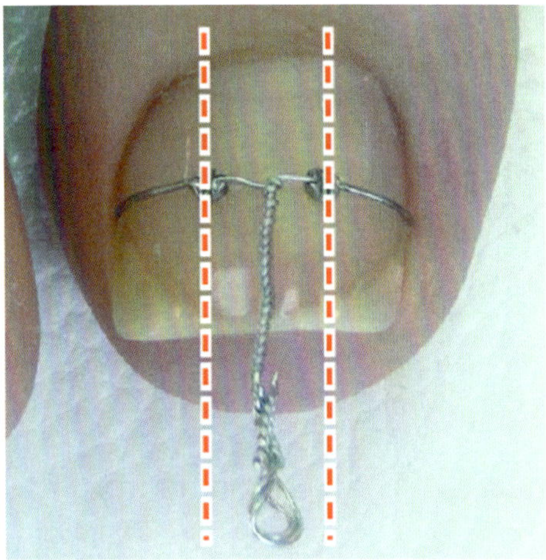

Image 5.128

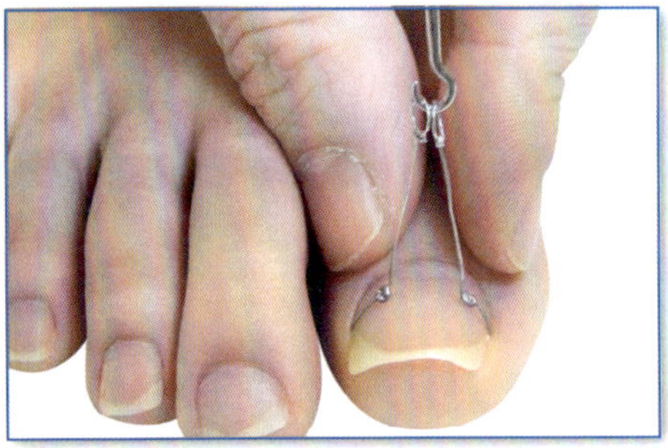

5

Press both brace plates on the nail with your finger. Grab both wire loops of the two wires with a winding hook twisting them over the centre of the nail. Make sure that the wire points upwards. Always leave a small gap between the nail surface and the centre of the connected wires to prevent breakage.

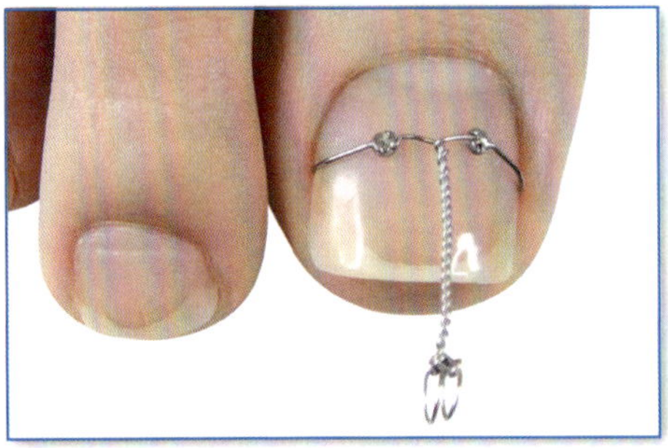

6

Twist the wires until they become one straight line. Bend the twisted wire piece towards the tip of the nail so that it lies on top of the nail surface and twist until both side pieces of the brace are tightened. Check if the tension is adequate; otherwise apply more tension by twisting the wire a few more turns.

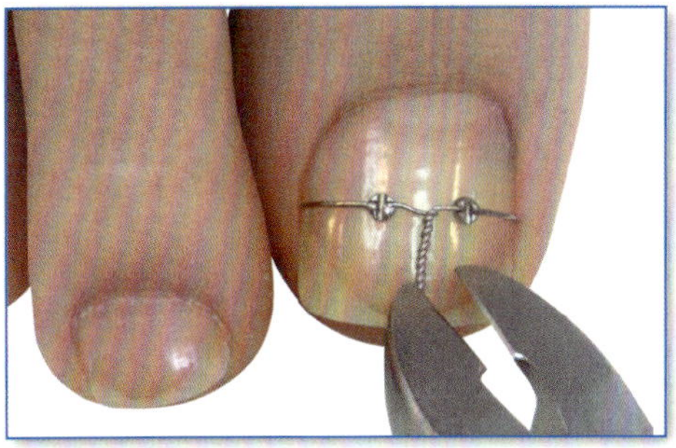

7 Cut off the unused wire and clean the nail surface with an anti-grease solution.

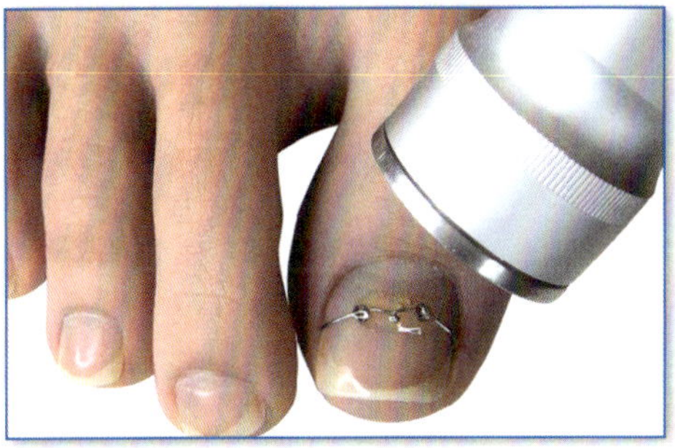

8 Secure the brace on the nail surface with Blue Light gel and cure with Blue Light (LED) for approx. 20 seconds or apply nail compound or Unguisan as a sealant.

All Corectio titanium images courtesy of Reflepro.

Complications

If the applied tension is too strong, it can cause the nail to fracture or detach from the nail bed. The centre of the twisted wire must be pointing towards the tip of the nail, thereby preventing the formation of a subungual clavus.

Important information for the patient

- The brace must be checked every night.
- In the event that the nail becomes painful, the brace loosens or for any other problems that might occur, visit the podiatrist.
- See the podiatrist for a follow-up visit within one to two days.

5.11 COMBIped brace

This brace is a combination of spring wire and adhesive brace. It is used to correct deformed, painful, ingrown and convoluted nails and can be applied to and be effective on one or both sides of the nail. Its design allows the single-sided application of a wire brace.

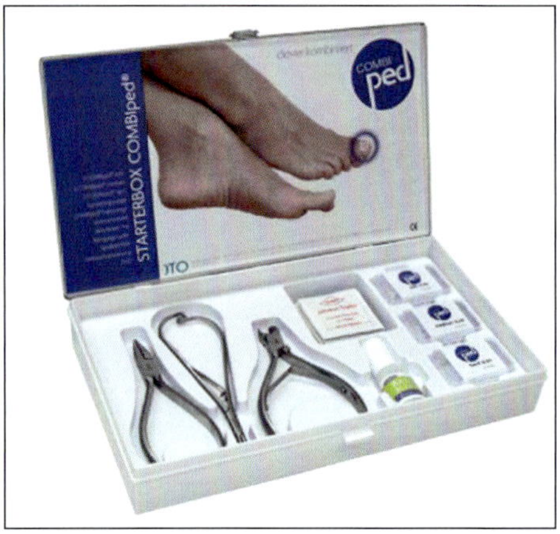

Image 5.129 The starter set contains all required instruments and products

Materials

- braces in three different diameters
- adhesive with brush
- alcohol swabs for cleaning the nail and the brace
- combination bending pliers
- fixation pliers
- side-cutting pliers
- sanding file

Effectiveness

The reset force of the spring wire has a gentle bending effect on the nail. Even severely deformed nails can be corrected. The strength of the force can be controlled by choosing the appropriate wire diameter and by pre-shaping the wire.

Indications

- unguis convolutus
- unguis incarnatus
- clavi in the sulcus
- onychophosis
- paronychia
- granulation tissue

Preparation

Prior to applying the brace, clean the nail fold with a probe and disinfect the area (images 5.140 and 5.141).

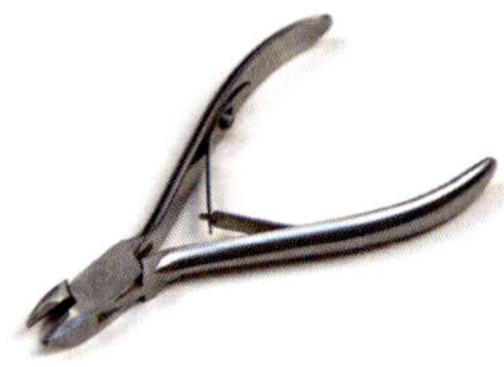

Image 5.130 Side-cutting pliers

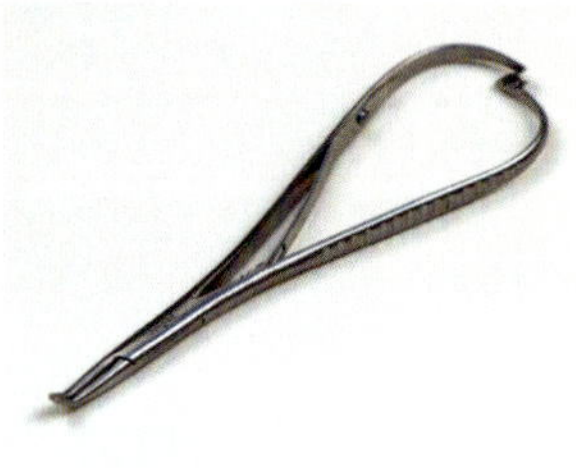

Image 5.131 Holding forceps

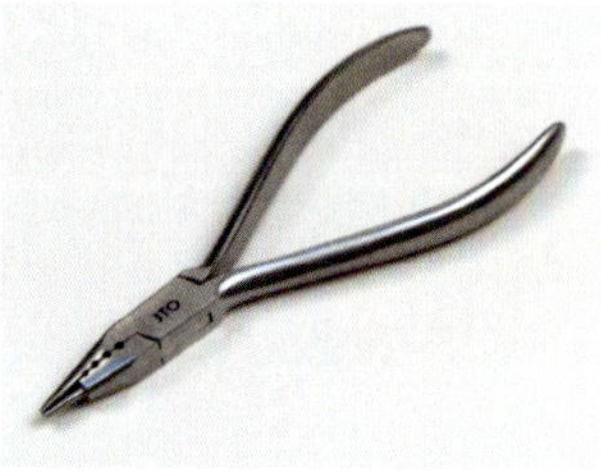

Image 5.132 Combination bending pliers

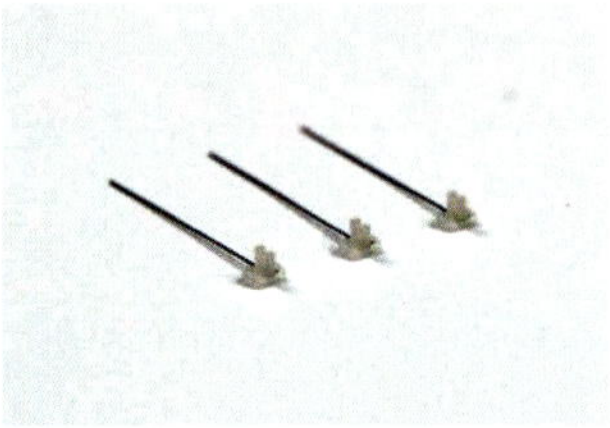

Image 5.133 Braces

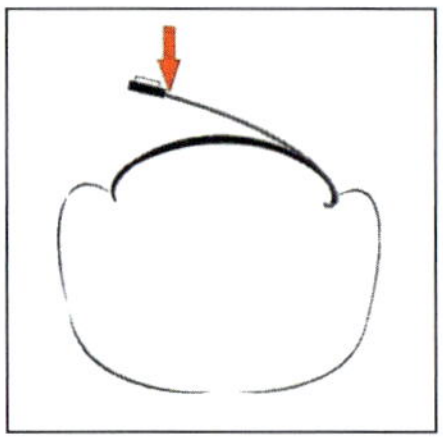

Image 5.134 The more the nail is curved, the greater the applied force of the brace

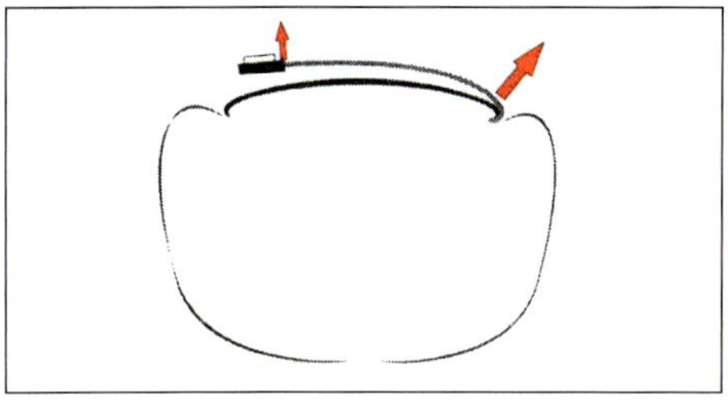

Image 5.135 The brace generates a stronger force on the side of the wire and less on the side of the brace plate

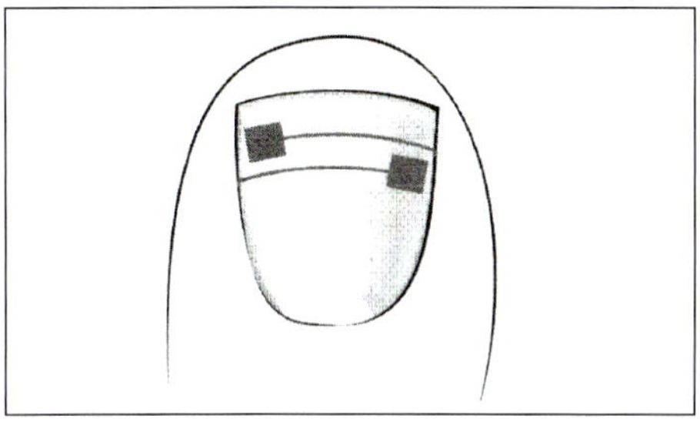

Image 5.136 If the brace is supposed to affect both sides of the nail, the brace must cover the entire width of the nail. It is also possible to place two braces with different wire thickness next to each other.

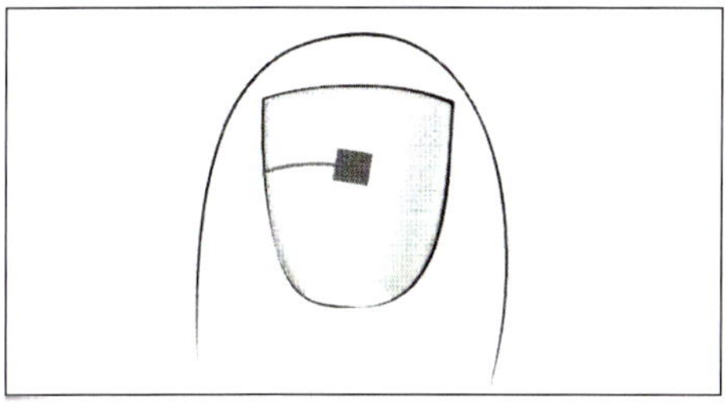

Image 5.137 For a one-sided effect, prepare a shorter brace and glue the brace plate in the centre of the nail. The force is then concentrated on one side.

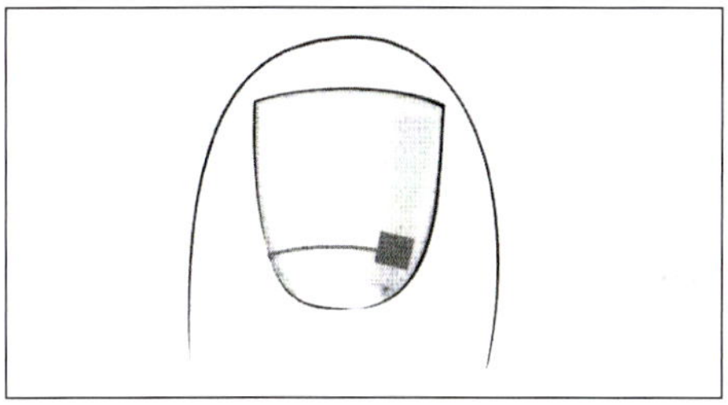

Image 5.138 To correct a severely convoluted nail, place the brace in the lunula area

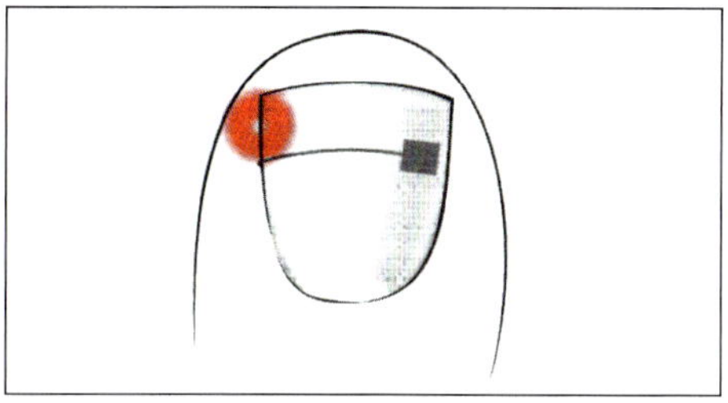

Image 5.139 Position the brace approx. 2 mm below a painful area

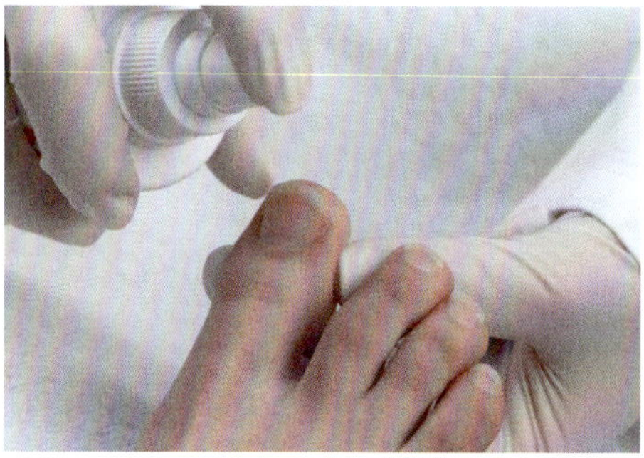

Image 5.140

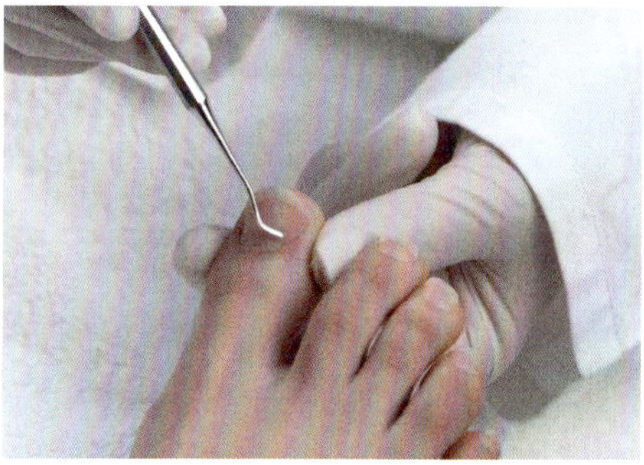

Image 5.141

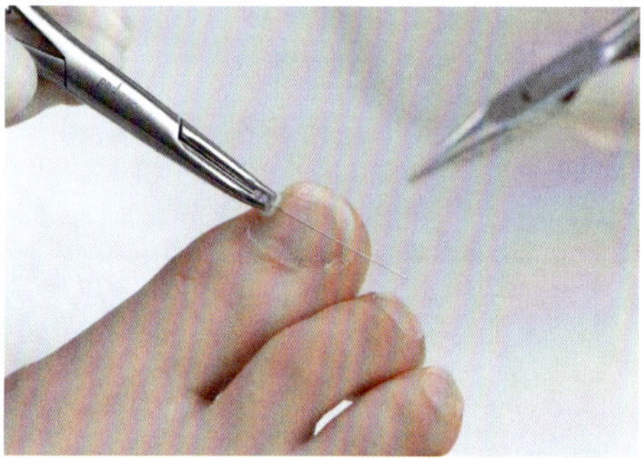

Image 5.142 Keep a gap between the brace plate and the fixation pliers to ensure that the brace stays flexible

The brace can be applied even with existing infections and granulation build-up. Suppuration in the nail fold must be treated prior to applying the brace. Consult with a physician. Prepare the nail and thoroughly clean the nail fold. Remove any loose particles from the nail surface. Smooth extremely rough nails or roughen very shiny nails with a sand file.

Wipe the brace wire with an alcohol swab prior to shaping the hook and before inserting it under the nail.

Choose the diameter of the brace wire according to the thickness of the nail (required force) (image 5.142).

Soft: Wire diameter 0.25 mm for soft and normal nails.
Medium: Wire diameter 0.30 mm for normal and thick nails.
Hard: Wire diameter 0.35 mm exclusively for extremely thick nails.

CAUTION: Use "soft" and "medium" for most cases. If the brace is too tight it might cause the nail to detach from the nail bed. Applying moderate tension is, therefore, the safest option.

If the tension is too tight and causes the patient pain, then it must be replaced by a less forceful brace.

Brace preparation

Fix the brace on both pins using fixation pliers. The length of the brace is determined by the width of the nail.

Use the combination pliers and bend a hook at the defined spot (images 5.143 to 5.146).

Use one of the four holes in the pliers to measure the hook size. The holes and, therefore, the hooks are smaller towards the tip of the pliers.

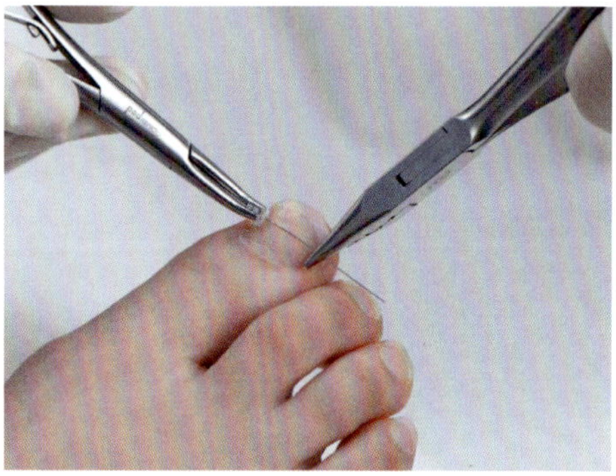

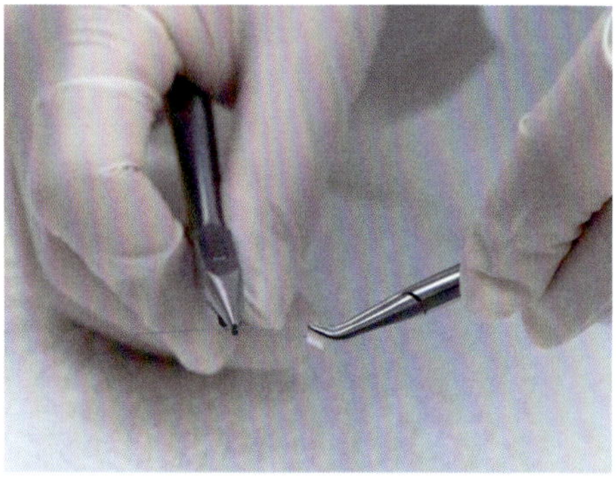

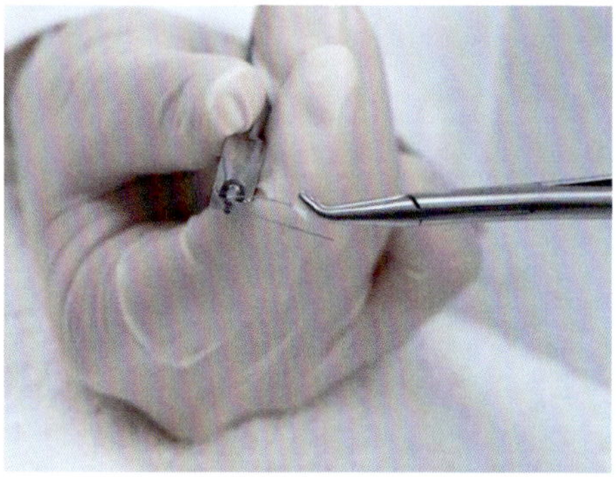

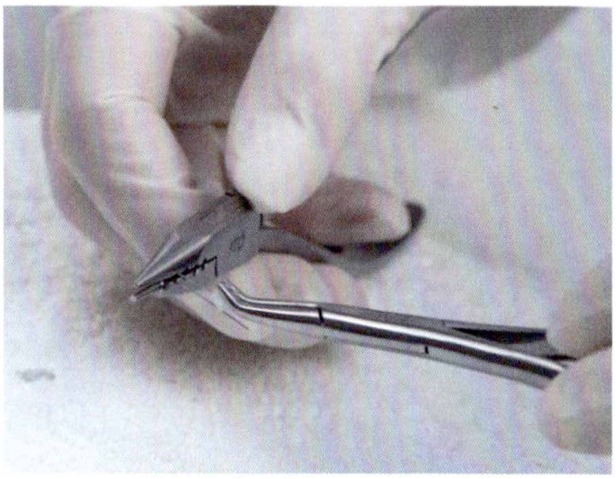

Images 5.143 to 5.146 (top to bottom)
Always bend the wire around the round part of the combination pliers

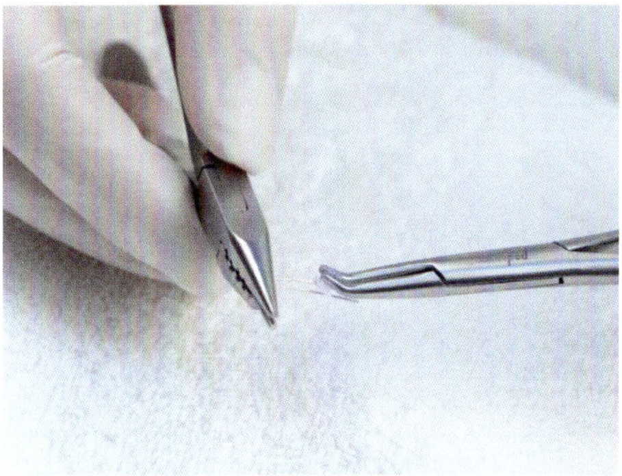

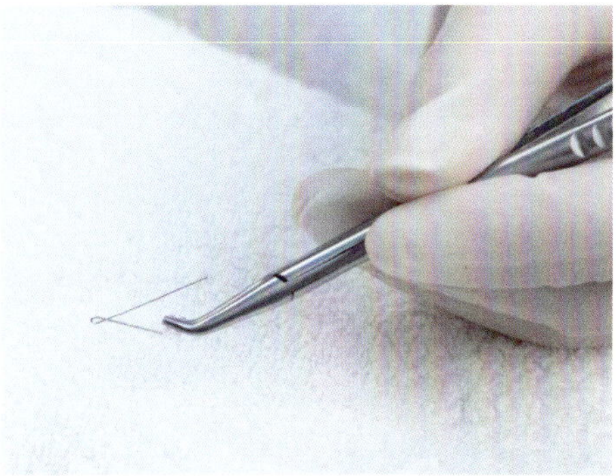

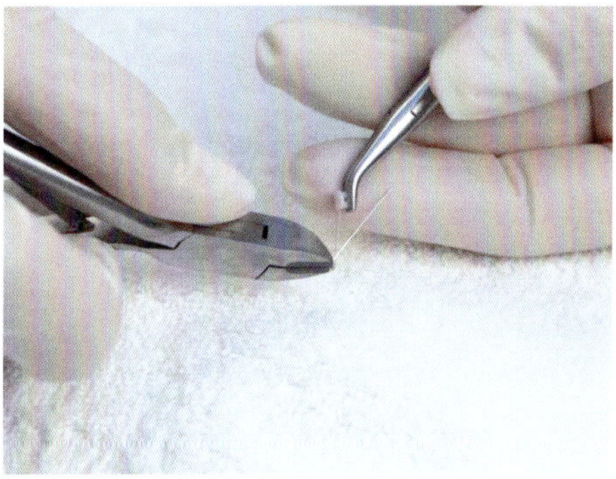

Image 5.147 bis 5.149 (top to bottom)

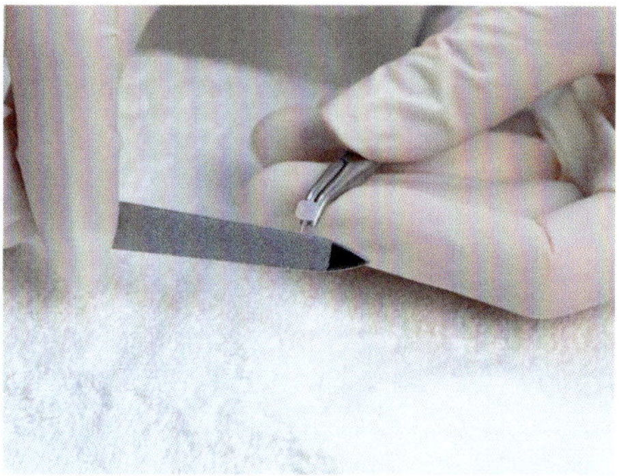

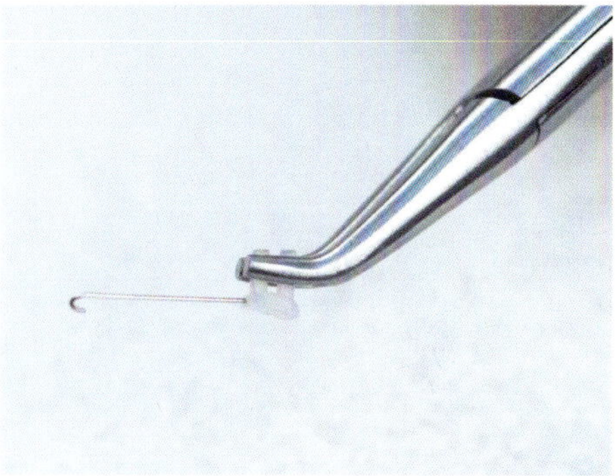

Image 5.150 and 5.151 (top to bottom)

Place the pre-bent hook into the appropriate hole of the combination pliers and firmly press the arms of the pliers together. The hook must not protrude on the other side of the pliers. Prevent unwanted bends in the hook by turning the closed pliers slightly counterclockwise. Trim the hook with side-cutting pliers. The flat side of the side-cutting pliers points to the remaining hook piece. Always ensure that you and the patient wear safety glasses to protect the eyes from pieces of wire. Debur the hook with a diamond nail file. Support the wire with your finger during filing (imagcs 5.147 to 5.151).

Positioning and fixation

Check the brace's tension and adjust if required. Do not preshape the brace wire; leave it straight for now. Insert the hook in the nail fold and attach it under the nail. Press the brace plate on the nail with the fixation pliers and gently pull the wire to keep the tension steady, otherwise the hook might detach from under the nail. If the tension is too tight, the wire will come out of the brace plate and the function of the brace will be destroyed. Adjust the brace's tension so that the patient feels comfortable.

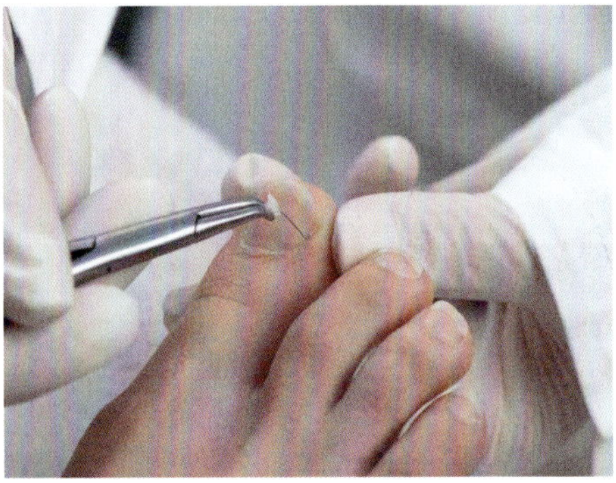
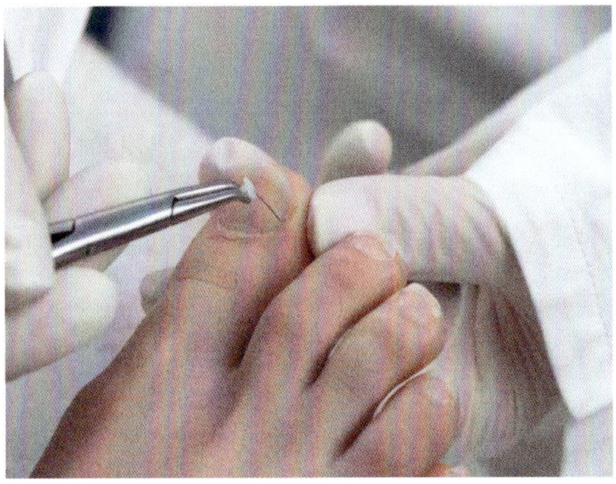

Image 5.152 and 5.153 (top to bottom)

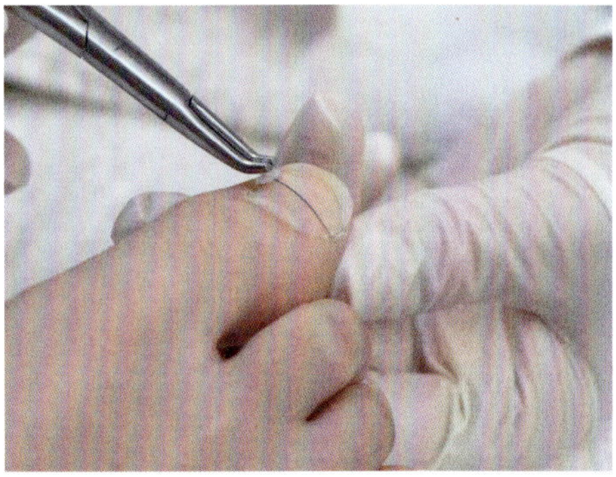
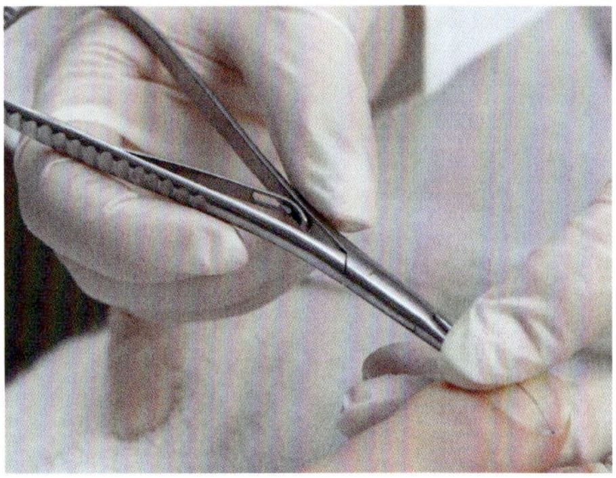

Image 5.154 and 5.155 (top to bottom)

If the tension is too tight for the patient, prebend the wire carefully with your finger or the pliers. It is always recommended to choose a less strong brace than to bend the wire! Clean the nail, brace and the brace plate with an alcohol swab and let dry completely before applying a thin layer of adhesive onto the adhesive surface of the brace plate with a brush. Be careful not to apply too much adhesive. Wipe the top of the small adhesive bottle clean with an alcohol swab after each use. Hook the brace under the nail's edge and gently pull it with the pliers, preventing the hook from detaching. Place the brace on the nail with fixation pliers, then increase the pressure by pressing slightly with your finger on the fixation pliers for approximately one minute. Holding the pliers correctly is important. Do not hold the pliers straight upwards since this will prevent proper bonding contact between the brace plate and the nail surface (images 5.152 to 5.155).

Cut each locking pin off the brace plate individually and sand the plate with a sand paper file (images 5.156 to 5.159).

Sealing (only if required) and follow-up care

Cover sharp adhesion edges with sealant gel such as PediGel. Sealing is also recommended for adolescents and very active patients.

Apply a drop of antiseptic Dolerma nail fold oil with a tamponade in the nail fold where the hook has been placed.

To remove the brace cut it off the nail with side cutting pliers.

Remove the adhesion residue and smooth the nail. Replace the brace every four to eight weeks until the desired result is achieved.

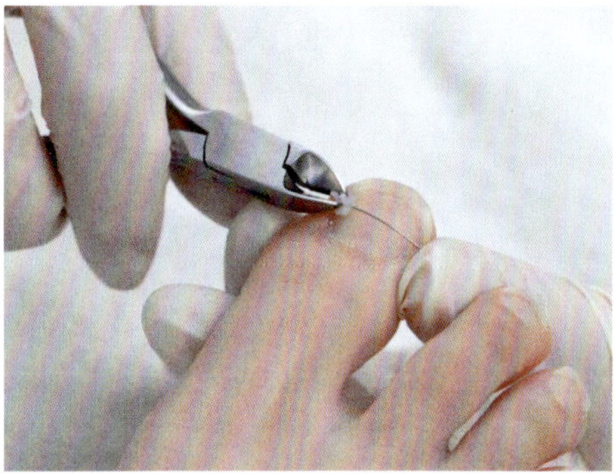

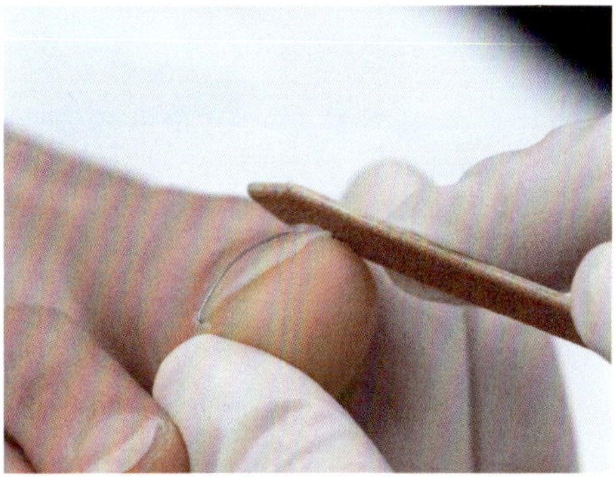

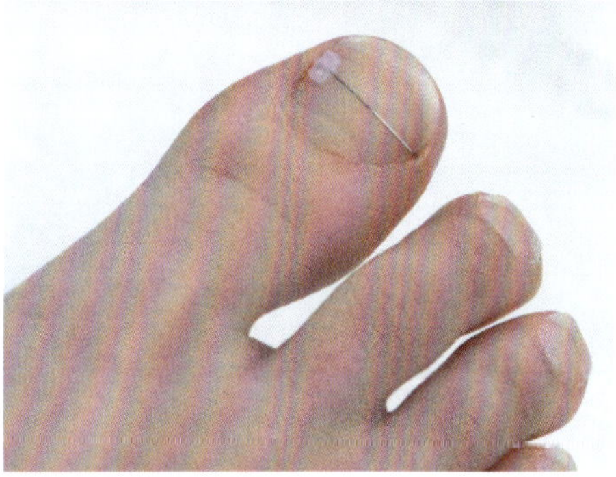

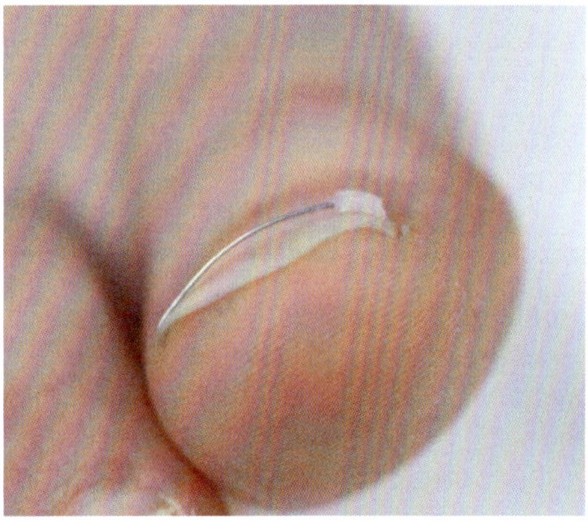

Image 5.156 and 5.159 (top to bottom)

General treatment information

If the patient feels uncomfortable, the brace must be removed.

If an infection is present, treat the infection and apply a dressing.

Once the nail has adjusted to the shape of the brace, the brace can loosen or detach. It is recommended to remove the brace and replace it with a new brace placed proximal to the previous position.

Depending on the severity of the case, schedule a follow-up visit:

- severe cases after one to three days
- mild cases after three to six days

Important information for the patient

Inform the patient about the effect the brace has on the nail, what it is supposed to accomplish and potential complications. Discuss the cause for ingrown toenails and offer recommendations on how to prevent this condition from reoccurring in the future.

After the successful treatment, it is advisable to apply the podofix active adhesive brace to promote straight nail growth. It also helps stabilize the nail and prevents ingrown and convoluted toenails.

5.12 Goldstadt professional full and half brace

Material (image 5.160)
Gold-plated stainless steel. This brace is available in three variants.

- **adhesive brace:** fixation with adhesion
- **half brace:** a hook is attached on one side and the brace is glued onto the nail
- **brace with fixation hooks:** hooks are attached on both sides of the nail; generating a plaster model is recommended

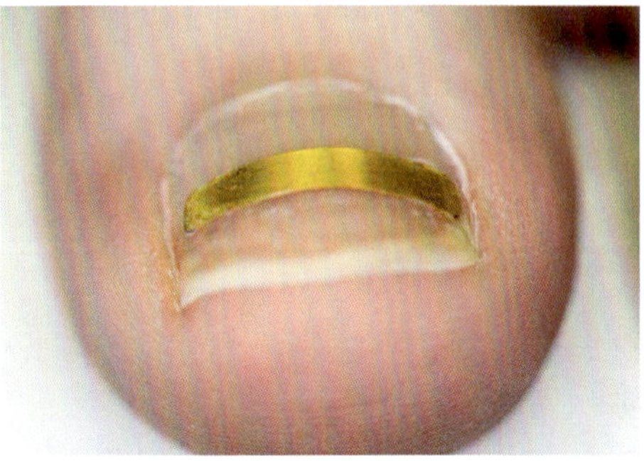

Image 5.160 Photo: Hellmut Ruck

Work materials

- brace
- brace applicator
- round-nosed pliers
- side-cutting pliers
- scissors
- contact glue
- acetone
- tamponade

Effectiveness
Leverage and tensile force are enhanced by the material's flexibility. The longer the suspension travel, the stronger the tensile force. Is the suspension travel larger than double the thickness of the nail, the brace has adequate tensile force and can function properly.

Indications

- unguis convolutus
- unguis incarnatus
- clavi in the sulcus
- onychophosis
- nail correction after partial nail resection if no free lateral nail wall is available
- keeping the shape of the nail in cases where the lateral nail margins were removed

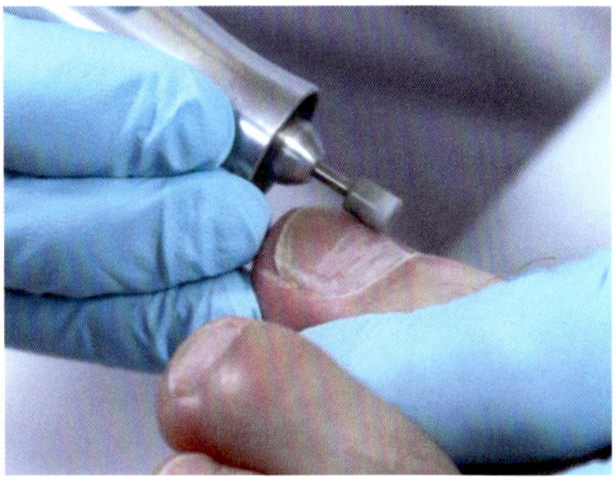

Image 5.161 Sanding the nail surface

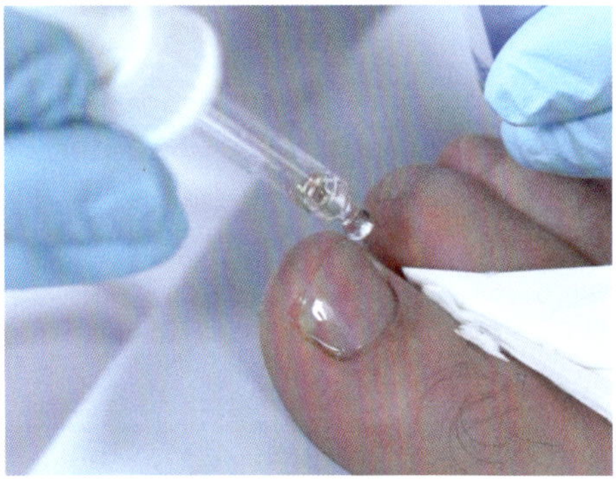

Image 5.162 Tamponade application

Preparation (image 5.161)
Clean the nail fold with a gauge blade or nail lifter, trim the tip of the nail, sand the nail surface and clean the surface with nail correction cleaner.

Tamponade application (image 5.162)
Apply peclavus pre-treatment to the nail fold and allow to take effect for 5 to 8 minutes. To expand the nail fold, insert a Copoline tamponade.

Measuring aid – determining the correct size for the full brace (image 5.163)
Insert the brace in the nail fold, mark the 0-point on the nail plate, measure each side up to the 0-point and add. Example: left side 10 mm, right side 13 mm = brace 23 mm.

Measuring aid – determining the correct size for the half brace (image 5.164)
Use the measuring aid to determine the length to the opposite nail fold. IMPORTANT: the shorter the brace, the stronger the effect. The length of the brace must be determined by the desired effectiveness.

Fixation of the full brace
(images 5.165 and 5.166)
Shape the brace's end pieces with round tier pliers. Position the brace on one side of the nail and gently push it onto the nail with the applicator. Position the second side and push both sides onto the nail. The basic tension increases with movement, therefore, it is important that the patient does not feel pain while the brace is fitted onto the nail. Clean the nail surface with an anti-grease solution and protect the nail fold with a tamponade.

Fixation of a half brace
Shape the brace's end piece with round tier pliers. Clean the nail plate and brace with an anti-grease solution and insert the tamponade. Apply the adhesive on the underside of the brace, hook the brace under the nail and secure it with your finger, then press down on the adhesive part of the brace for 20 to 40 seconds. Apply the activator and remove adhesive residue. Tip: do not press too hard since the adhesive will squeeze out from the sides of the brace, preventing the brace from bonding properly to the nail surface.

Sealing (image 5.167)
Brush UV-gel Pedique silver PLUS+ over 80 per cent of the nail plate. It can touch the tamponade. Cure with a curing light

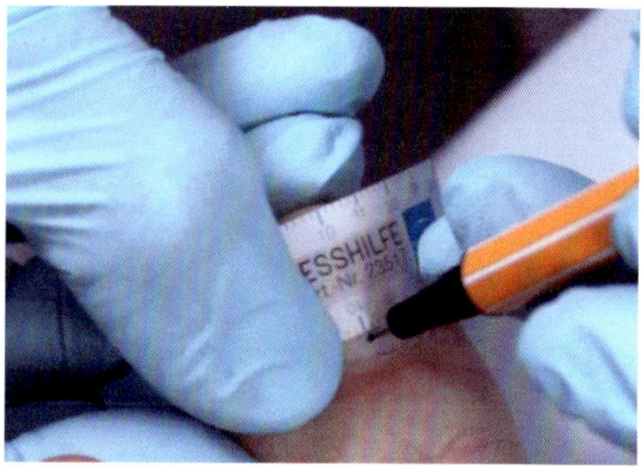

Image 5.163 Measuring aid for the full brace

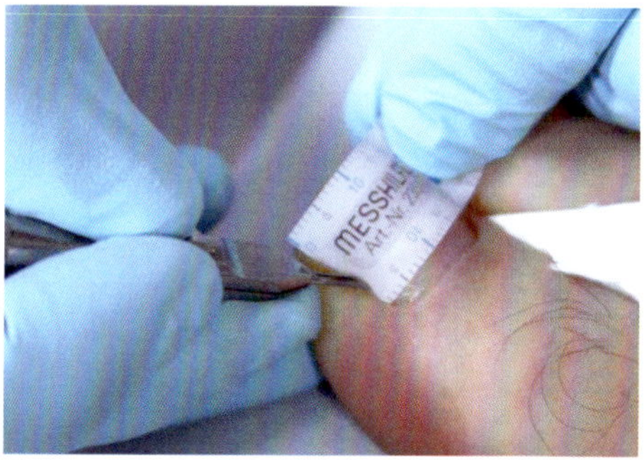

Image 5.164 Measuring aid for the half brace

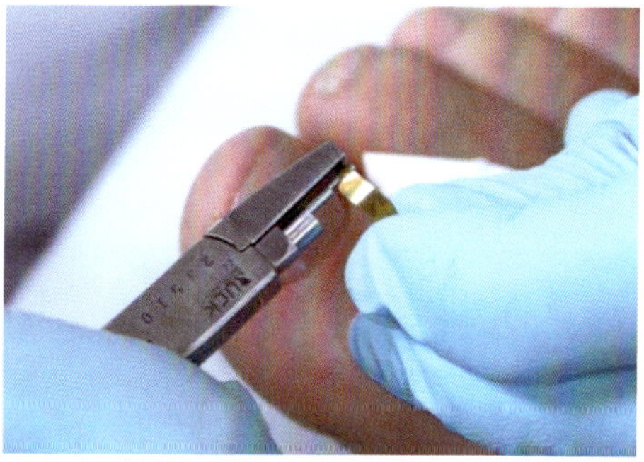

Image 5.165 Shaping the brace's end pieces

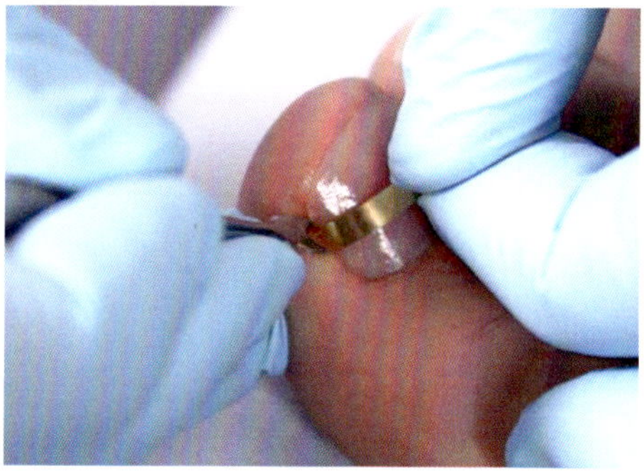

Image 5.166 Fixating the brace

for approx. two minutes. Remove the dispersion layer with cleaning solution. Close the gel container immediately after use and clean the brush. Remove the tamponades.

Finishing work (image 5.168)
Replace a soiled tamponade with one that has been impregnated with peclavus post-treatment or Anti-MYX silver which has a soothing effect.

Important information for the patient
- The brace must be checked every night.
- In the event that the nail becomes painful, the brace loosens or for any other problems that might occur, visit the podiatrist.
- See the podiatrist for a follow-up visit within one to two days in an acute case, otherwise in four to six weeks.
- The brace will be repositioned after four to six weeks.

Documentation is obligatory.

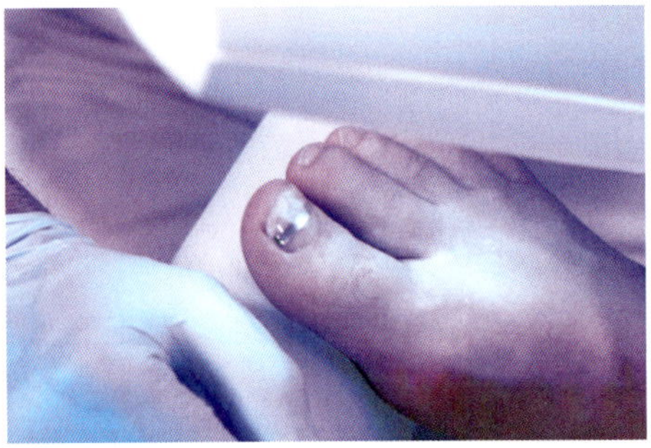

Image 5.167 Light curing

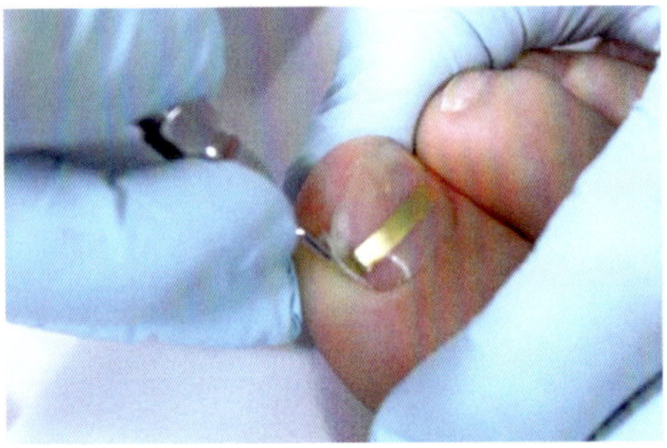

Image 5.168 Aftercare

5.13 Goldstadt Professional Classic

Material
Gold-plated stainless steel for optimal adhesion. Hypoallergenic.

It comes in four 100 mm long strips that are 3 mm wide and 0.1 mm thin. It functions as a full, half or adhesive brace, depending on the required application.

These predefined braces (see chapter 5.12), besides their time efficient application, have the advantage of having the end pieces of the full and half braces are entirely gold-plated. This is a big advantage since gold is known to have an anti-inflammatory and anti-allergenic effect.

With the Goldstadt Classic brace, a small portion of the gold is removed during trimming.

The Classic brace is applied when a particularly long brace is needed.

Work materials and application process are identical to the Goldstadt professional full and half brace (see chapter 5.12).

Individually cutting the Goldstadt professional Classic brace

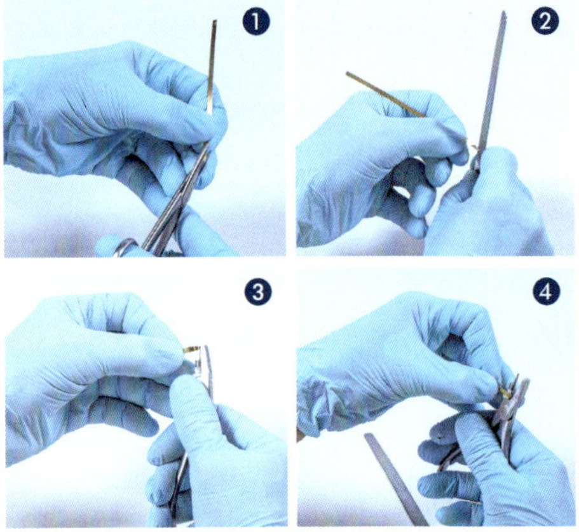

1. Cut the Classic brace to the desired length;
2. deburring;
3. shape the end hooks with round tier pliers;
4. verify the fit on the nail.

Images courtesy of Hellmut Ruck GmbH

5.14 Goldstadt professional adhesive brace

Applied on extremely thin nails or if the nail fold is inflamed.

Material

Gold-plated stainless steel adhesive brace.

Work materials (image 5.169)

- brace of five different widths
- brace applicator
- round tier pliers
- double-ended nail fold instrument
- brace applicator
- flat gel model brush
- activator
- Cleaner
- measuring aid
- adhesive
- Pedique silver PLUS+ gel

Effectiveness

Leverage and tensile force are enhanced by the material's flexibility. The longer the suspension travel the stronger the tensile force. Is the suspension travel larger than double the thickness of the nail, the brace has adequate tensile force and can function properly.

Indications

- unguis convolutus
- unguis incarnatus
- clavi in the sulcus
- onychophosis
- nail correction after partial nail resection if no free lateral nail wall is available
- keeping the shape of the nail in cases where the lateral nail margins were removed

Preparation

Prior to applying the brace, ensure that the nail fold is clean and does not show any sign of inflammation. Clean the nail surface with an anti-grease solution and moisten it lightly.

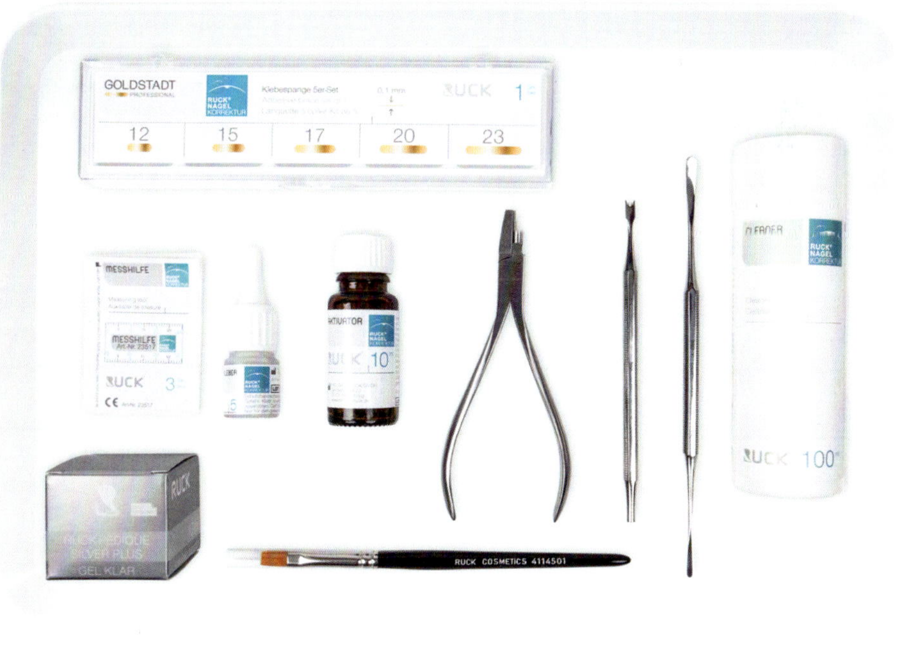

Image 5.169 Adhesive brace starter set

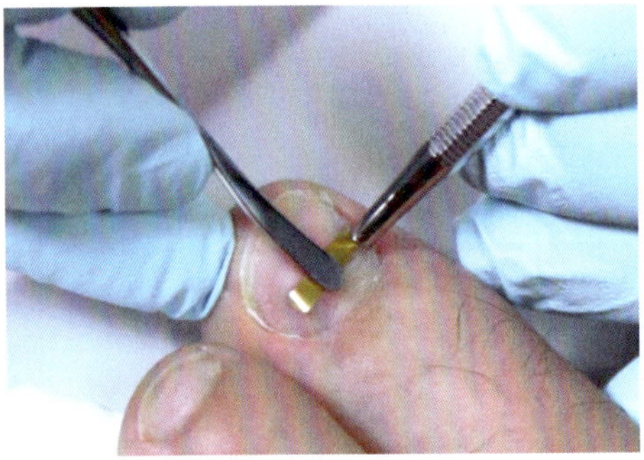

Image 5.170 Positioning the brace

Brace preparation (image 5.170)
Measure the nail surface with the measuring aid. Prebend the brace to conform to the nail curvature.

Clean the brace with anti-grease solution and apply the activator to half of the nail surface. Apply the adhesive on the bottom of one half of the brace. Position the brace and press it on the nail with the brace applicator for 20 to 40 seconds. Apply the activator to the second half of the brace and press down creating tension. Remove the adhesive residue. Brush UV-gel Pedique silver PLUS+ over 80 per cent of the nail plate. It can touch the tamponade. Cure with a curing light for approximately two minutes. Remove the dispersion layer with cleaning solution. Close the gel container immediately after use and clean the brush. Remove the tamponades.

Important information for the patient

- The brace must be checked every night.
- In the event that the nail becomes painful, the brace loosens or for any other problems that might occur, visit the podiatrist.
- See the podiatrist for a follow-up visit within one to two days in an acute case, otherwise in four to six weeks.
- The brace will be repositioned after four to six weeks.

Documentation is obligatory.

5.15 BS brace Classic

Material
Adhesive brace made of synthetic fibreglass material.

Material properties
The brace, made of a special synthetic fibreglass material, is ground with the precision of two thousandths of a millimeter. This material complies with the specific criteria of stability and elasticity, as well as in terms of individually fitting by trained podiatrists. Computer-supported testing of its bending strength and frequent verification of its adhesiveness by the manufacturer are standard procedures.

Work materials
braces
multi applicator
quick-drying adhesive
brush-on adhesive
cleaning solution

Effectiveness
This brace consists of Duroplast, strengthened with fibreglass. It is applied on the entire width of the nail and works like a leaf spring according to the physical law of pressure and counter pressure. The resulting resetting forces at the brace's ends lift the side edges of the nail out of the nail fold. The generated counter pressure automatically positions itself at the correct part of the nail, at exactly the highest point. It conforms to the individual shape of the nail. By bonding the brace to the nail with adhesive, pressure and counterpressure are distributed evenly over the nail. The strongest tensile force occurs at the ends of the brace and decreases continually up to the 0-value of the line of force. Then the counterpressure increases again up to the highest point of the nail, applying tensile force on the opposite side of the brace.

The tensile forces can be adjusted by targeted grinding, particularly on the ends of the brace. This achieves optimal and pain-free nail correction results. The brace complies to the classic physical principle: less flexure = less force, more flexure = stronger force.

Indications

unguis convolutus
unguis incarnatus
calvi in the sulcus
onychophosis
paronychia
granulation tissue

Preparation

Start by grinding extremely thick nails thinner (image 5.171). Footbaths and the use of a disinfectant just before brace applications must be avoided. Clean the nail by applying one drop of degreasing solution (image 5.172) and dry afterwards with a dry swab.

Brace selection

The brace is most effective if it covers the entire width of the nail and is positioned 1 to 2 mm behind the area causing the pain. Ensure that the brace does not come into contact with the skin and choose the size of the brace accordingly.

Precise measuring

Position the brace on the right edge of the nail; if you are left-handed, start on the left side. It is important that you start where the brace will be fixed later. Then press the brace over the width of the nail to the opposite side with the steel applicator, ensuring that it does not shift.

If the brace is too short or too long, exchange it for the correct size.

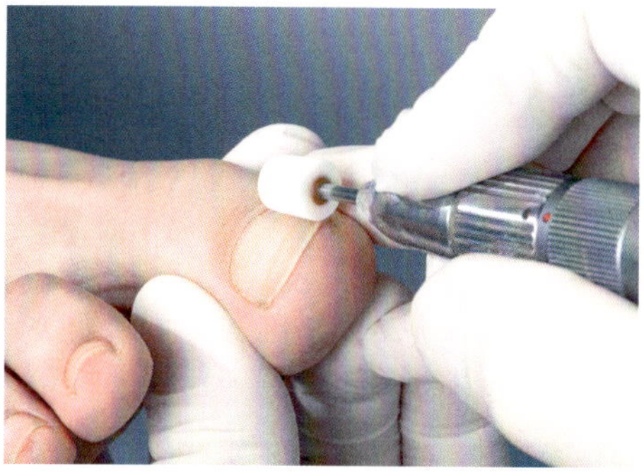

Image 5.171 Grind down extremely thick nails

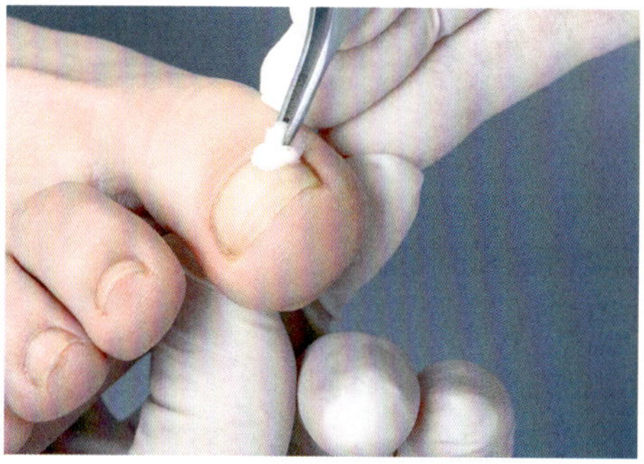

Image 5.172 Clean the nail surface

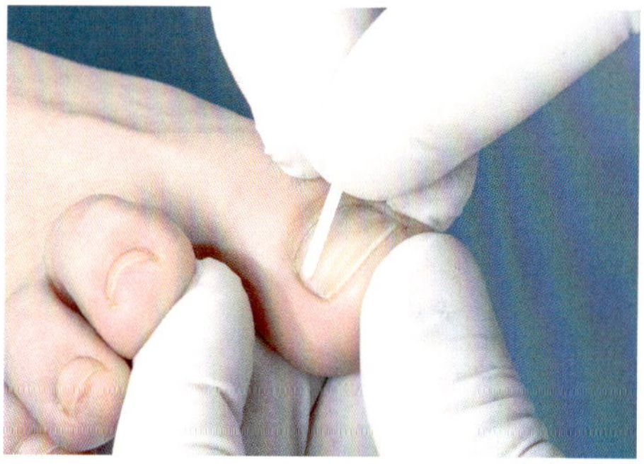

Image 5.173 Measure the width of the nail

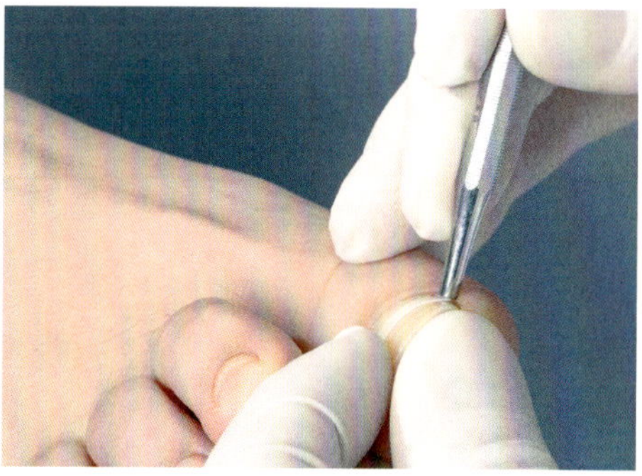

Image 5.174 Select the correct brace size

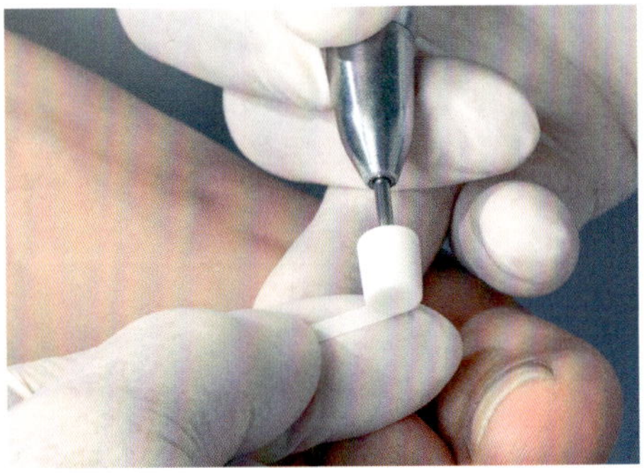

Image 5.175 Grind the ends of the brace

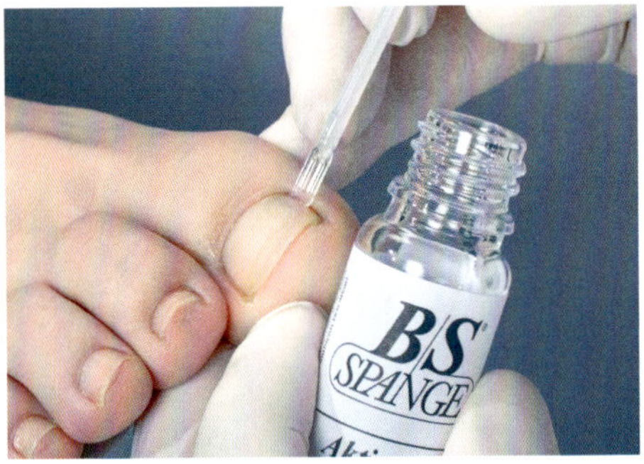

Image 5.176 Apply the activator

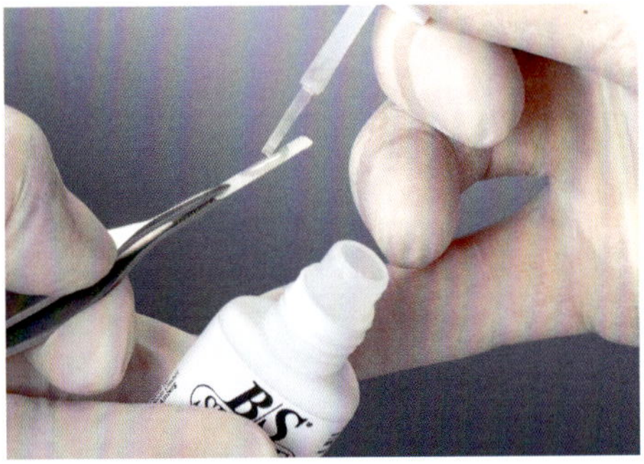

Image 5.177 Apply the adhesive

Brace preparation (image 5.175)
Place the brace rough side up on one finger and then carefully grind the brace's ends a little thinner with a diamond bur or a corundum grinder. CAUTION: the rough side is the non-glossy side.

Adhesive component application
(images 5.176 and 5.177)
This is a quick-drying adhesive. Apply the activator to the left and right lateral edge of the nail, not to the entire nail. Apply a drop of base adhesive in the centre of the rough side of the brace. It is also possible to apply activator to the brace and base adhesive on the entire nail surface. Hold the brace with tweezers during the process. This is quick-drying adhesive, so make sure that you do not wipe off the applicator brush on the bottle neck!

Positioning (images 5.178 to 5.180)
Position the brace in the centre of the nail with a steady hand by supporting your hand with the finger of the other hand and wait 7–10 seconds. Next, use the applicator to press one of the brace ends on to one side edge of the nail, holding it in place for another 10 seconds. Repeat this process for the other side of the brace.

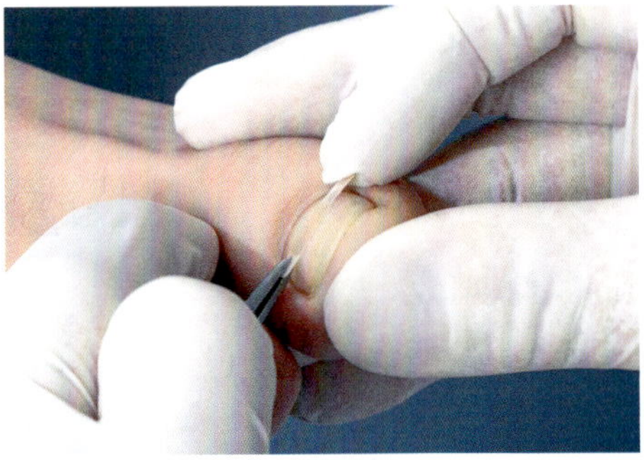

Image 5.178 Position the brace in the center of the nail

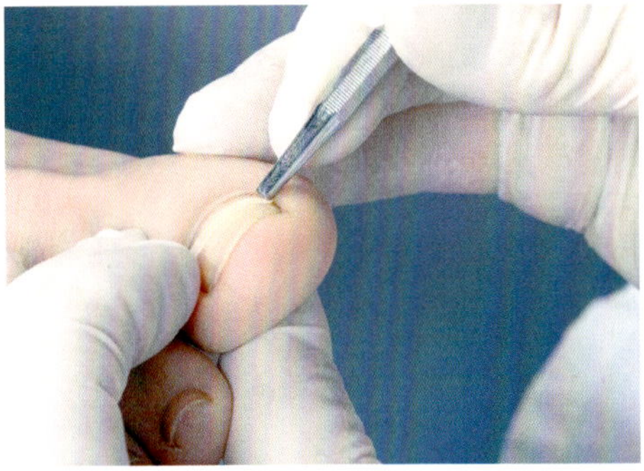

Image 5.179 Press down on the right side of the nail

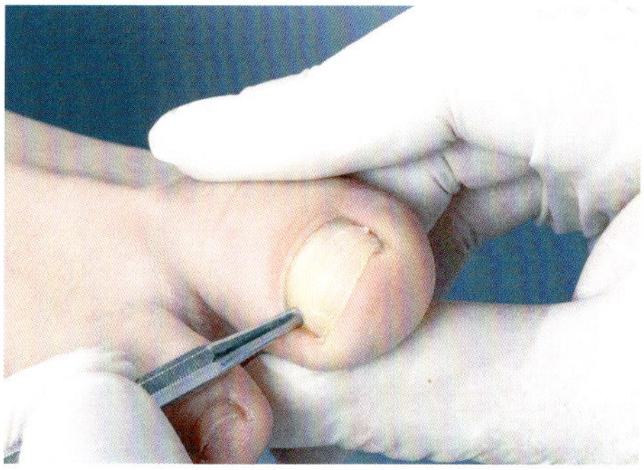

Image 5.180 Press down on the left side

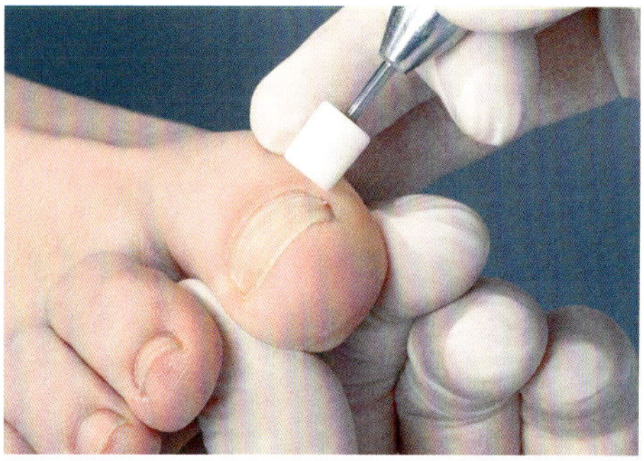

Image 5.181 Grind the transition of the brace margin to the nail

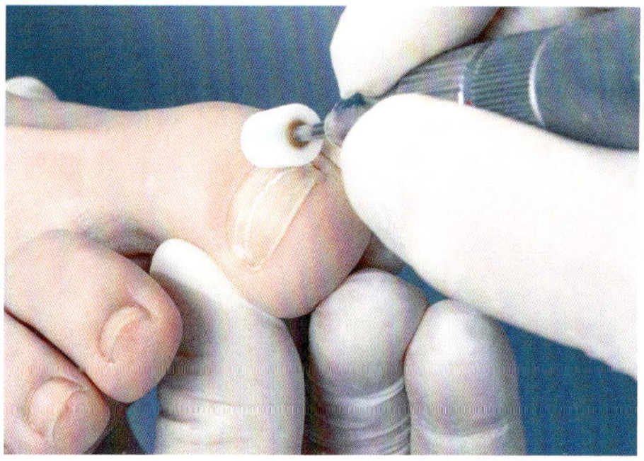

Image 5.182 SCorrect the tensile force by grinding

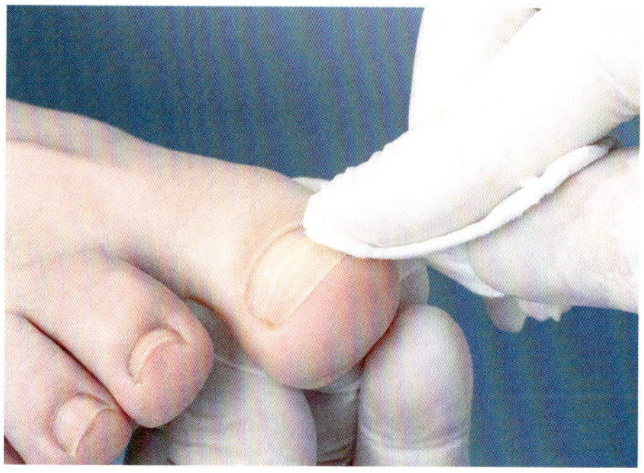

Image 5.183 Clean before sealing

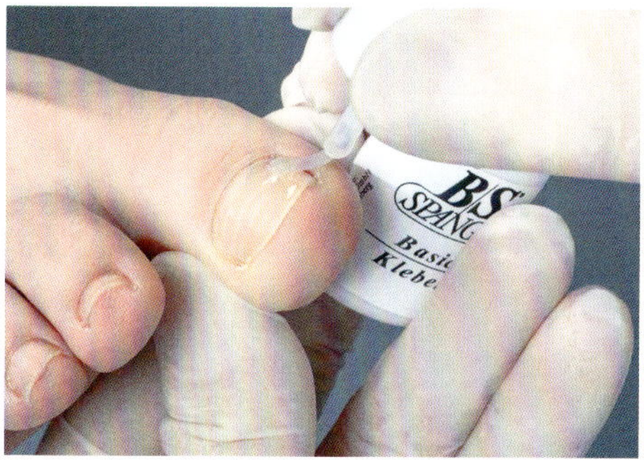

Image 5.184 Sealing

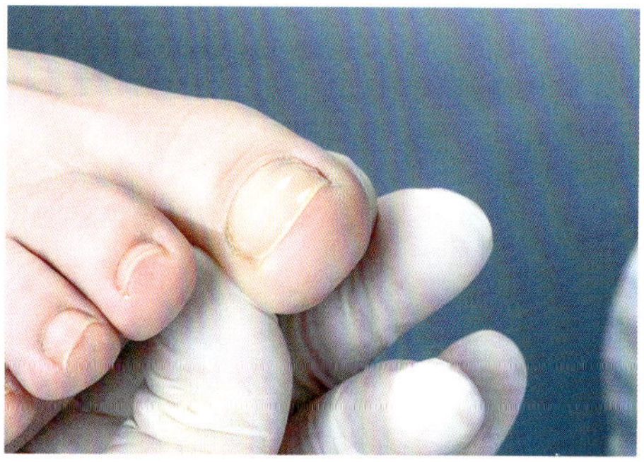

Image 5.185 The finished result

Individual tensile force setting
(images 5.181 and 5.182)
First clean the nail surface and the brace with cleaning solution and dry with a dry swab. The tensile force setting is ideal if the patient feels none or very little tension. Be sure to ask the patient as it is easy to regulate the tensile force. If it is too strong, then grind the ends of the brace thinner. If that is not sufficient, then carefully grind the transition of the margins of the brace to the nail thinner.

Sealing (images 5.183 to 5.185)
Apply the brush-on adhesive over the entire nail surface. This secures the brace and ensures that it is protected against water and moisture. The application is similar to nail polish application whereby the brush-on adhesive acts as a sealant. Once

dry, usual nail treatment, such as disinfecting, applying tamponades or ointment, can be performed.

Beautifying finish (images 5.186 to 5.188)
The nail is ready to be beautified with nail polish or special nail applications. For removal of the nail polish, use regular nail polish remover or the cleaning solution.

Important information for the patient
Synthetic material applies less tensile force than stainless steel. This brace is, therefore, ideal for the correction of thin and brittle nails and works well on toes with inflamed nail folds.

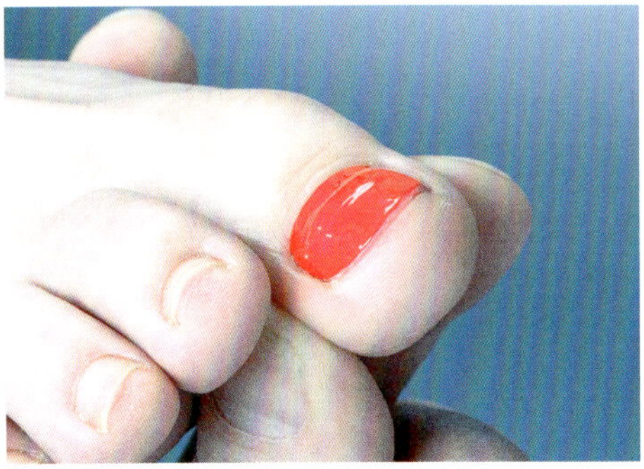

Image 5.186 Polished nail with brace

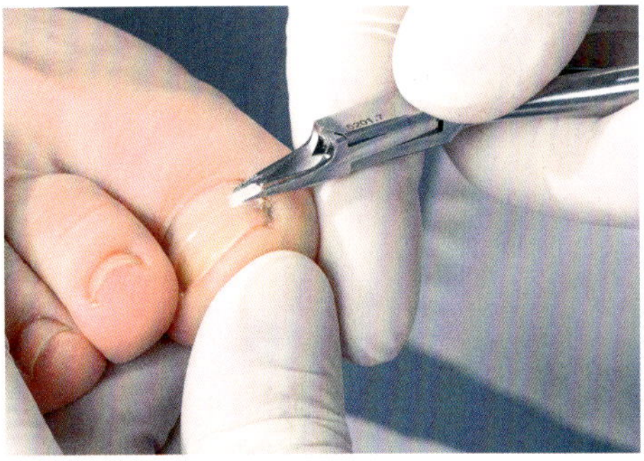

Image 5.187 Removing the brace, step 1

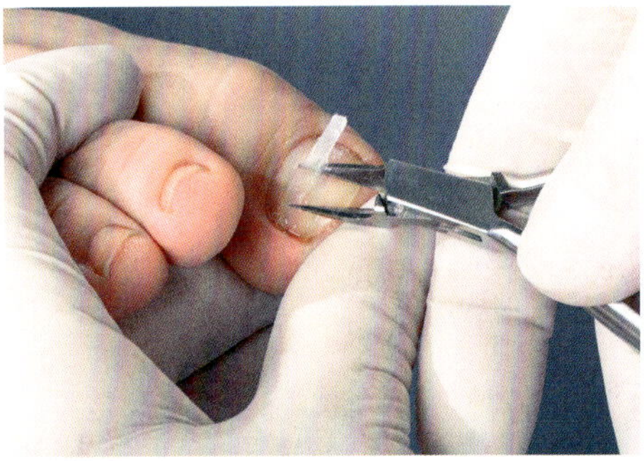

Image 5.188 Removing the brace, step 2

5.16 BS brace Classic+

The standard width of the BS brace Classic is 3 mm. For the new Classic+ the width has been increased to 4 mm.

Because the width of the Classic+ variant is 30 per cent greater, its adhesive surface has also increased by 30 per cent causing the brace's tensile force to increase by 30 per cent.

Indications
- Unguis convolutus.
- Unguis incarnatus.
- Clavi in the sulcus.
- Onychophosis.
- Paronychia.
- Granulation tissue.

In the case of the Classic+ the change has no effect on the familiar BS brace application method. It is simply an enhancement of the corrective treatment of extremely thick ingrown nails. However, due to the increased tensile force that this brace applies, it is important to ensure that the patient is not subjected to tension pain or any other discomfort.

The BS brace Classic+ is only available in the magnetic version. But it can also be easily applied with the steel applicator because, during the final cleaning, the magnetic point is automatically removed.

Preparation and procedure are performed according to the methods described in chapter 5.17.

5.17 BS brace with magnetic applicator

Material
Adhesive brace made of synthetic material.

Work materials
- Braces.
- Pencil.
- Tweezers.
- Magnetic applicator (image 5.189).
- Instant adhesive.
- Nail degreaser (e.g., Acetone).
- Fine grinding bur.

Effectiveness
This brace consists of Duroplast, strengthened with fibreglass. It is applied on the entire width of the nail and works like a leaf spring according to the physical law of pressure and counterpressure. The resulting resetting forces at the brace's ends lift

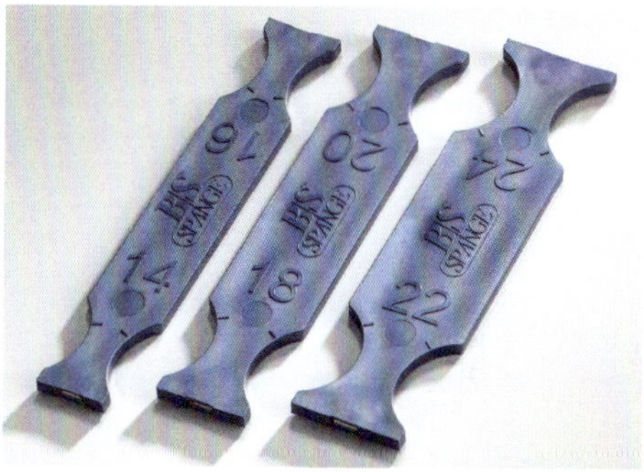

Image 5.189

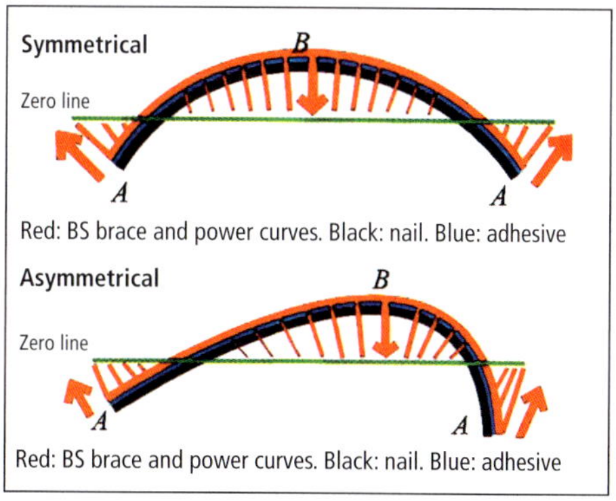

Image 5.190

the side edges of the nail out of the nail fold.

The generated counterpressure automatically positions itself at the correct part of the nail, at exactly the highest point. It conforms to the individual shape of each nail. By bonding the brace to the nail with adhesive, pressure and counterpressure are distributed evenly over the nail. The strongest tensile force occurs at the ends of the brace and decreases continually up to the 0-value of the line of force. Then the counterpressure increases again up to the highest point of the nail, applying tensile force on the opposite side of the brace.

The tensile forces can be adjusted by targeted grinding, particularly on the ends of the brace. This achieves optimal and pain-free nail correction results. The brace complies with the classic physical principle: slight bending = slight force, strong bending = strong force.

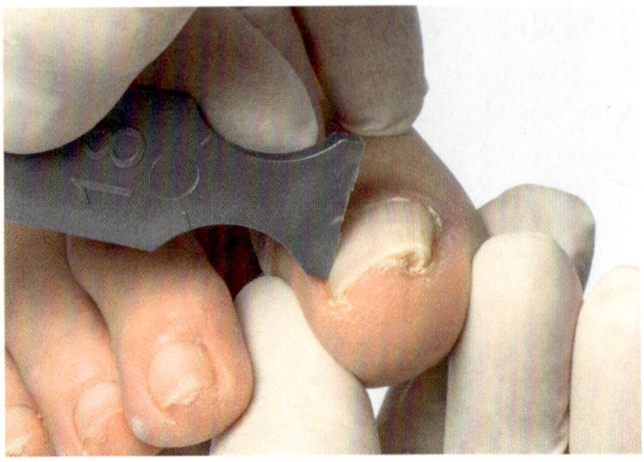

Image 5.191 Measuring from one side of the nail …

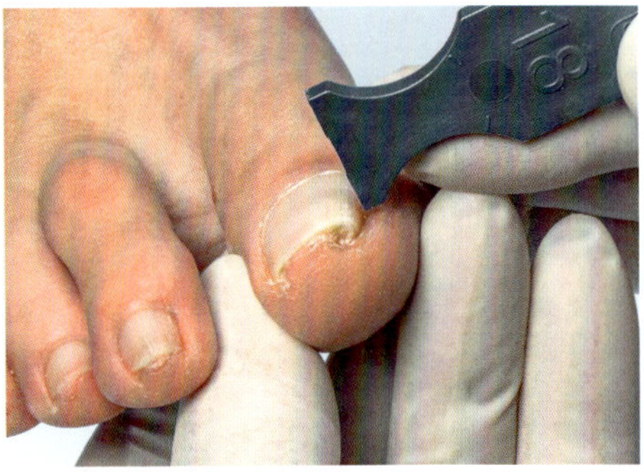

Image 5.192 … to the other side

Indications

- unguis convolutus
- unguis incarnatus
- clavi in the sulcus
- onychophosis
- nail correction after partial nail resection if no free lateral nail wall is available
- keeping the shape of the nail in cases where the lateral nail margins have been removed

Preparation

Footbaths and the use of a disinfectant just before brace applications must be avoided. Clean the nail by applying one drop of degreasing solution and dry afterwards with a dry swab.

Choosing the right size of the brace and sticking it across the whole nail 1–2 mm behind the part which is causing pain is the best way to achieve the best effect. The brace must not come into contact with the skin. Place one tip of the applicator exactly at the edge of the nail where the brace is to be fixed. Roll the magnetic applicator, without shifting, across the width of the nail to the opposite side. The width of the nail determines the correct length of the brace (images 5.191 and 5.192).

Brace preparation

Once the correct brace size has been determined, grind the brace's ends thinner on the side that does not display magnetic points (image 5.193). This can be done with the brace placed on one finger or on the magnetic applicator.

Place the brace on the magnetic applicator so that the magnetic point faces the applicator (image 5.194). This secures the brace on the magnetic applicator and facilitates handling and precise positioning of the brace on the nail. Distribute the adhesive on the brace and apply the activator to the nail surface (images 5.195 and 5.196). Do not apply the adhesive too thinly.

As the adhesive has a setting time of 2 minutes, immediately apply the brace which adheres to the magnetic applicator on the entire width of the nail (images 5.197 to 5.200). If you are right-handed, work from left to right and, if you are left-handed, work from right to left. This way you are not blocking the work field. Afterwards, clean the nail and brace with a swab moistened with cleaning solution. This removes the magnetic point from the brace and the activator from the nail plate (image 5.201). Then smooth out the transition between brace and nail with a diamond bur or corundum grinder.

Individual tensile force setting

The tensile force setting is ideal if the patient feels none or very little tension. Be sure to ask the patient as it is easy to regulate the tensile force. If it is too strong, then grind the ends of the brace thinner (image 5.202). If that is not sufficient, then carefully grind the transition of the margins of the brace to the nail thinner. Seal nail and brace with adhesive.

Sealing for a functional finish

Seal the brace and the nail with adhesive to make sure it is secure and water resistant. This is similar to applying nail polish (image 5.203).

However, should adhesive be applied to the nail instead of the activator, then it is no longer necessary to apply a final sealant. In this case, before smoothing out the transition of the brace edges to the nail or making any necessary corrections to the tension, it is essential to wait for the adhesive to dry. This takes about four minutes. Once the adhesive is dry, wipe off the magnetic point using a swab moistened with cleaner. It is still possible to apply a sealant if desired.

Finishing

Once it is dry, usual nail treatment, such as disinfecting, applying tamponades or ointment, can be performed. Nail polish can also be applied.

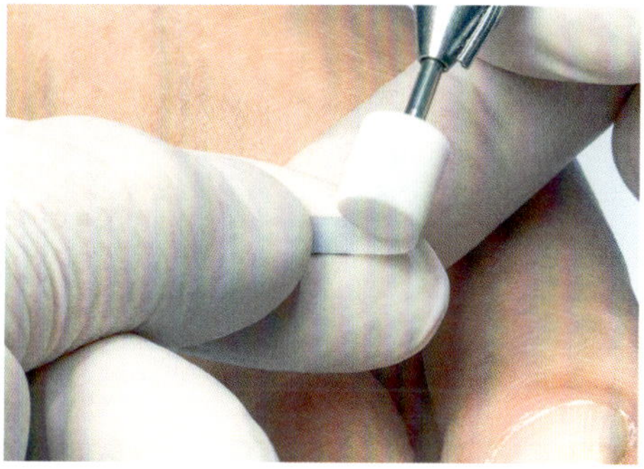

Image 5.193 Thin out the brace's ends

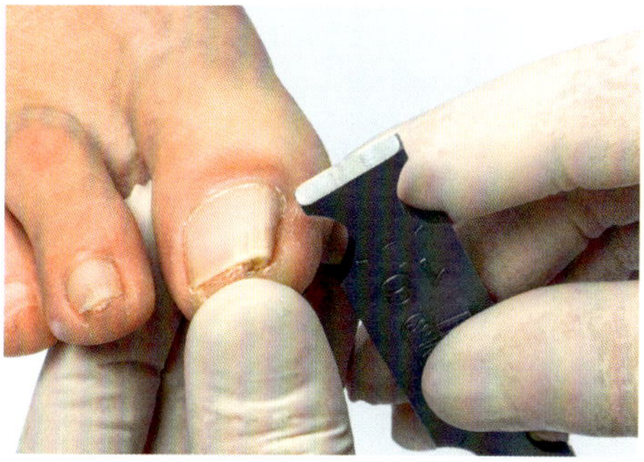

Image 5.194 The brace on the applicator

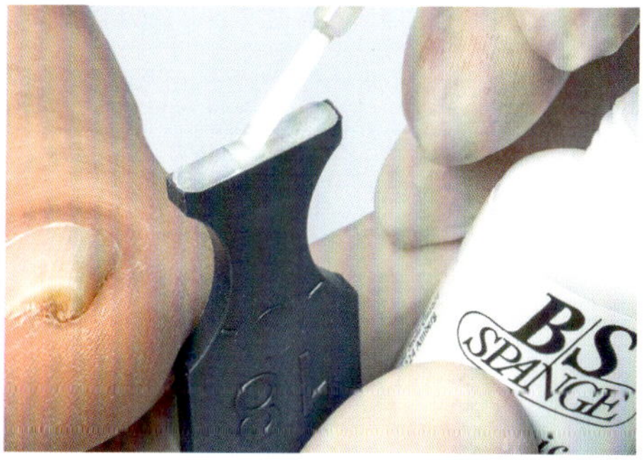

Image 5.195 Apply adhesive to the brace

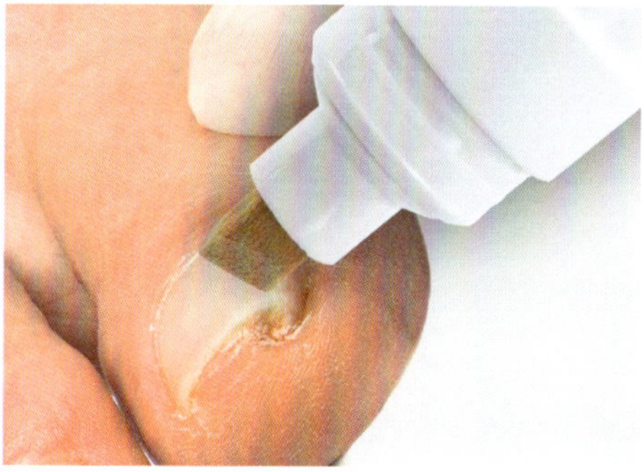

Image 5.196 Apply activator to the nail surface

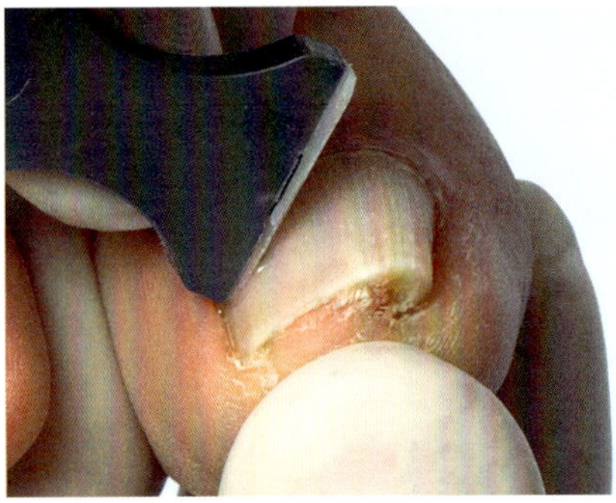

Image 5.197 Apply the brace on the left side and press down for approx. 7 seconds

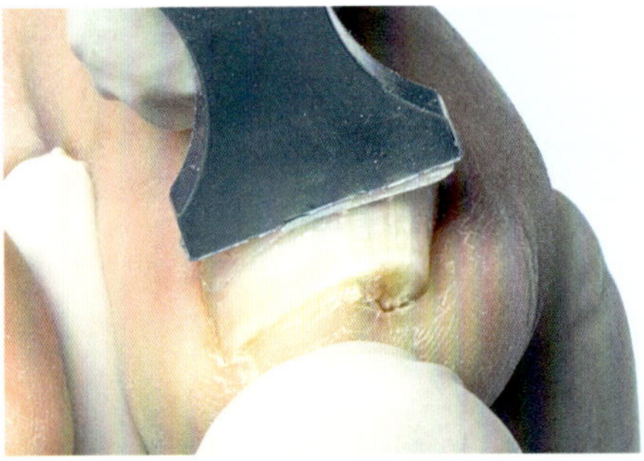

Image 5.198 Apply over the width of the nail

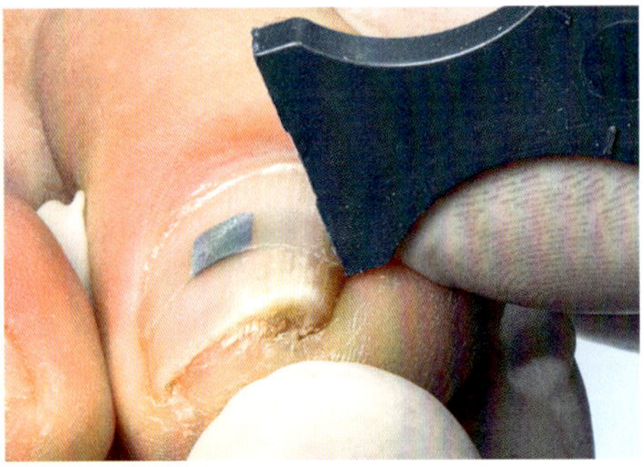

Image 5.199 At the right nail edge, press down for approx. 7 seconds

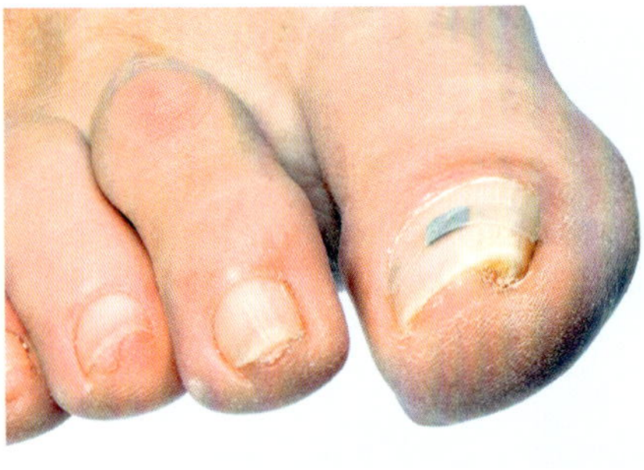

Image 5.200 The nail with brace

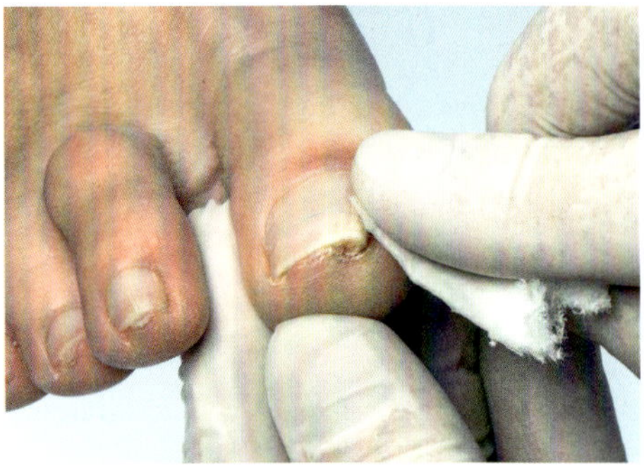

Image 5.201 Final cleaning

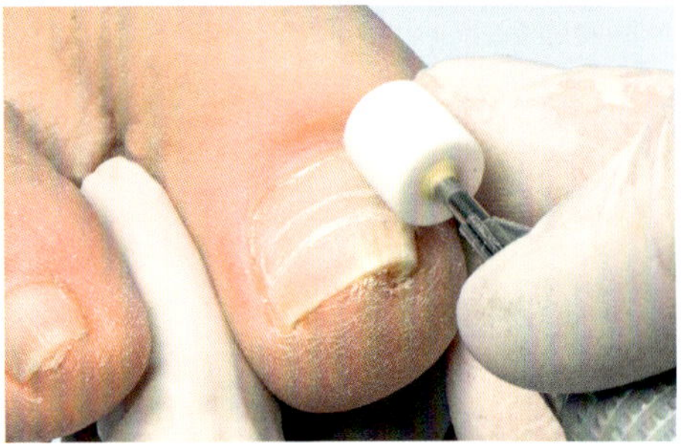

Image 5.202 Grind the ends of the brace thinner to reduce tension

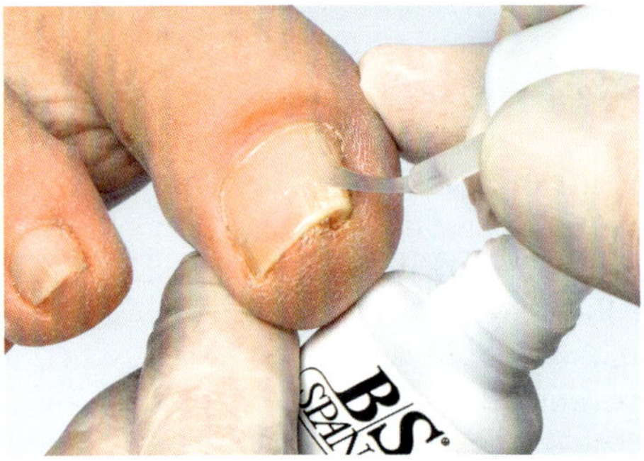

Image 5.203 Sealing

5.18 BS Quick brace

This brace can be applied to almost all ingrown toenails. It is especially suitable for diabetics, after partial resections, dry hyper-granulation, clavi in the sulcus, inflamed and purulent ingrown nails.

Material

Adhesive brace made of synthetic material.

Work materials

- braces
- multi applicator
- quick-drying adhesive
- brush-on adhesive
- cleaning solution

Effectiveness

This brace consists of Duroplast, strengthened with fibreglass. It is applied on the entire width of the nail and works like a leaf spring according to the physical law of pressure and counter pressure. The resulting resetting forces at the brace's ends lift the side edges of the nail out of the nail fold.

The generated counterpressure automatically positions itself at the correct part of the nail, at exactly the highest point. It conforms to the individual shape of the nail. By bonding the brace to the nail with adhesive, pressure and counterpressure are distributed evenly over the nail. The strongest tensile force occurs at the ends of the brace (A) and decreases continually up to the 0-leven of the line of force. Then the counterpressure increases again up to the highest point (B) of the nail, applying tensile force on the opposite side of the brace.

The tensile forces can be adjusted by targeted grinding, particularly on the ends of the brace. This achieves optimal and pain-free nail correction results. The brace complies with the classic physical principle: slight bending = slight force, strong bending = strong force.

Indications

- unguis convolutus
- unguis incarnatus
- clavi in the sulcus
- onychophosis
- paronychia
- granulation tissue

Preparation

Prepare the nail by drying moist areas in the nail fold and wipe any sweat of the nail. Foot baths, oil or cream application as well as disinfectants must be avoided before applying the brace. The same applies for grinding the nail with a wet grinder. Oil and water compromise proper adhesion.

Grind extremely thick nails to the desired thickness and roughen the surface of thin nails prior to applying the brace (image 5.204).

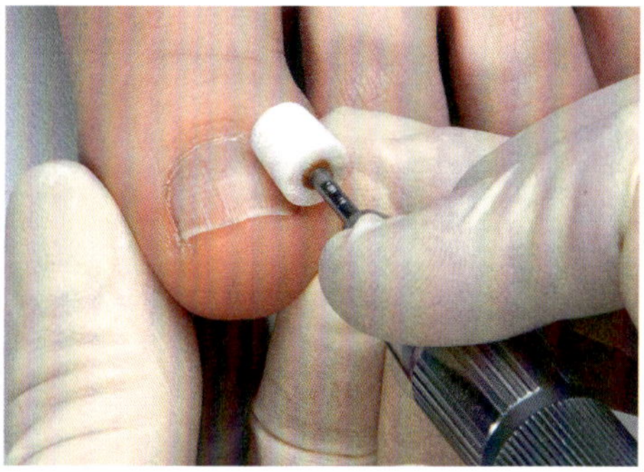

Image 5.204 Grind the nail

It goes without saying that the usual measures for treating an ingrown toenail must be performed before applying the brace. Then choose the correct width of the brace by placing the stencil across the nail. The correct length is determined when the lines match the edges of the nail (image 5.205).

Cut off the brace and the carrier foil lengthwise, leaving a short and long tab. Be sure not to use the helpful measuring stencil first (image 5.206). Do not touch the brace or remove it from the foil.

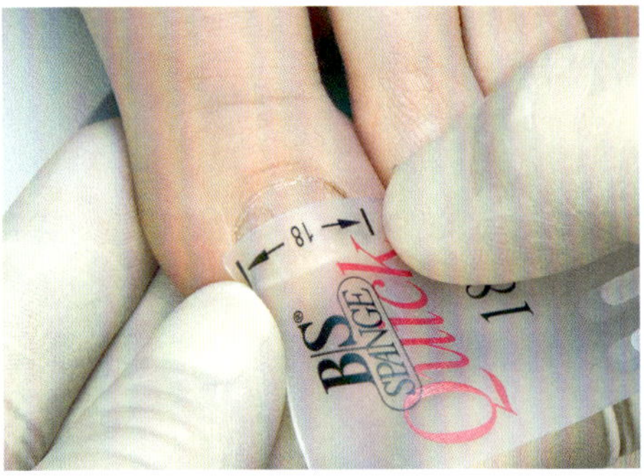

Image 5.205 Measure the nail

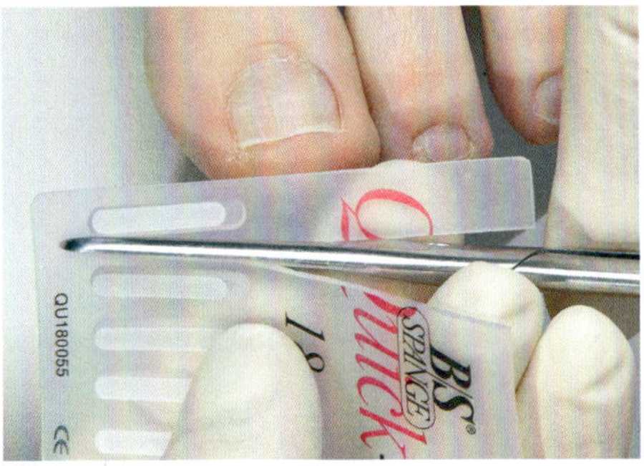

Image 5.206 Cut off the carrier foil with the brace

The brace can be positioned anywhere on the nail, right up to the nail root. However, the best result is achieved when the brace is placed about 1–2 mm behind the part of the nail area that is causing pain. Grinding the brace thinner prior to application is recommended (image 5.207).

As with the BS brace Classic, it is possible to adjust the BS Quick brace before or after application in order to reduce tensile force. If the nail is badly rolled, then this is done beforehand by grinding the brace thinner or, if the patient complains about tension pain, the brace can be ground thinner while it is already applied to the nail.

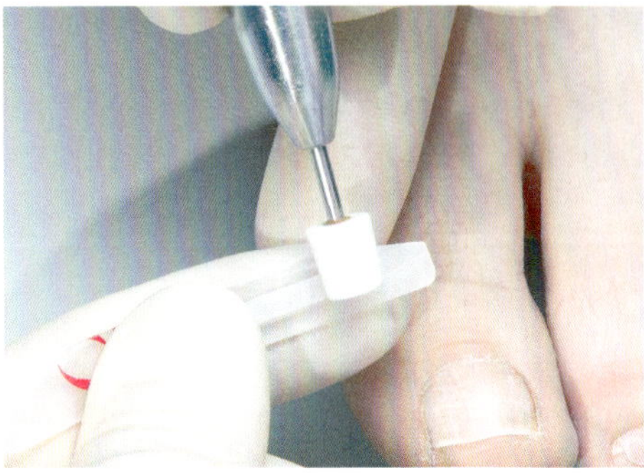

Image 5.207 Grind the BS Quick brace thinner before applying it

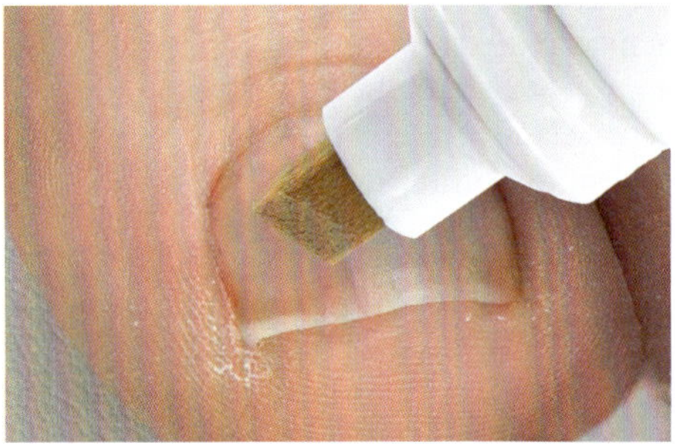

Image 5.208 Apply the activator to the nail surface

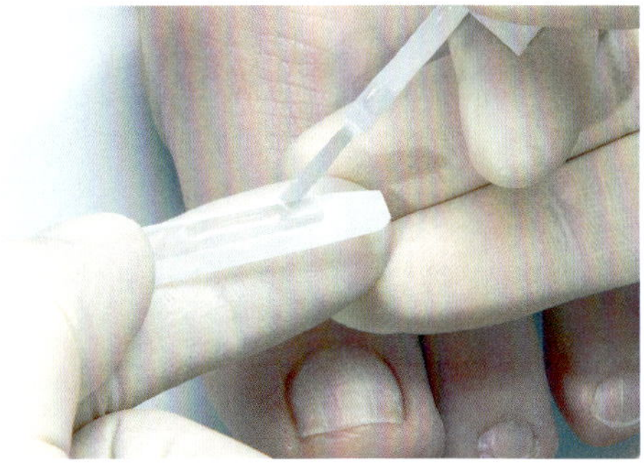

Image 5.209 Apply adhesive to the brace

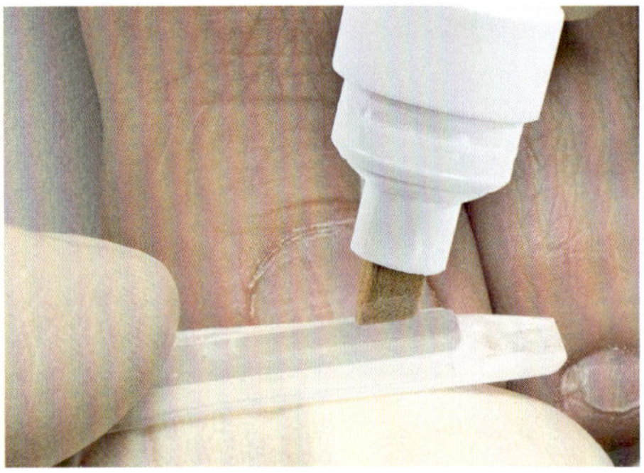

Image 5.210 Apply the activator to the brace

Degrease the nail plate before applying the brace. Do not degrease the brace! In order for the adhesive to stick immediately, once the cleaner is dry, apply the activator on the entire nail surface (image 5.208).

Place the brush with the adhesive on the brace and stroke it lightly across the brace to the opposite end, applying a thick layer of adhesive (image 5.209).

Alternatively, as seen in images 5.210 and 5.211, you can do the following: apply the activator to the brace first and then brush adhesive over the nail. The adhesive has a setting time of two minutes.

Now grab the long tab of the carrier foil holding the correct-sized brace and place the short tab with the end of the brace on the side edge of the nail, holding it firmly in place with one finger for about three seconds (image 5.212).

Without letting go, press the brace slowly across the nail to the opposite edge. Wait about five seconds before removing the carrier foil from the brace (images 5.213 to 5.215).

Use a diamond bur or corundum grinder to smooth the transition between the brace and the nail. If necessary, reduce the tension by grinding the ends of the brace thinner (image 5.216). Ask the patient if he/she feels any tension. Ensure that the patient feels comfortable.

Finally, seal the nail plate, including the brace, with adhesive which is resistant to nail polish remover. Prior to sealing, the nail plate and the brace must be cleaned with cleaner. Simply wipe with a moistened swab.

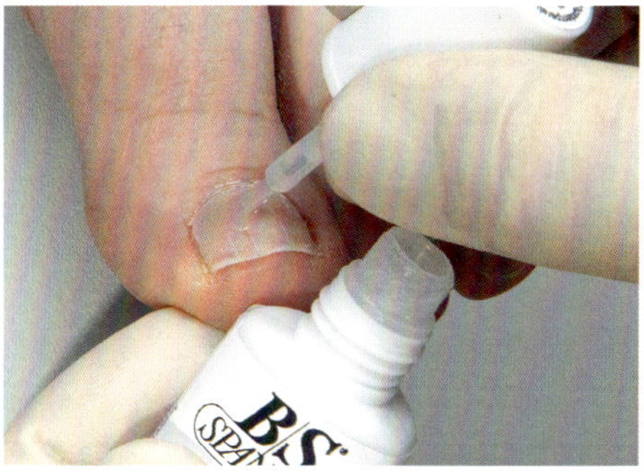

Image 5.211 Apply adhesive on the nail

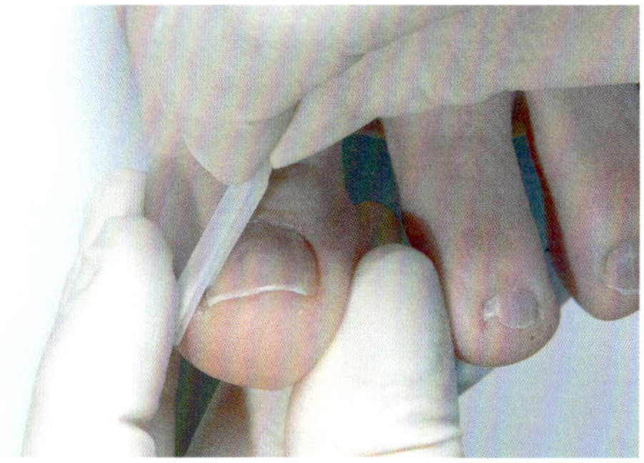

Image 5.212 Position the brace on the nail

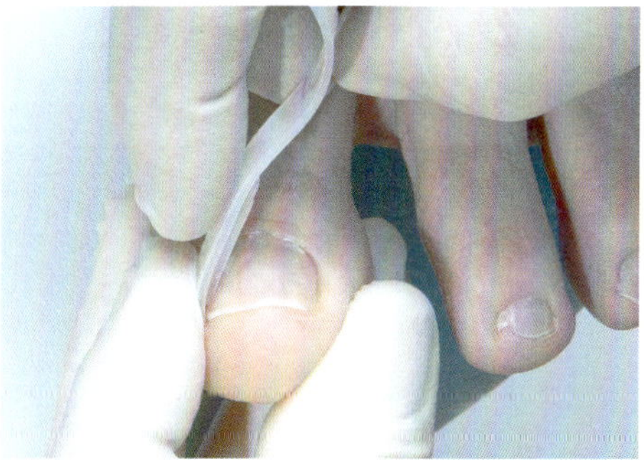

Image 5.213 Press the brace on the nail

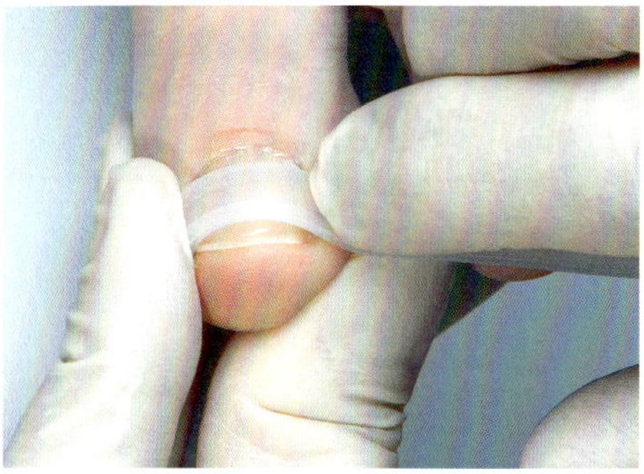

Image 5.214 Hold for 5 seconds – done

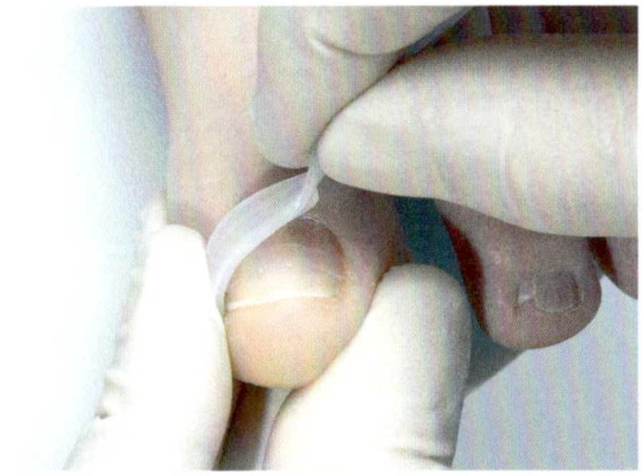

Image 5.215 Remove the carrier foil

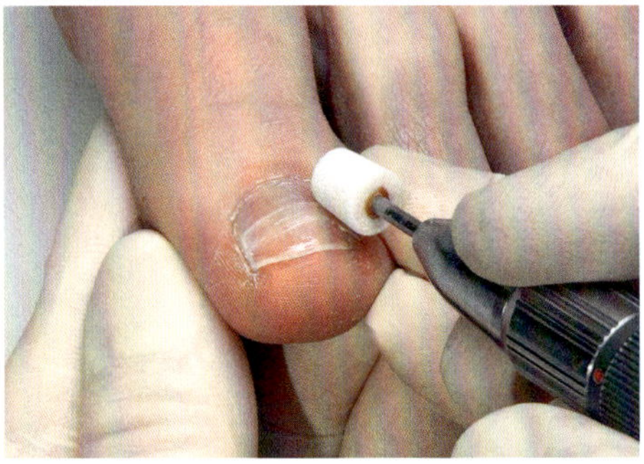

Image 5.216 Correct tensile force by grinding the brace's end pieces

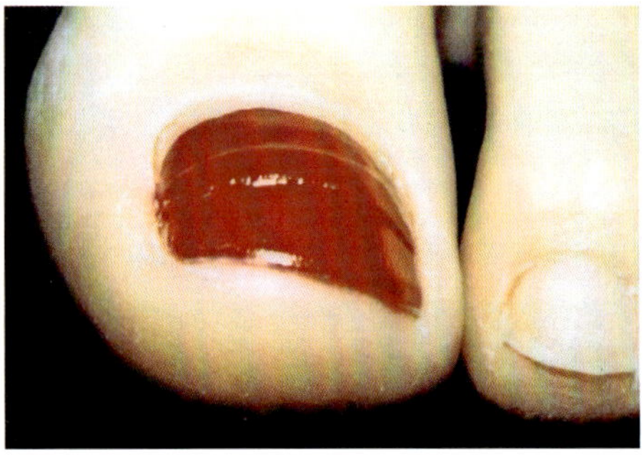

Image 5.217 Nail with brace and nail polish

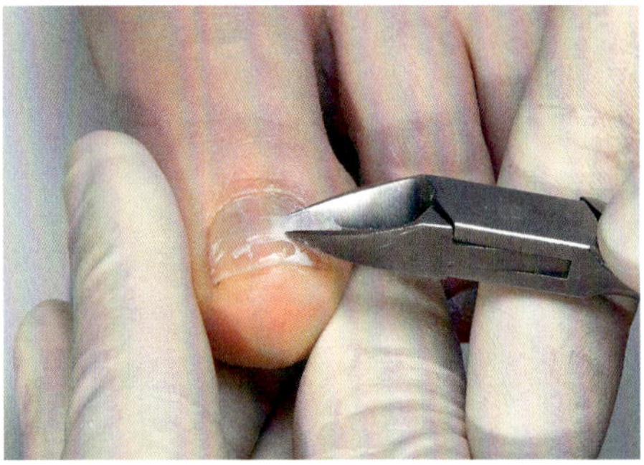

Image 5.218 Brace removal

Once the sealant has dried, the nail can be treated as usual with a disinfectant, tamponade and ointment application. Nail polish can also be applied. Use nail polish remover or the BS cleaner to remove nail polish (image 5.217).

The brace works for about four weeks. After this time, either remove the brace and apply a new one or place a second brace behind the first one. Removing the brace is easy. Cut the side edge of the brace with pointy nail pliers to separate it from the nail. Then carefully peel the brace off (image 5.218).

5.19 Onyclip brace

Onyclips are versatile applicable plastic-coated nail correction braces with precisely adjustable tension force. Especially applicable to ingrown toe nails. The application process is simple, the brace is comfortable to wear and can be used on any nail shape.

Material (image 5.219)
Epoxy-coated flexible stainless steel strip with adhesive gel.

Work materials
- standard strip measuring 10 cm long, 4 mm wide and 0.1 or 0.15 mm thick
- round-nosed pliers
- measuring tape
- side-cutting pliers
- applicator
- tweezers

Effectiveness
Nail correction system with precisely adjustable tensile force.

Indications
- unguis incarnatus
- unguis convolutus
- callositas

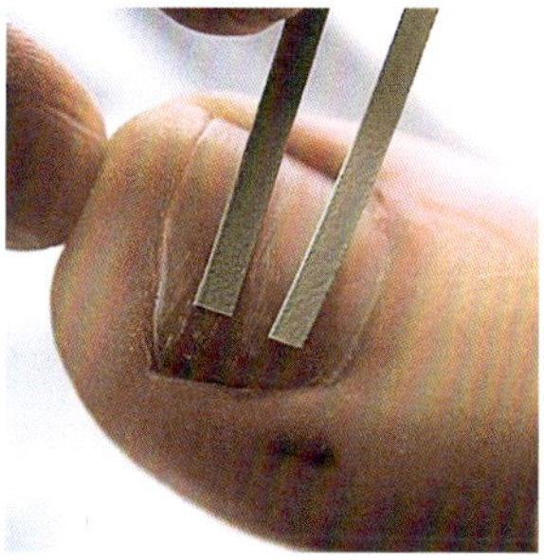
Image 5.219
Foto: Erkodent

- hyperkeratosis
- clavus in the sulcus or beneath the nail plate

Contraindication
Paronychia (attaching the brace causes pain).

Preparation (image 5.220)
As with all adhesive braces, smooth, clean and degrease the nail plate.

Brace preparation/positioning/fixation (images 5.221 to 5.227)
- Measure the width of the nail with the measuring tape.
- Cut the Onyclip strip to the desired length (strips come in two different thicknesses).

Images 5.220 to 5.227 courtesy of Erkodent

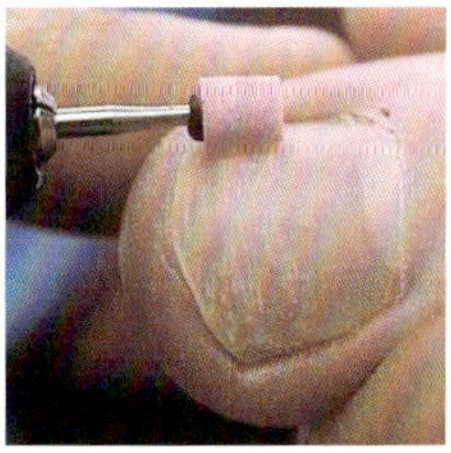
Image 5.220

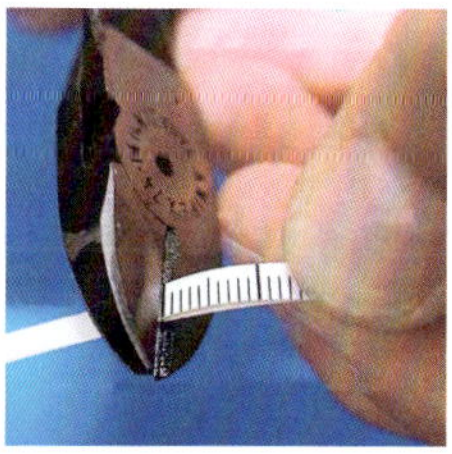
Image 5.221

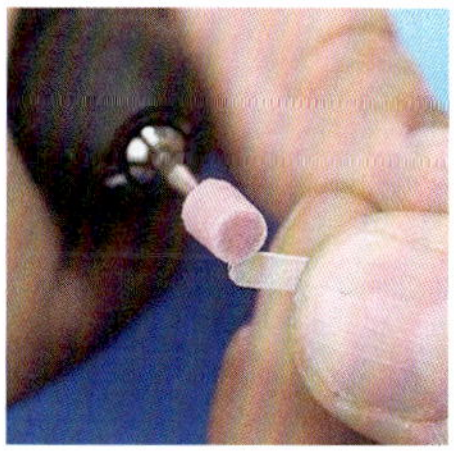
Image 5.222

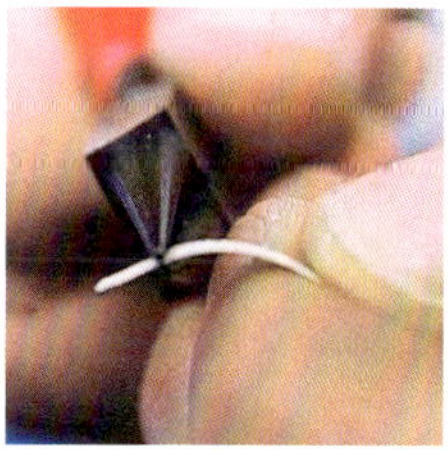
Image 5.223

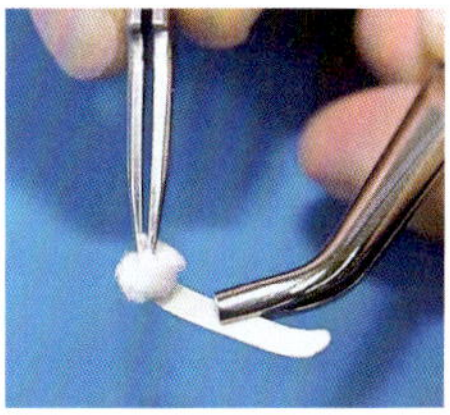
Image 5.224

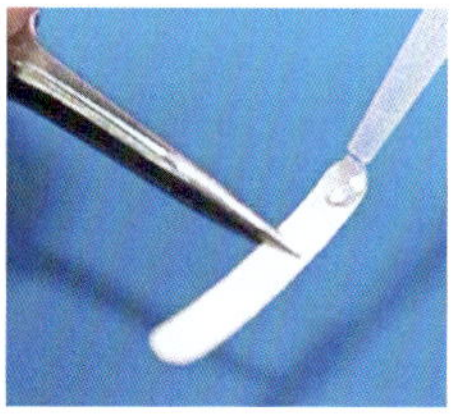
Image 5.225

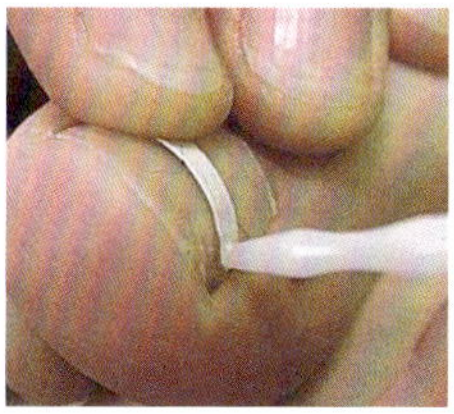
Image 5.226

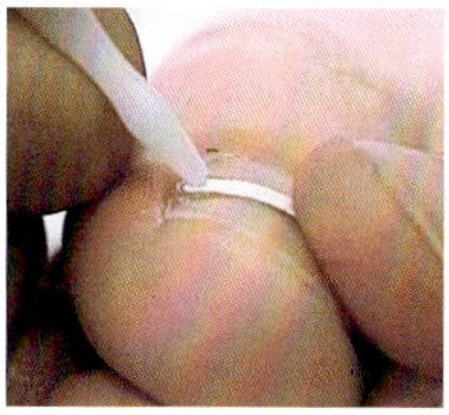
Image 5.227

- Soften the edges to prevent injuries to the nail fold.
- Prebend the brace with round-nosed pliers to fit the shape of the nail and adjust the tensile force by bending the sides (max. 2 mm).
- Degrease the nail surface and the brace.
- Apply a small dot of adhesive to the right side of the brace and fixate on the nail.
- Repeat the same on the left side after about one minute.

Important information for the patient

- The brace must be checked every night.
- In the event that the nail becomes painful, the brace loosens or for any other problems that might occur, visit the podiatrist.
- See the podiatrist for a follow-up visit within one to three days.
- Schedule a visit within four to six weeks with the podiatrist to reposition and align the brace.

5.20 Podofix active adhesive brace

Material (image 5.228)
The brace consists of a flexible plastic pad and an activation wire that applies tensile force after the brace has been glued to the nail.

Work materials (image 5.229)
The brace is available in four sizes:

mini:	9–12 mm
S (small):	16 mm
M (medium):	19 mm
L (large):	22 mm

- alcohol swabs for cleaning nail and brace
- side-cutting pliers for cutting the wire
- active adhesive gel
- Tension instrument for brace activation
- PediGel for sealing the brace
- micro light for curing PediGel
- spatula for PediGel application

Image 5.228

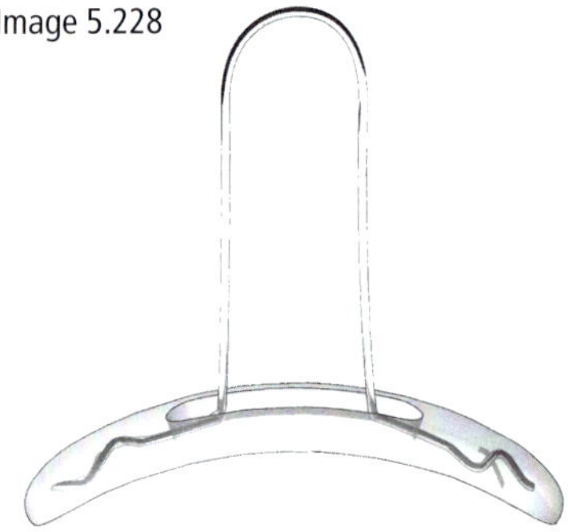

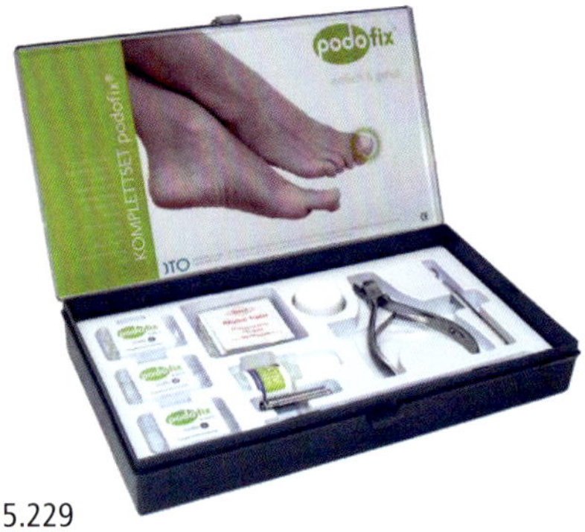

Image 5.229

- sharp instrument for cleaning the adhesion pipette
- needle for opening the adhesion pipette

Effectiveness

The podofix active adhesive brace can be used for nearly all forms of deformed and painfully ingrown or enrolled nails and it has shown to be very effective in the treatment of hypergranulation and clavi in the nail fold.

This brace is also suitable as a pre-treatment prior to the application of the 3TO brace or any other wire brace in the event that the nail fold is too narrow to receive wire hooks.

It is also useful as post-treatment after a wire brace has been removed since it supports the corrected growth of the nail and prevents ingrown toe nails from reoccurring.

Indications

- unguis convolutus
- unguis incarnatus
- clavi in the sulcus
- onychophosis
- paronychia
- granulation tissue

Preparation (image 5.230)

Clean the nail

Prior to applying the brace, clean and degrease the nail thoroughly with an alcohol or isopropyl swab. Afterwards, allow the nail to dry completely (approx. 30 seconds).

Brace preparation (image 5.231)

Fitting the brace

- Choose the appropriate size. The size must be chosen so that the brace can be fixed as close to the ingrown nail edge as possible.
- Position the brace on the side of the nail that is most affected by an ingrown nail.
- Bend the brace with your finger to fit the patient's nail.
- Bend the brace slightly more than the curvature of the nail; this will ensure a closer fit. This is important for the end pieces of the brace.
- For very small nails, shorten the brace by cutting out 3 mm in the centre of the strip (only recommended for experienced users).

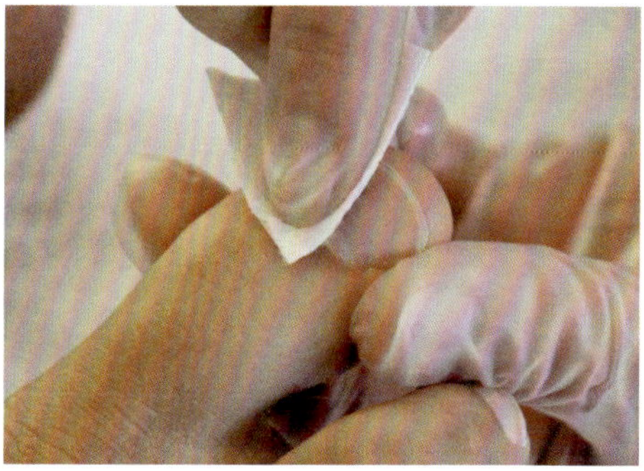

Image 5.230

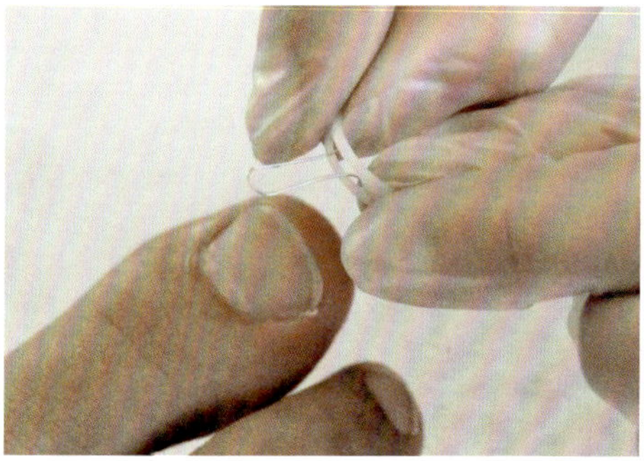

Image 5.231

Cleaning the brace

Degrease the brace with an alcohol swab and allow to dry for approximately 30 seconds.

Positioning/fixation (images 5.232 to 5.240)
Place the brace in or below the area that is painful. Position the brace as close as possible to the edge of the nail that is causing pain without protruding the nail edge.

If the tensile force of one brace is insufficient, then two braces can be placed one after another.

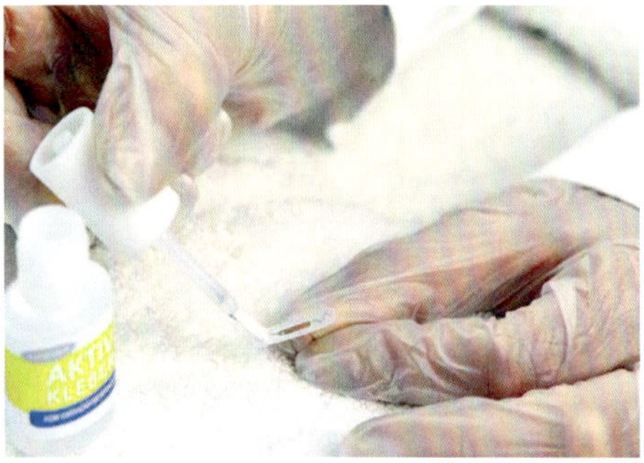

Image 5.232 Apply the adhesive

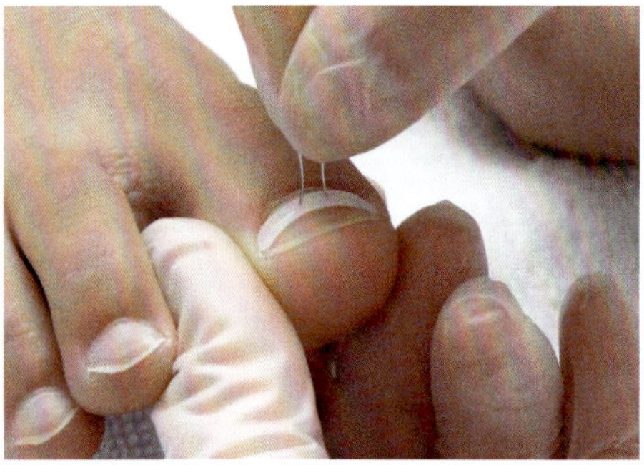

Image 5.233 Position the brace

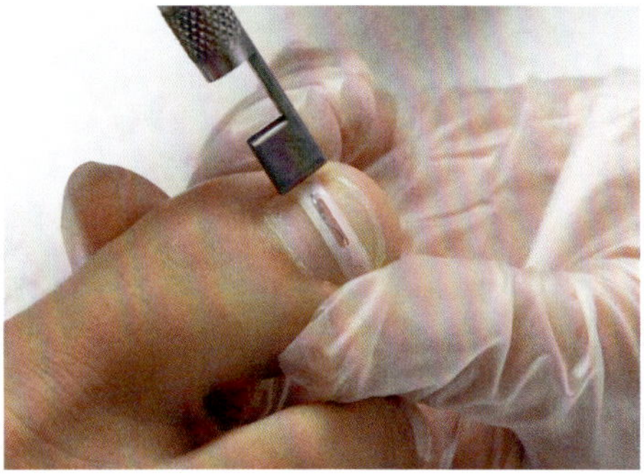

Image 5.234 Press it in place with the tension instrument

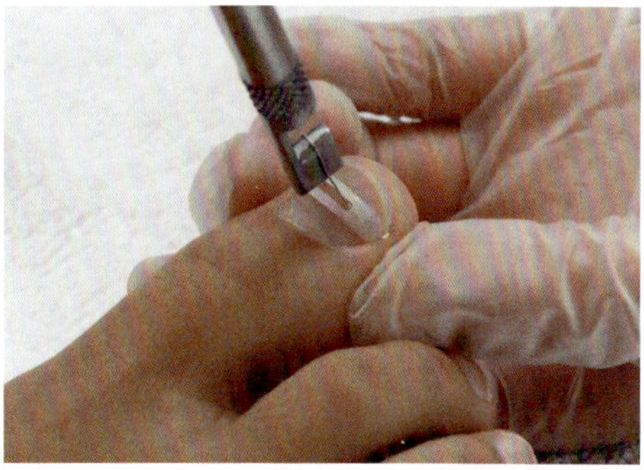

Image 5.235 Activate the brace

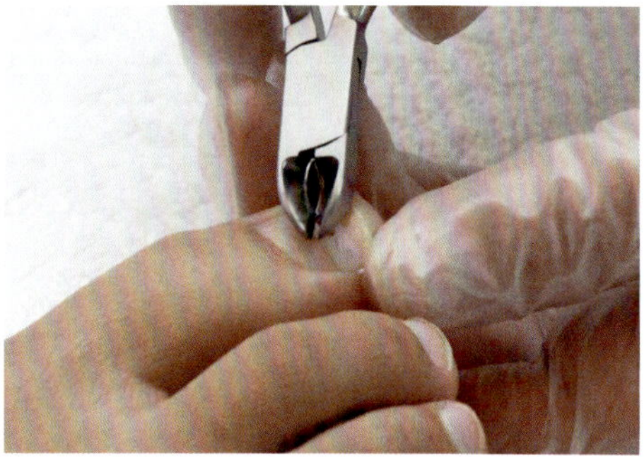

Image 5.236 Cut off the tension wire

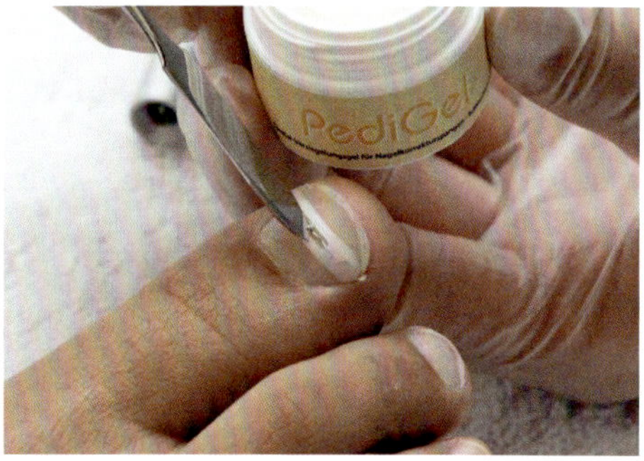

Image 5.237 Seal the brace

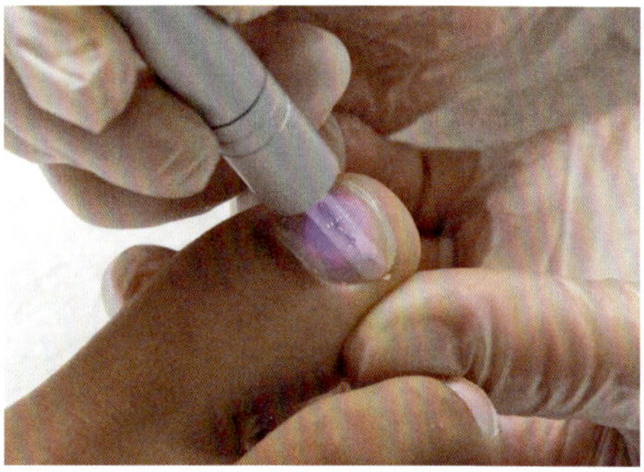

Image 5.238 Curing with a curing light

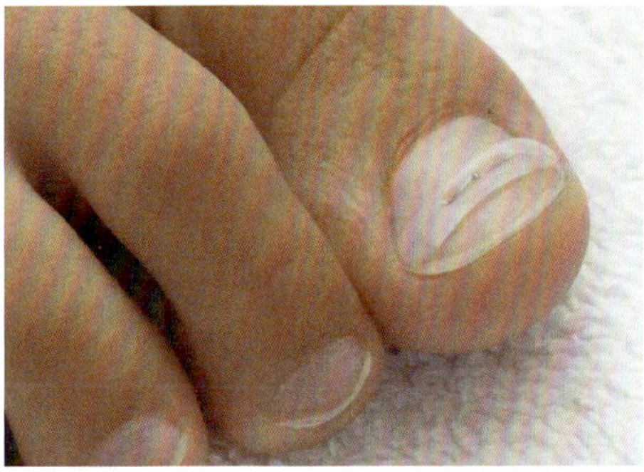

Image 5.239 The finished brace on the nail

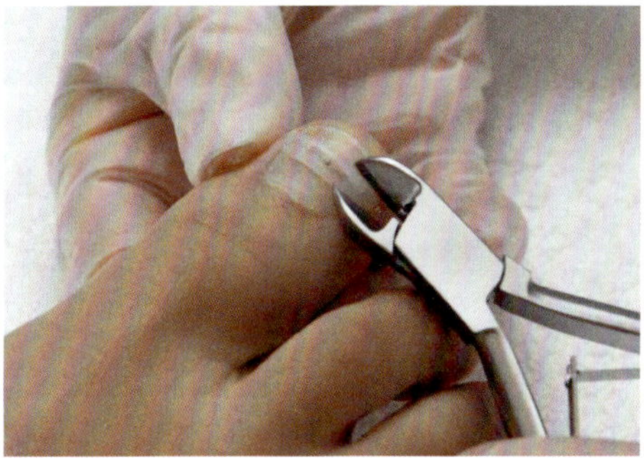

Image 5.240 Brace removal

All photos are courtesy of 3TO

Adhesive application

Using too much adhesive will impair proper bonding. Wipe the brush off on the inside of the bottle and apply a thin layer on the brace. One brush stroke, starting at the centre of the brace towards the end pieces of the brace, is sufficient. Also apply the adhesive to the brace's margins.

Positioning the brace

- Position the brace on the side with the more severely ingrown nail.
- Grab the brace at the wire and carefully position the brace on the nail.
- Press the adhesive side of the brace on the nail for 15 seconds with your finger. Pull the brace's ends in each direction close to the nail fold, causing the centre of the brace to lie close to the nail surface.
- Use the tension instrument to press down the margin areas of the brace without shifting it.
- Wait at least one minute before activating the brace since the adhesive must first harden.

Twisting the wire loop

- Place the tension instrument in the wire loop.
- Turn the tension instrument once, maximum twice, until the desired tension is achieved. Turning the activation wire by more than two turns can cause the wire to break, rendering the brace useless. Pull the tension instrument slightly upwards while turning.
- Remove the tension instrument.

Cutting off unused wire

- Cut off the wire loop with side-cutting pliers by placing the pliers flat on the brace and cut the wire loop with one cut.
- Smooth the wire ends with a diamond nail file.
- Remove the filing dust by blowing on the area or with a soft brush.

Sealing the connection wire

- Apply a drop of PediGel on the brace with a spatula and distribute it on the brace.
- Activate the microlight by turning the front part of the light clockwise. The PediGel will be hard after 20 seconds. Hold the microlight a maximum of 5 mm from the area to be sealed.
- Wipe the brace with an alcohol swab once the PediGel has completely hardened. Cover any protruding wire pieces with another layer of PediGel.

Removing the brace

Detaching the brace

Detach the end pieces of the brace with side-cutting pliers.

Cleaning the nail

Clean adhesive residue with a file or grinding bur.

Treatment period

The brace stays on the nail for a period of two weeks to two months and is replaced by new braces until the desired treatment success has been achieved.

Preventing complications

To prevent failure, the following guidelines must be followed:

The nail is too soft

The nail must not be soft prior to applying the brace. Avoid foot baths, the application of disinfectants or cuticle softener prior to the treatment.

Too much adhesive

The brace does not bond to the nail surface if too much adhesive has been applied.

Working with latex gloves

Handling the brace with latex gloves or finger cots is recommended to prevent fingers from sticking to the brace and to avoid getting grease on the nail surface.

Important information for the patient

- The brace must be checked every night.
- In the event that the nail becomes painful, the brace loosens or for any other problems that might occur, visit the podiatrist.
- See the podiatrist for a follow-up visit within one to three days.
- Schedule a visit within two weeks to a month with the podiatrist to replace the brace.

Additional information

- During transport, the brace's activation wires can get slightly bent. This does not affect the quality of the brace. After positioning the brace, rebend the wire to facilitate placement of the tension instrument.
- Please note that the side-cutting pliers included in the set are only suitable to cut the soft podofix wire and not the hard wire of other braces.

5.21 Erki technique

Material

Adhesive hook elements, rubber rings.

Work materials

- Erki adhesive hook elements
- rubber ring
- tubing
- tweezers
- special adhesive

Effectiveness

The Erki plastic hook elements are glued to each side of the nail and are connected with a rubber ring. The different sizes of rubber rings determine the applied tensile force.

Indications

- unguis convolutus
- unguis incarnatus
- clavi in the sulcus
- onychophosis
- paronychia
- granulation tissue

Preparation

Degrease and roughen the areas of the nail where the hook elements are supposed to be attached.

Positioning/fixation (images 5.241 to 5.249)

Use tweezers to position and glue the hook elements on each lateral nail edge. Then hook the correct rubber ring onto one hook element and, with a crochet hook, pull the rubber tubing over the rubber ring for protection. Now hook the rubber ring in the hook element on the other side. Both hook elements are pulled together by the rubber ring which is fixed on the nail plate with adhesive. The tensile force is adjusted by choosing differently sized rings.

Image 5.241

All photos courtesy of Erkodent

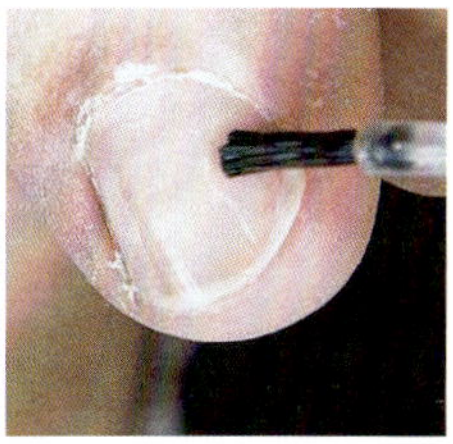

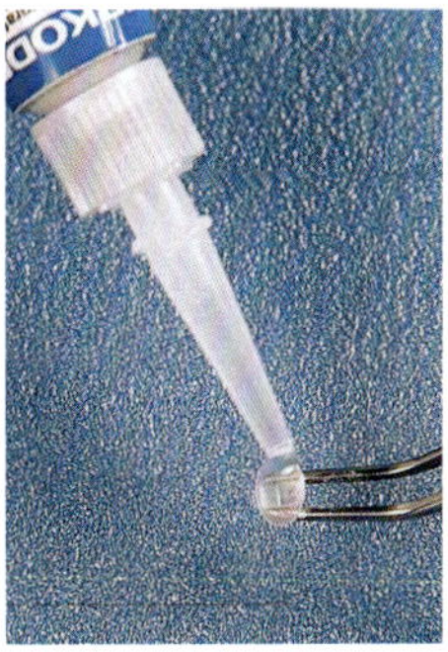

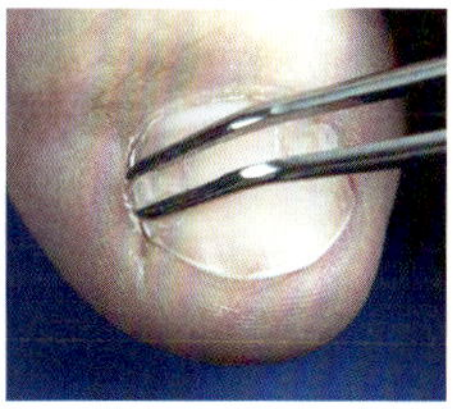

Image 5.242

Image 5.243

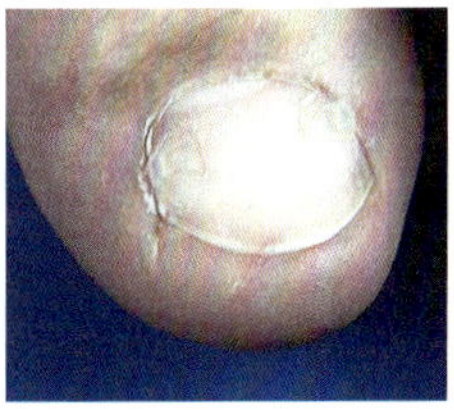

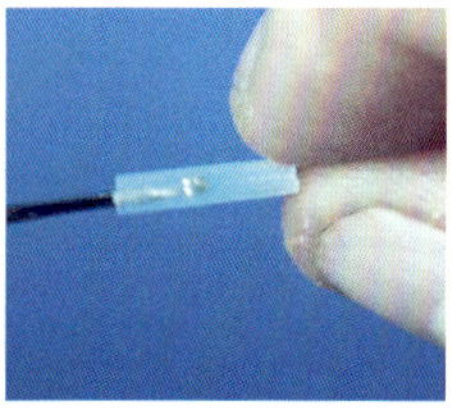

Image 5.244

Image 5.245

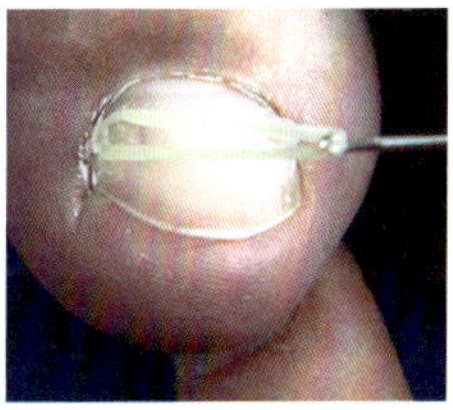

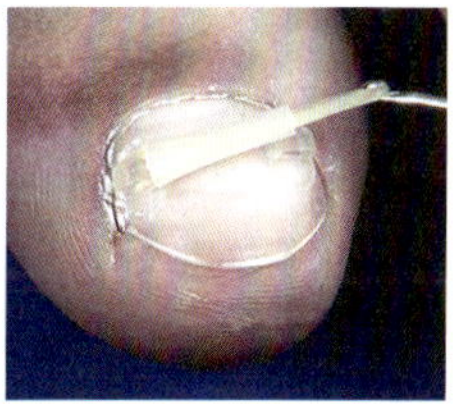

Image 5.246

Image 5.247

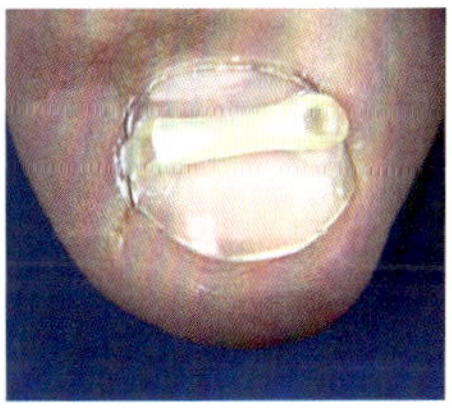

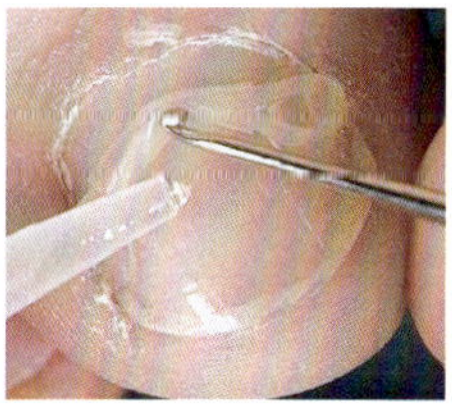

Image 5.248

Image 5.249

Important information for the patient

- The brace must be checked every night.
- In the event that the nail becomes painful, the brace loosens or for any other problems that might occur, visit the podiatrist.
- See the podiatrist for a follow-up visit within one to three days.
- Schedule a visit within four to six weeks with the podiatrist to reposition and align the brace.

5.22 Unguisan Blue Light

The Unguisan Blue Light system secures braces with a light curing material. It consists of a gel in a dosing syringe and a high performance LED light.

Blue Light technology
Compared to other UV materials, the Unguisan polymerization process is triggered by blue light. It works fast, is harmless and has been used by dentists for a long time.

Blue light gel
Accurate to dose and easily pliable, the final hardness was optimized specially for orthonyxia applications, meaning that the material's flexibility enables the nails and brace to move.

Blue light lamp
The high-performance LED light was developed to combine efficient processing with maximum reliability. The battery-powered light can be applied everywhere, which is especially useful in mobile podiatry. Constant current control ensures consistent brightness via battery power.

Application
- Apply the gel very precisely with the dosing syringe.
- Cure with the LED light for 20 seconds.

The most important advantages:
- suitable for all types of wire braces
- only two work materials are needed, the light and the syringe
- a short curing time of 20 seconds due to the high performance LED light (1.3 watts, battery-powered).
- one syringe lasts for 100 applications; there is no wasteful material residue since only the exact amount of material needed is used
- blue light instead of harmful UV rays
- accurate to dose, easily pliable, no additional instruments needed
- no offensive odour

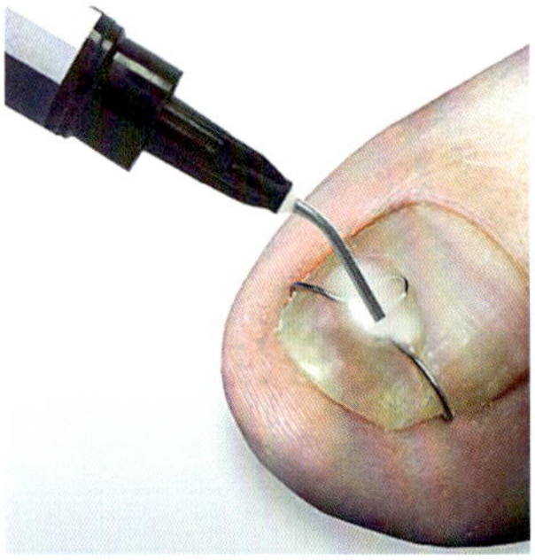

Image 5.250

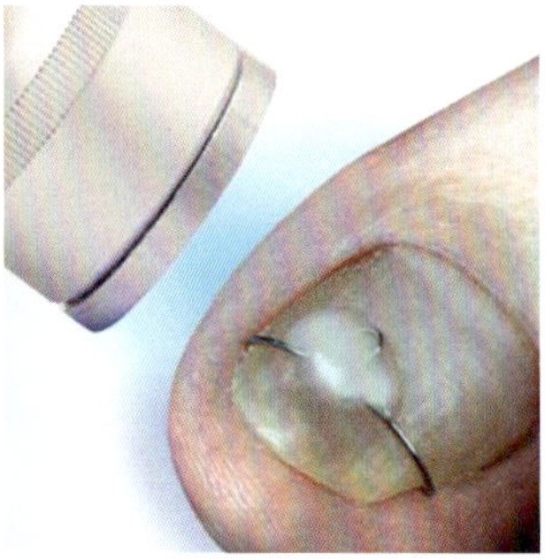

Image 5.251

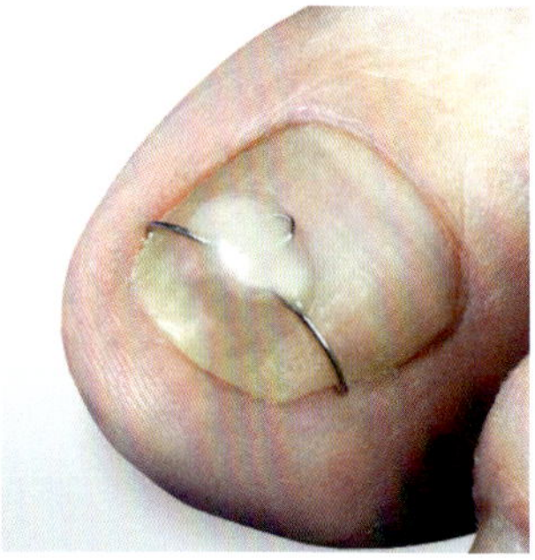

Image 5.252
All photos courtesy of Hellmut Ruck

5.23 3TO PLUS+ brace

The 3TO PLUS+ brace is an advanced version of the original 3TO brace. It consists of two spring steel wire arms with partially preformed hooks and an innovative PLUS+ pad which fixes the wire arms on the nail.

The PLUS+ pad is glued to the nail with Ortho Glue. Afterwards, the wire arms are hooked underneath the nail edge and clipped under the PLUS+ pad.

A special training course is not obligatory to purchase or apply this product. A comprehensive training DVD explains step-by-step how to fix the brace correctly on the nail.

Work materials (image 5.253)

- wire arms made of spring steel wire with partially preformed hooks (0.25 or 0.30 mm)
- PLUS+ pad
- combination pliers
- side-cutting pliers
- holding forceps
- Ortho Glue®
- PediGel®
- microlight
- spatula

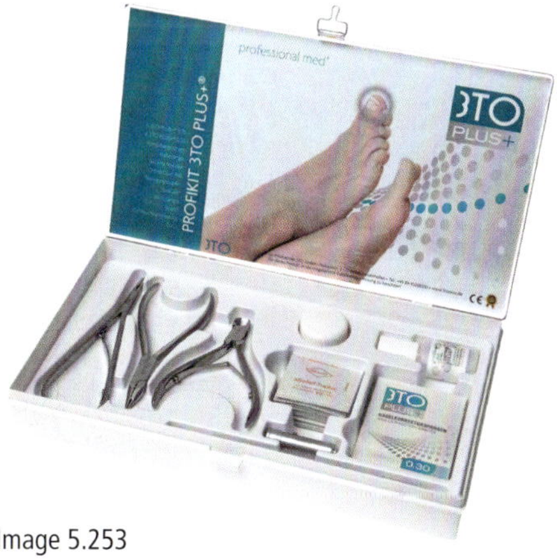

Image 5.253

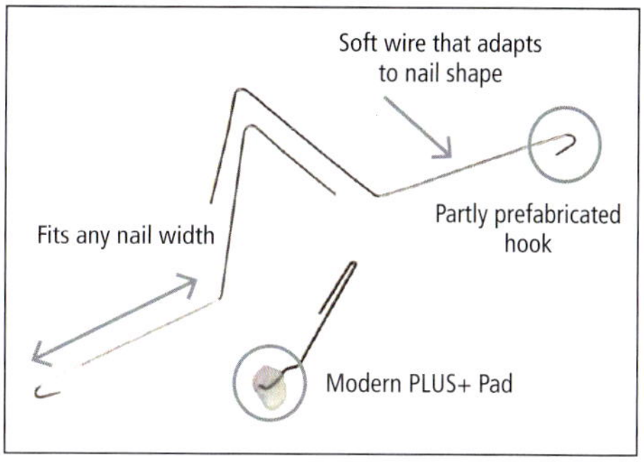

Image 5.254 Parts of the 3TO PLUS+ brace

Effectiveness

The brace works through the spring force of the wire by continuously and gently pulling the nail edges upwards. The nail is gently guided towards healthy nail growth. To increase effectiveness, there are two different wire strengths to choose from: 0.25 mm and 0.30 mm (image 5.254).

Indications and preparation the same as with the 3TO brace

Function

The brace consists of a PLUS+ pad which is carefully glued in the centre of the nail plate with Ortho Glue and two flexible wire arms. The wire arms come with small hooks and are hooked carefully underneath the edge of the nail and clipped under the PLUS+ pad on the nail.

The spring force of the wire causes the nail edges to lift slightly and immediatcly relieves the surrounding often painful tissue. The constant force on the nail promotes healthy and straight nail growth.

Treatment process

Choose the correct wire strength and adjust the shape of the prebent hooks with combination pliers. Glue the PLUS+ pad on the nail with Ortho Glue. Then secure the small hooks underneath both nail edges and fix the wire under the pad. Seal short wire pieces with light curing Pedi Gel.

The application of the brace takes only a few minutes and the patients barely feel anything.

As soon as the brace is activated, it lifts the nail edges slightly which immediately relives pain. This also has a positive impact on healing inflammation.

Due to the high comfort level, the patient can wear this brace, without limitations, to work, at school or while doing sports and, of course, in shoes.

This brace system is suitable for all age groups and types of patients.

Additional information
The 3TO PLUS+-brace has a permanent effect on the nail. Every 6 to 10 weeks (depending on nail growth) the brace is replaced by a new one to ensure that it is optimally positioned. The brace must be placed at the beginning of the front third of the nail.

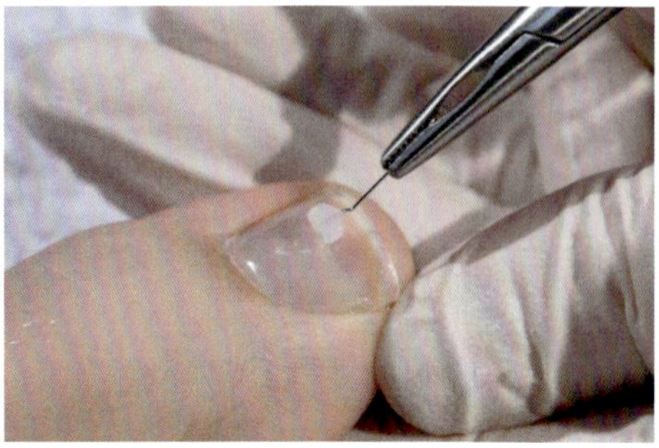

Image 5.255 The PLUS pad that holds the wire arms is simply glued to the nail

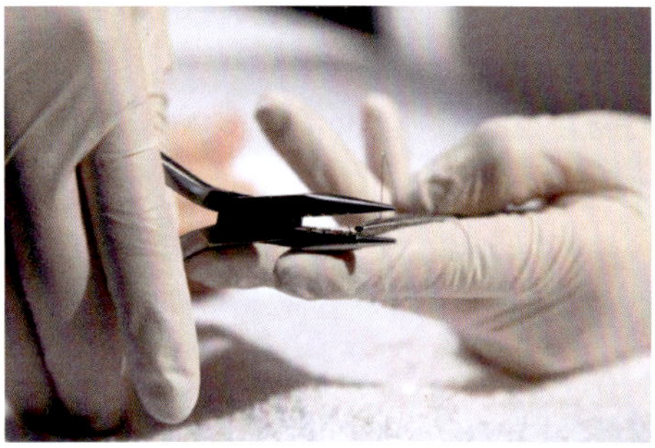

Image 5.256 The partially prepared hooks are easily adjusted to the individual nail thickness

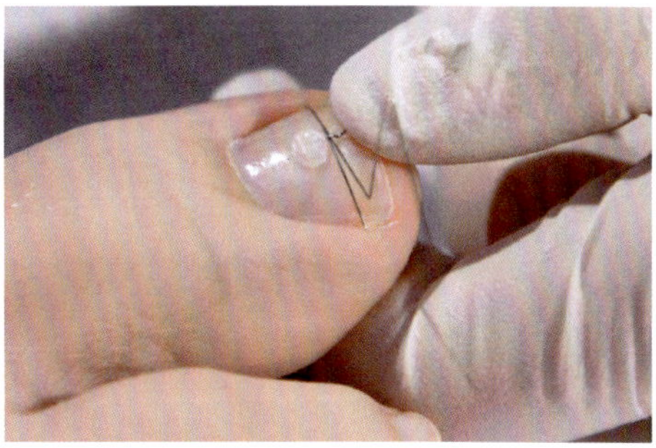

Image 5.257 The wire arms are gently hooked underneath the nail edges and fixated under the PLUS pad

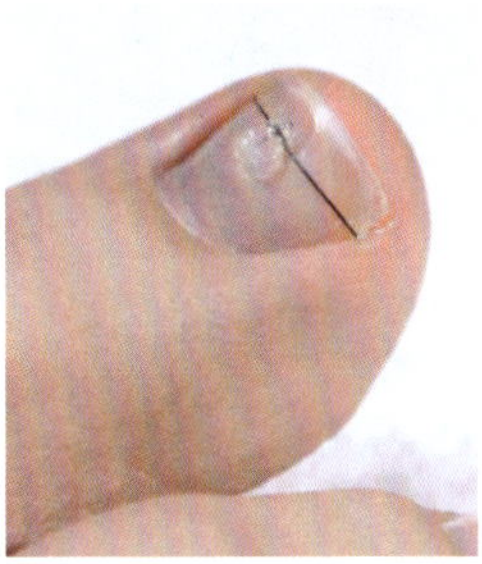

Image 5.258 Finally the wire ends are sealed with PediGel®. The brace is effective for several weeks due to the applied spring force.

5.24 Onyfix®

The Onyfix® nail correction system is a versatile product for the pain-free treatment of pincer and ingrown toe nails (unguis incarnatus). It can be used to treat almost all types of pincer or deformed nails. The system consists of a primer (bonding agent), a soft and a hard composite.

After more or less proximal fixation of this nail correction system using a hardened composite, a pincer or ingrown nail will be shaped into a natural nail shape through normal growth. It thus works like a standard nail brace, but without the pain from metal wires hooked laterally or the tension by pulling.

Work materials (image 5.259)
- Onyfix® Primer
- Onyfix® Hard correction composite
- Onyfix® Soft correction composite
- ceramic or carbide burs
- spatula
- probe
- bent needles fort he soft composite
- cotton swabs
- LED blue light lamp
- cleaners
- disposable cotton buds

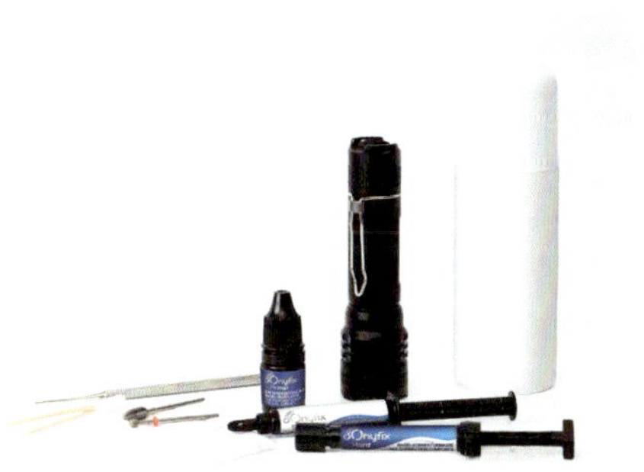

Image 5.259 Items required for preparation and application of the Onyfix nail correction system. Additionally needed are various burs, cotton swabs, LED blue light lamp, probe, cleaners and disposable cotton buds.

Preparation
- Smooth and roughen the nail with ceramic or carbide burs. Sand any thickened or arched areas of the nail plate until you have a broadly uniform nail surface.
- Prepare the nail folds. Cut out the corners of the nail as far as required. Remove any areas of keratosis or deposits from the nail folds.
- Degrease the nail and surrounding skin, paying particular attention to the nail folds. At the same time, thoroughly clean away any nail dust using a cotton swab and standard disinfectant. Leave the nail to dry (60–120 seconds).

Applying the composite

Step 1: Place a drop oft he primer in the lid of the primer bottle or a small bowl (image 5.260). Wet a cotton bud with a little bit of the primer. Do not use too much primer, as this can cause the composite to slip on the nail (image 5.261). Place the disposable cotton bud in the middle of the nail and work the primer evenly into the nail (image 5.262). Ensure that the primer is not applied to the nail folds. Depending on the temperature of the room, the primer requires about 5 minutes to dry. It can sometimes be helpful to dry the primer for 10 seconds using the LED blue light lamp (image 5.263). The primer must be completely dry. See images next side.

Step 2: Place the composite in the required position on the prepared nail. The hard composite can be used for large and severely deformed nails. The soft composite is intended for use on very thin, small nails and children's nails. Hard composite: squeeze a little of the composite from the syringe onto a spatula (image 5.264). Using the spatula, apply the hard composite to the nail in the required position and shape it to an appropriate shape (images 5.265 and 5.266). Soft composite: attach a bent needle to the soft composite syringe and apply the required amount in the re-

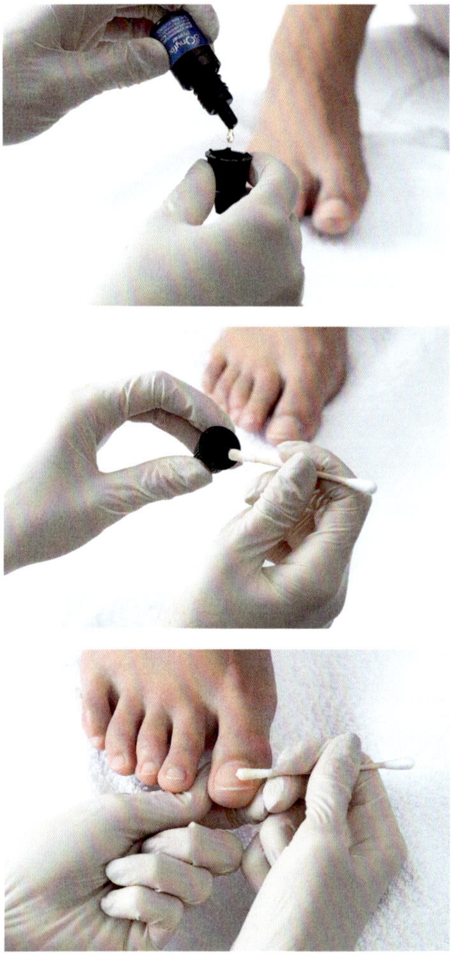

Images 5.260–5.263 The individual steps for preparing the nail

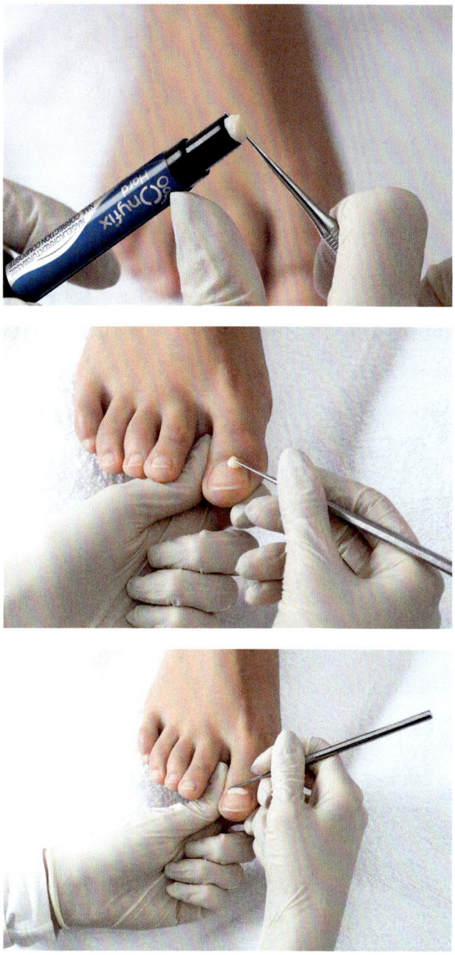

Images 5.264–5.266 Dispensing and shaping the hard composite

quired position on the nail (image 5.267) Shape the composite using a spatula (image 5.268).

For best results, both composites should be applied with a thickness of about 2 mm! **Step 3:** Polymerise the composite using an LED blue light lamp (image 5.269) held close to the composite for 20 to 30 seconds. Ensure that the whole of the nail is exposed to the blue light.

Step 4: Once the nail correction system has hardened, remove the dispersion layer using the cleaner.

The patient should not go swimming or bathe for 24 hours! The composite can remain on the nail until nail growth brings it to the distal end of the nail.

Other options for using the composite

Lifting the nail: For best results, the composite can also be removed after a few months (either using a bur or with nippers) and a new nail correction systems applied at the proximal end of the nail (image 5.270). For faster results, an Onyfix® nail correction system can be applied to the distal end of the nail (either on its own or together with a proximal Onyfix® sys-

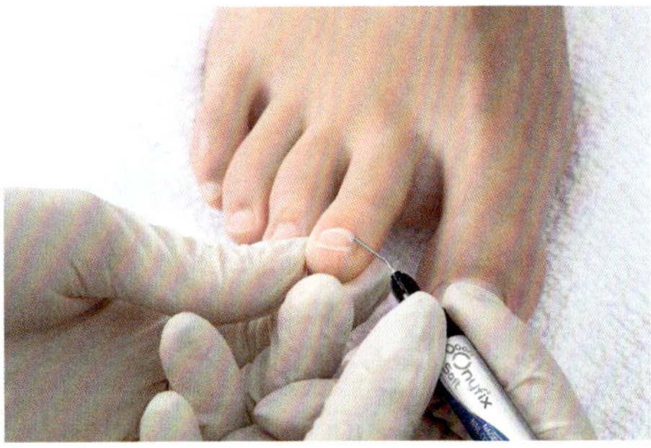

Image 5.267 Dispensing the soft composite using a needle

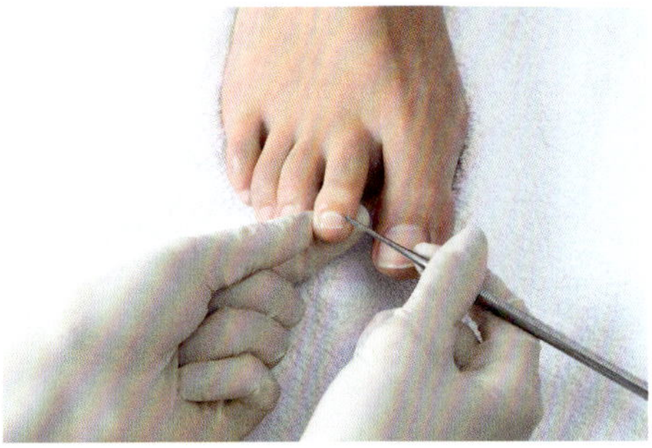

Image 5.268 After shaping the composite

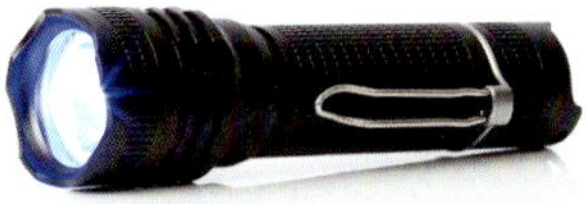

Image 5.269 LED blue light lamp for polymerizing the composite

tem) whilst lifting the nail using a probe. This can be achieved by placing packing under one or both corners of the nail if required (image 5.271).

Using the composite in combination with a wire: For severely pincered or ingrown nails, it may be helpful to generate tension by combining the composite with a wire brace (images 5.272 and 5.273).

The nail is prepared as described above. Then prepare (stretch, bend) the metal brace. Shape a wire (which should have a small omega-shaped bend in the middle)

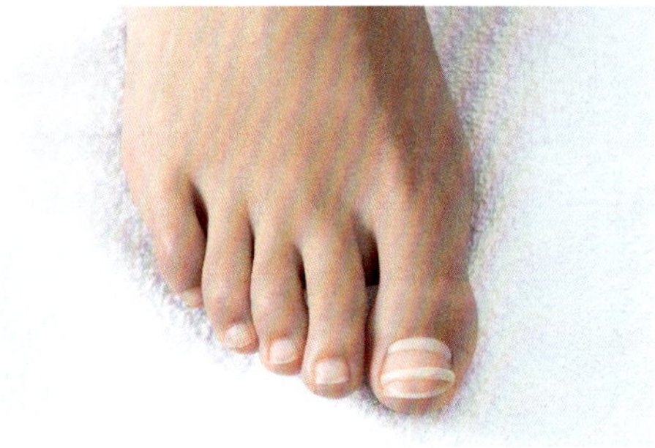

Image 5.270 Nail with two nail correction systems. The two corners of the nail should be lifted during hardening of the distal composite.

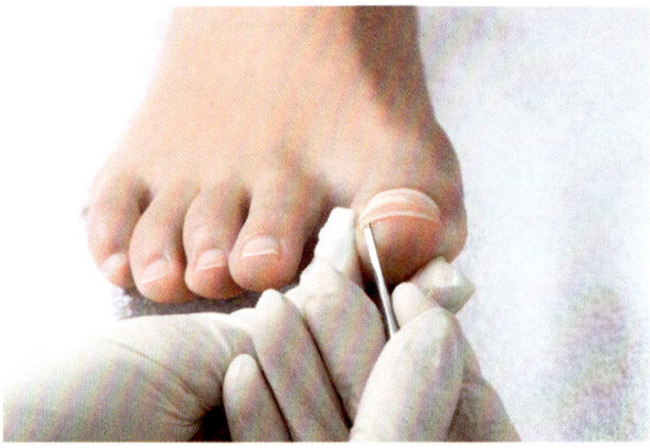

Image 5.271 Lifting the nail during polymerisation

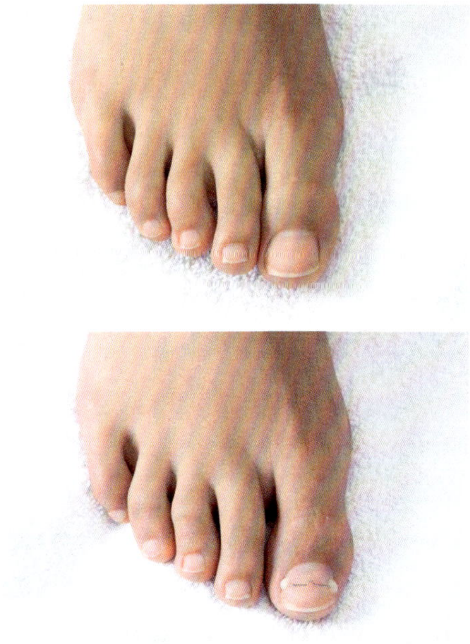

Images 5.272 and 5.273
Onyfix® composite used in combination with a wire brace, before and after

to the target shape of the prepared nail. To attach the wire, apply a spot of the hard composite to one end of the wire after placement on the nail (image 5.274). Ensure that the end of the wire in the composite is still easily visible. To enable you to attach the wire to the other side, harden this spot of composite for about 20 to 30 seconds using the LED blue light lamp (image 5.275). Now harden the second spot using the LED blue light lamp. The wire will then be firmly attached to the nail (image 5.276). The omega-shaped bend can be activated using pliers if required, generating the required tension (image 5.277).

Using the hard composite as a nail correction system for one half of the nail only: If the nail is pincered on one side only, you should apply the nail correction system to just half of the nail (image 5.278), which should be prepared as described above. Once you have shaped the nail correction system on the nail, lift the affected side using a spatula. Keeping the nail lifted, use the LED blue light lamp to harden the composite whilst retaining the required shape.

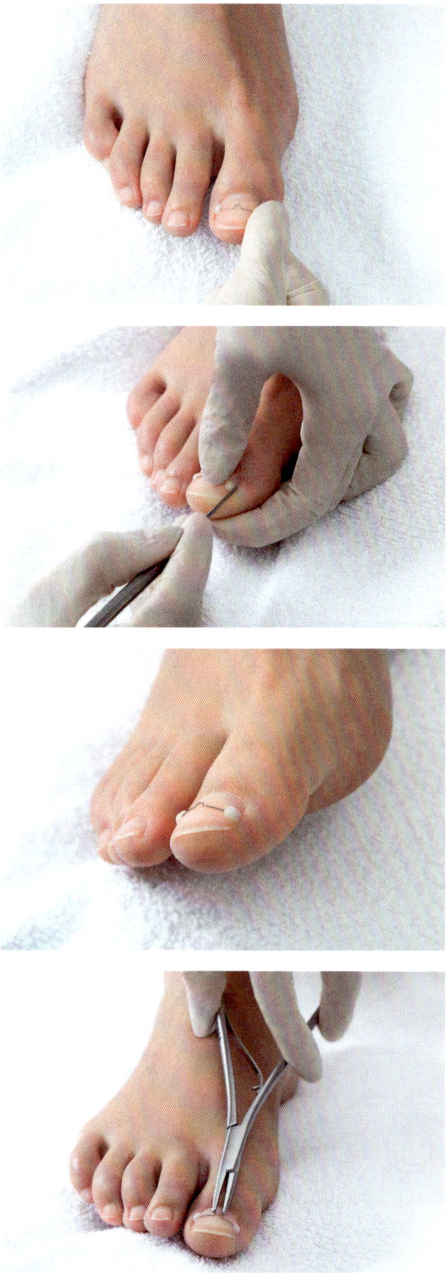

Images 5.274–5.277 The steps described above, using the product in combination with a wire

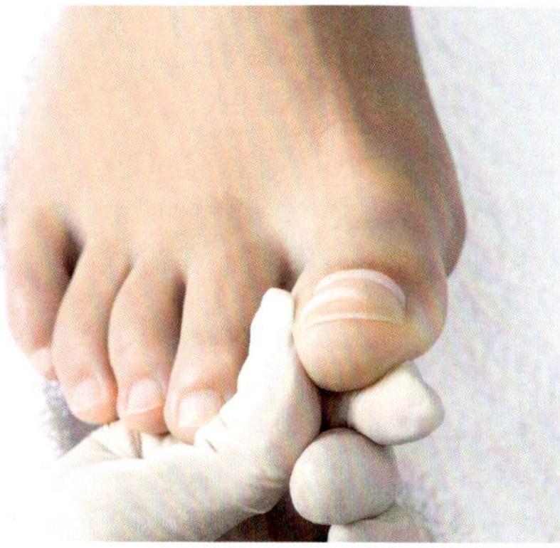

Image 5.278 Onyfix® nail correction system applied to one half of the nail only

5.25 Tools used for the preparation of wire braces

Brace	Description	Design	Wire	Loop/Omega	Side wires	Hooks	Activation and hook width adjustment	Helpful tools	Cutting the wire	Fixation
Fraser	bilateral brace with two end loops, produced with a plaster model	the omega is the pivot point	0.5 or 0.4 mm spring wire	round-nosed pliers, nail correction pliers or Rading tier pliers	round-nosed pliers	round-nosed pliers	flat-nosed pliers	holding forceps, anvil, hammer (100g), file	side cutting pliers	Onycholit, Unguisan® or gel-technique
3TO	stainless steel three-part brace, open design concept	two side wires plus one centre loop	prepared spring wire brace in different thicknesses plus centre wire		combination bending pliers	combination bending pliers	combination bending pliers	holding forceps, winding hook, file	side cutting pliers	Onycholit, Unguisan® or gel-technique
3TO PLUS	three-part brace with preshaped hooks	two spring side wires with PLUS+Pad	0.25 or 0.3 mm spring wire			combination bending pliers		holding forceps, alcohol swabs	side cutting pliers	Gel and adhesive
VHO-Osthold	stainless steel three-part preshaped brace	two side wires plus one centre loop	prepared spring wire in different thicknesses plus centre wire in different width		round-nosed pliers or needle-nosed pliers	reshaping with round-nosed pliers	flat-nosed pliers or needle-nosed pliers	holding forceps, winding hook	side cutting pliers	Onycholit, Unguisan® or gel-technique
Ortogrip	stainless steel preshaped brace with plastic holder	two side wires plus one centre loop	prepared spring wire in different thicknesses plus centre wire in different width		tier pliers	reshaping with tier pliers	tier pliers	winding hook, double-ended nail fold instrument, applicator, scissors, file, adhesion, cleaning agent, measuring aid	side cutting pliers	Onycholit, Unguisan® or gel-technique

5.25 Tools used for the preparation of wire braces
– continued –

Brace	Description	Design	Wire	Loop/Omega	Side wires	Hooks	Activation and hook width adjustment	Helpful tools	Cutting the wire	Fixation
SSO4U	three-part preshaped stainless steel nail correction brace	2 side wires plus 1 U-loop	preshaped spring wire brace, different thicknesses, centre wire		bending pliers	bending pliers	bending pliers	holding forceps, winding hook, file, 2 safety glasses	side cutting pliers	Onycholit, Unguisan® or gel-technique
ORa	preshaped spring stainless steel brace	2 side wires	preshaped spring stainless steel wire right/left		round-nosed pliers	round-nosed pliers	flat-nosed pliers with holes	needle holder, file	side cutting pliers	Onycholit, Unguisan® or gel-technique
Corectio Titanium	preshaped titanium brace	2 side wires	preshaped brace, different thicknesses		round-nosed pliers			holding forceps, winding hook	side cutting pliers	Onycholit, Unguisan® or gel-technique
COM-BI-ped	adhesive and wire brace combo	spring wire brace	spring wire brace, 3 different thicknesses		combination bending pliers	combination pliers	combination pliers	holding forceps, file, alcohol swabs, adhesive	side cutting pliers	Pedigel
Goldstadt professional	three preparation variants	with fixation hooks, half brace, adhesive brace	gold-plated stinaless steel up to 3 mm wide and 0.1 mm thick		tier pliers	tier pliers	tier pliers	scissors, file, side wire applicator, tweezers, nail fold instrument		activator, cleaning agent, gel model brush, adhesive, measuring aid, light-curing gel
Gorkiewicz Orthese Austria	bendable spring wire without a centre loop or omega	flat spring brace			round-nosed pliers	round-nosed pliers	flat-nosed pliers	holding forceps, file	side cutting pliers	Onycholit, Unguisan® or gel-technique

5.26 Overview of adhesive braces

Brace	Description	Material	Work material	Sealant
Goldstadt professional Classic	customized design, stainless steel, gold-plated for optimal adhesion, hypoallergenic	gold-plated stainless steel up to 3 mm wide, 0.1 mm thick, length 100 mm	round-nosed pliers, applicator double-ended nail fold instrument, applicator, scissors, file, adhesive, activator, cleaning agent, measuring aid	light-curing gel
Goldstadt professional	three preparation variants: with fixation hooks, half brace, adhesive brace	gold-plated stainless steel up to 3 mm wide, 0.1 and 0.15 mm thick	flat gel brush, tier pliers,double-ended nail fold instrument, activator, adhesive, applicator, cleaning agent, measuring aid	light-curing gel
BS brace	flat spring made of synthetic material	adhesive brace made of synthetic material	braces in different sizes, instant glue, brush-on adhesive, cleaning agent	sealing lacquer
Onyclip	versatile plastic coated nail correction system	epoxy coated spring stainless steel strip with adhesive gel	round-nosed pliers, scissors, file, side wire applicator, tweezers, measuring tape, gel adhesive	gel adhesive
podofix Active adhesive brace	brace consisting of a synthetic pad with activation wire that is tightened after adhesion	adhesive brace made of synthetic material	brace in different sizes, alcohol swabs, active adhesive, tightening aid	PediGel with micro lamp
Erki technique	adhesive brace with two holding elements with a rubber ring connection		holding elements, rubber ring, protective tubing, tweezers, holding hooks, special adhesive	special adhesive

5.27 Errors and consequences of incorrectly prepared nail correction braces

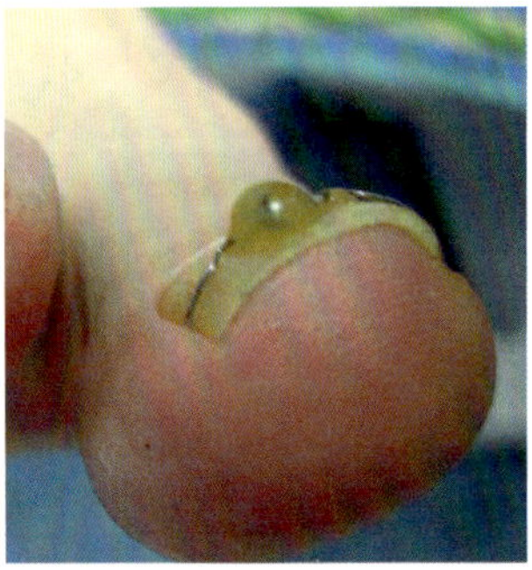

Image 5.279 Clavus risk due to too much sealant

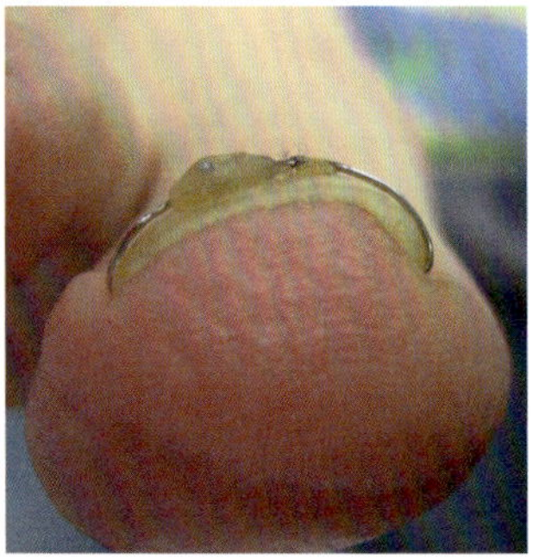

Image 5.280 Clavus risk due to incorrectly rounded wires. Pressure and tensile force are impaired.

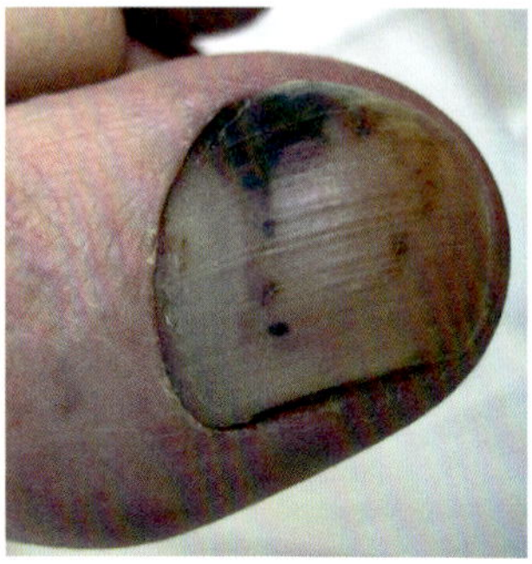

Image 5.281 Subungual hematoma due to too much tensile force

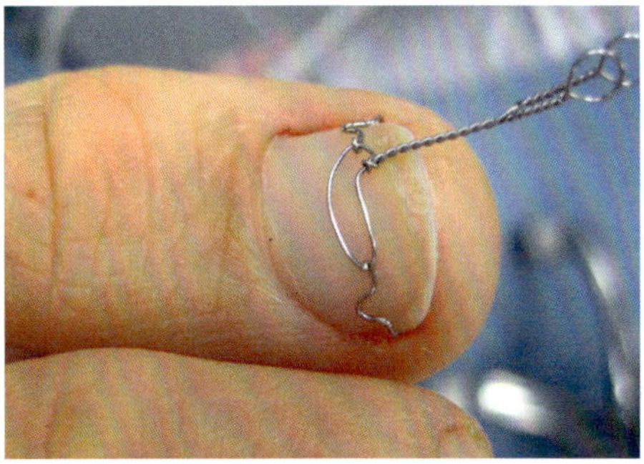

Image 5.282 Clavus risk. Concentrated pressure on the nail plus the center loop is not centered correctly resulting in uneven tensile force distribution.

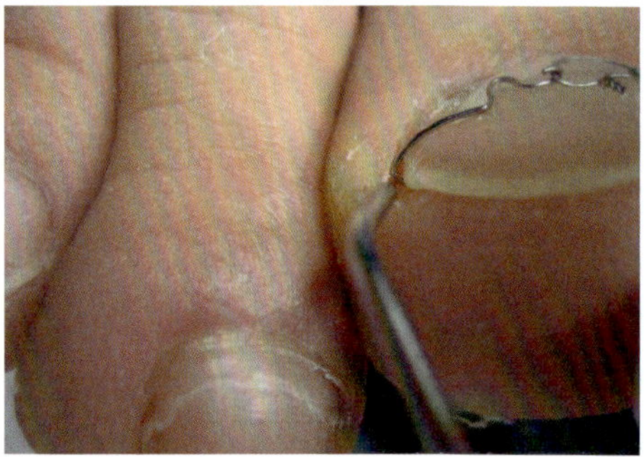

Image 5.283 Incorrect hook positioning causing sulcus irritation

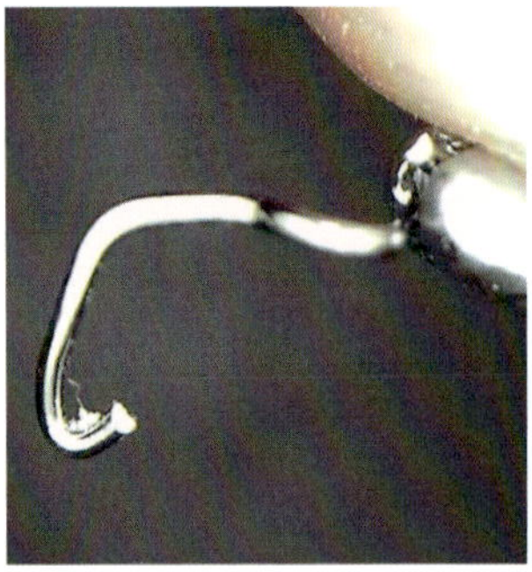

Image 5.284 Failure to trim the hook ends correctly can cause tissue injuries

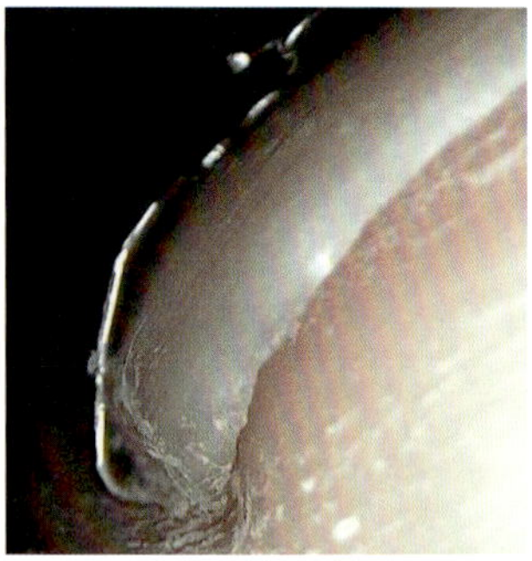

Image 5.285 Incorrectly bent wires

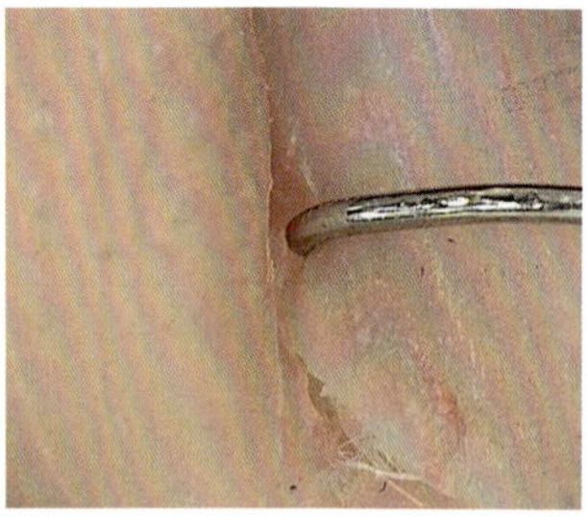

Image 5.286 Overactivation of the brace on a thin nail

6

Nail prosthetics

6 Nail prosthetics

The term nail prosthetics signifies the therapeutic effective replacement of damaged parts of the nail plate by placing an artificial nail or nail part over the affected area. This technique is also used to reinforce damaged nail plates.

Two different groups can be distinguished:

- as a temporary measure (subungual clavus or onycholysis)
- for the treatment of permanent damage, such as onychodystrophy or onychomadesis

The following techniques are suitable:

- casting technique
- plate prosthetics
- Impro System
- BS Nail
- light-curing technique
- acrylate material
- Unguisan technique
- brush application of synthetic materials

The most frequently used techniques are described below.

6.1 Casting technique

Materials

Cold-curing synthetic material (powder and liquid). The powder comes in three different colours: clear, pink and opal.

Work materials (image 6.1)

- dappen dish
- spatula
- tamponade
- probe/excavator
- pipette
- small spoon.
- Onycholit (Gerlach)
- Unguisan (Greppmayr)
- Paladur (Kulzer)

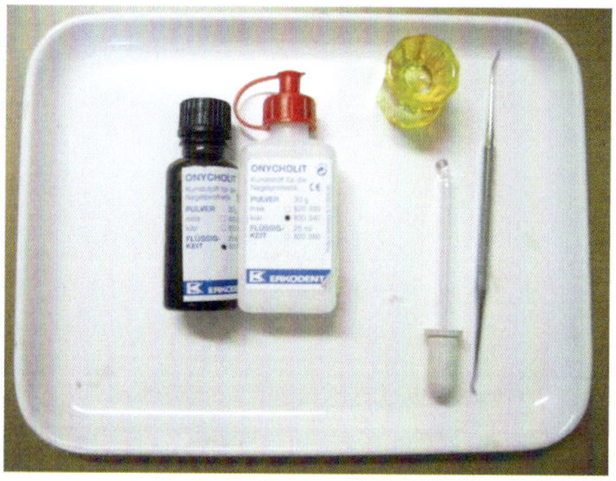

Image 6.1

Indications

- nail plate replacement
- partial nail plate replacement
- correction of a curved toe tip
- protection from friction
- fixation of an orthonyxia brace

Contraindications

- nail bed injury
- nail bed infection
- granulation tissue
- eczema in the nail bed area
- onychomycosis
- complete nail loss, can have different causes

Instructions (images 6.2 to 6.6)

Remove all hornification and brittle nail parts. Degrease the nail plate with acetone or benzene (do not use an alcohol con taining solution since it impairs adhesion). Apply tamponades to the nail fold. Combine a spoonful of powder with six drops of liquid (equates to five parts liquids and three parts powder) in a dappen dish and blend swiftly with a small spatula for about 15 to 20 seconds until the consistency of the mixture resembles liquid honey. Distribute the mixture evenly on the nail and reconstruct the nail. Placing cellulose film over the nail facilitates the contouring process. Remove the tamponade. After a curing time of five minutes the nail is ready for grinding.

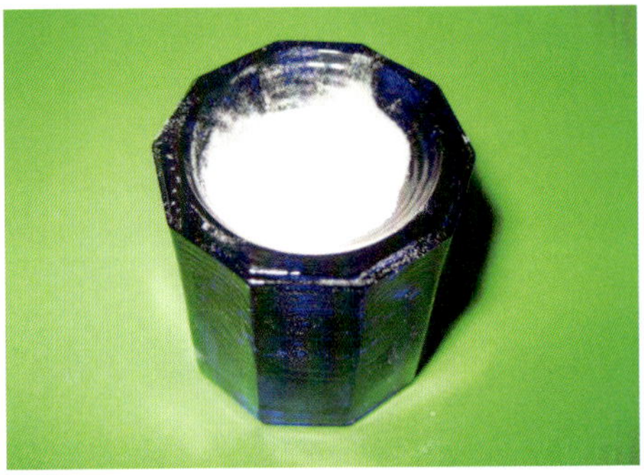
Image 6.2

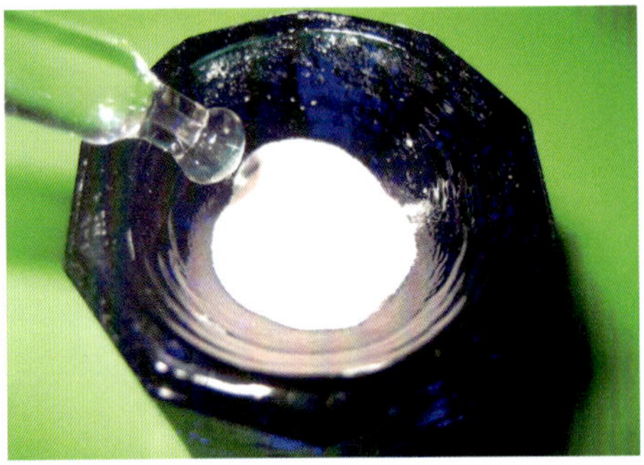
Image 6.3

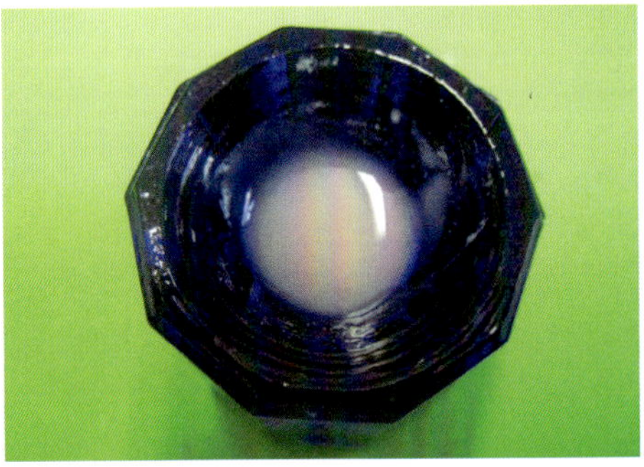
Image 6.4

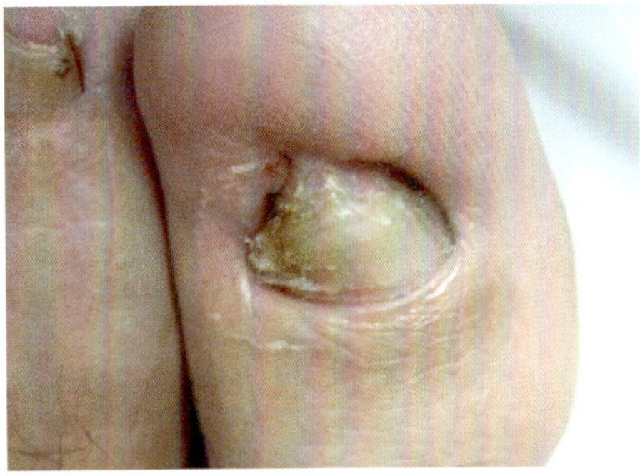
Image 6.5

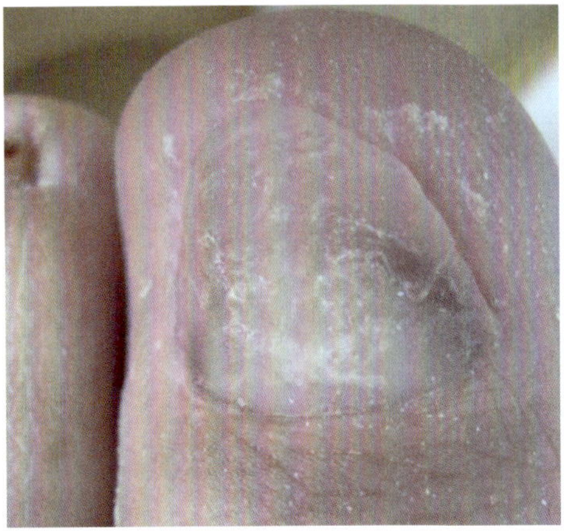
Image 6.6

Recommendations
Apply the mixture in layers preventing deformation and overheating (chemical reaction).

Store the materials at room temperature in brown bottles and protect them from sunlight.

6.2 Casting technique with rhodoid

Materials

- 0.5 millimeters thick clear, thermoplastic pliable cellulose-acetate (rhodoid) sheet.
- Cold-curing synthetic material (powder and liquid). The powder comes in three different colours: clear, pink and opal.

Work materials

- dappen dish
- spatula
- tamponade
- probe/excavator
- pipette
- small spoon
- Onycholit (Gerlach)
- Unguisan (Greppmayr)
- Paladur (Kulzer)

Indications

Correcting a nail bed too narrowly formed distally.

Contraindications

- nail bed injury
- nail bed infection
- granulation tissue
- eczema in the nail bed area
- onychomycosis
- complete nail loss, can have different causes

Instructions (image 6.7)

Cut an acute-angled triangle out of the sheet. The length of the triangle must be the same as the visible lateral nail margin and, to facilitate positioning of the splint, be at least 10 millimetres longer than the tip of the toe. Round off the triangle's edges with a corundum grinder. Bend the triangle and push it under the proximal lateral nail margin; the tip of the triangle must be positioned so that it is slightly lower than the original nail width. Press the distal part of the splint gently outward against the nail wall, widening the nail bed. Keep the splint in this position until

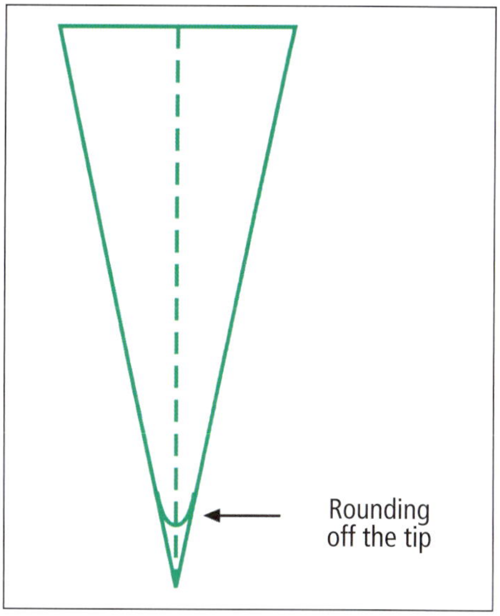

Image 6.7 Acute-angled triangle with center-line fold

Source: Klaus Grünewald, Theorie der medizinischen Fußbehandlung – tome 2, 3rd edition 2016, Verlag Neuer Merkur

the material has completely hardened. Combine a spoonful of powder with six drops of liquid (equates to five parts liquid and three parts powder) in a dappen dish and blend swiftly with a small spatula for about 15 to 20 seconds until the consistency of the mixture resembles liquid honey. Finally, grind off protruding edges and insert tamponade in the nail fold.

6.3 Plate prosthetics

Materials
Cold-curing synthetic material (powder and liquid). The powder comes in three different colours: clear, pink and opal.

Work materials (image 6.8)
- two plexiglass plates (5 to 10 mm thick)
- Leukotape P (BSN medical)
- dappen dish
- spatula
- tamponade
- probe/excavator
- pipette
- small spoon
- Onycholit (Gerlach)
- Unguisan (Greppmayr)
- Paladur (Kulzer)

Indications
- nail plate replacement
- correcting an upward pointing toe tip
- correcting a nail bed too narrowly formed distally

Contraindications
- nail bed injury
- nail bed infection
- granulation tissue
- eczema in the nail bed area
- Onychomycosis
- complete nail loss, can have different causes

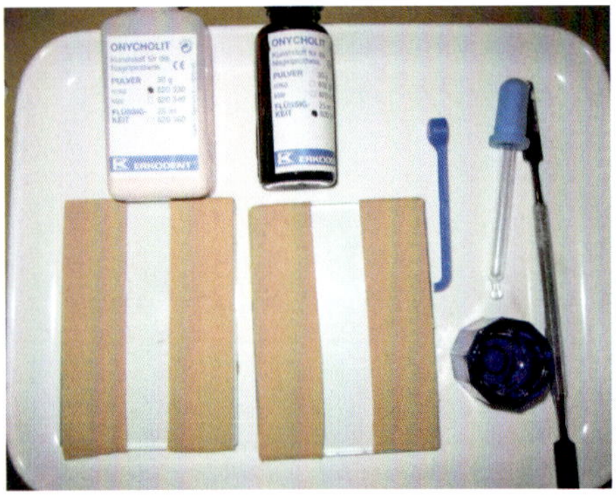

Image 6.8

Instructions (images 6.9 to 6.18)
- To produce an artificial nail plate, stick two Leukotape strips to one glass plate to create uniform spacing. Blend a small amount of synthetic material. Ensure that there is no bubble formation. Combine powder and liquid (five parts liquids and three parts powder) in a dappen dish and blend swiftly with a small spatula for about 15 to 20 seconds until the consistency of the mixture resembles liquid honey. Pour almost all material onto the plexiglass plate with the Leukotape strips and place the second plexiglass plate on top.
- Press both plates gently together ensuring an even distribution of the material.
- Once the material has hardened, the two plates are separated with a spatula.
- Since 1997 prefabricated transparent plates (PG190, Greppmayr) are available, plus 30 types of plate prosthetics that can be individually cut out with scissors.

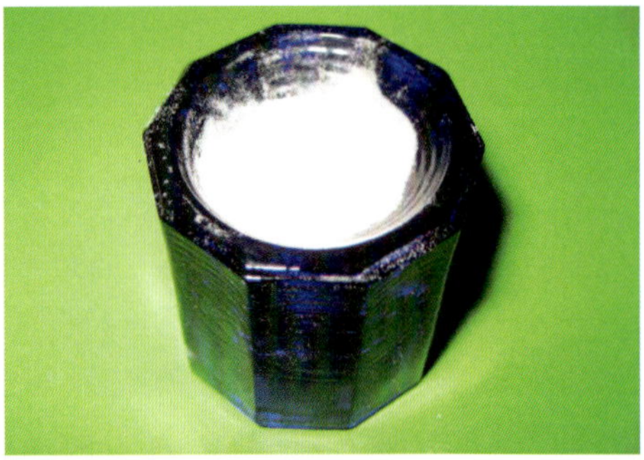

Image 6.9

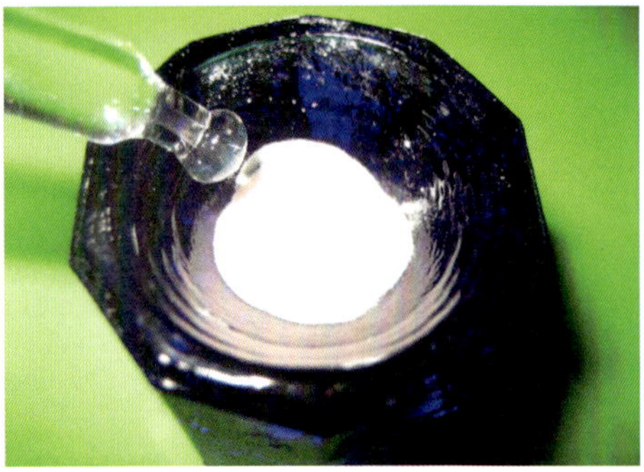

Image 6.10

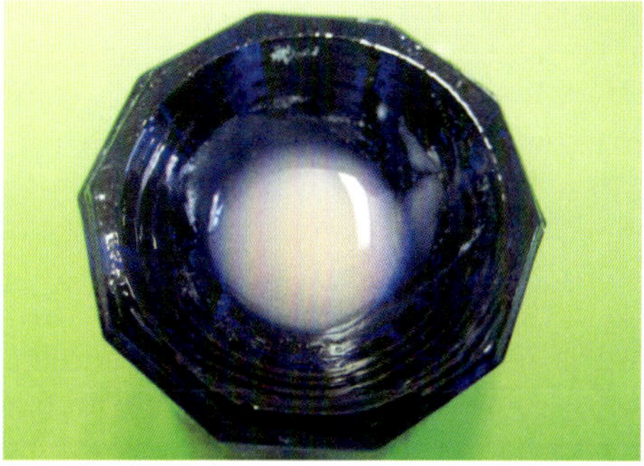

Image 6.11

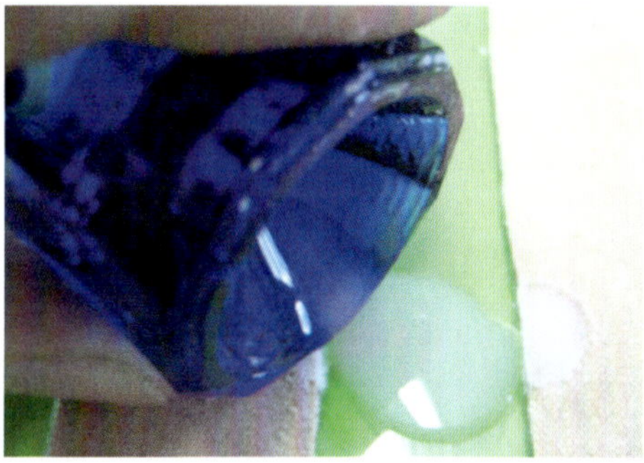

Image 6.12

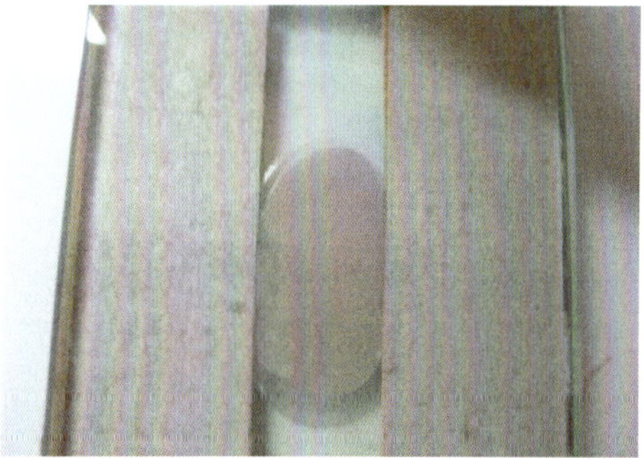

Image 6.13

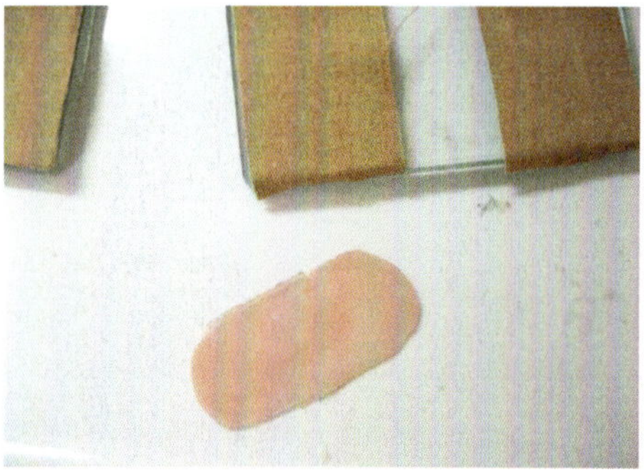

Image 6.14

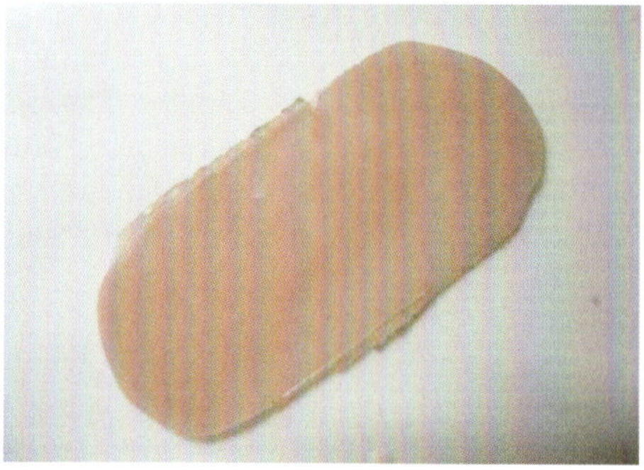

Image 6.15

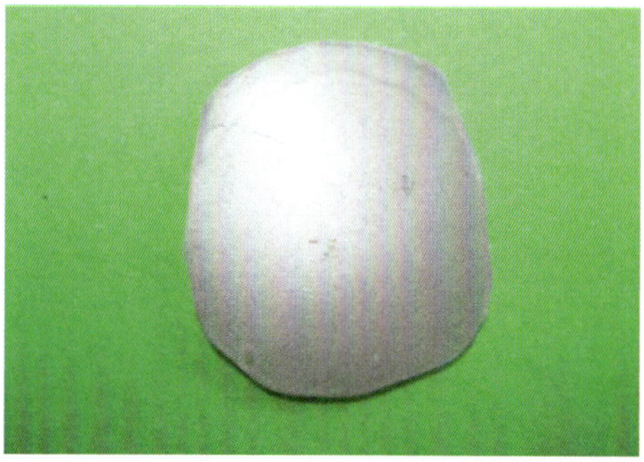

Image 6.16

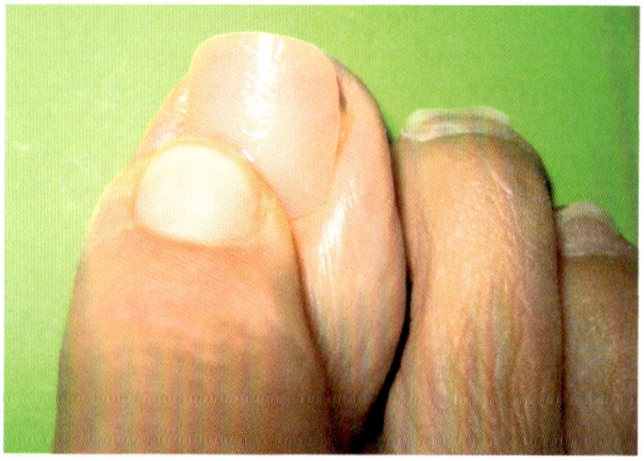

Image 6.17

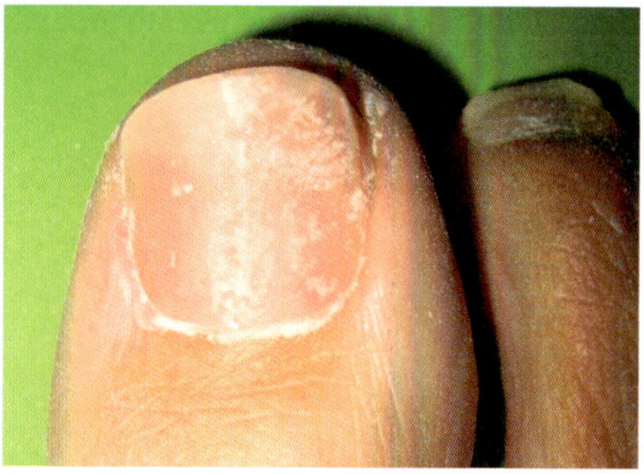

Image 6.18

Applying the plate prosthetic

- Warm the produced plate prior to cutting, then carefully cut out the original nail shape with scissors. Warming the plate makes the material more pliable and ensures that the prosthetic nail properly conforms to the transversal curvature of the nail bed.
- PG190 material is pliable even when cold and can be shaped with a round-nose-plier.
- Use the left-over material mixture to fixate the prosthetic nail.
- Distribute the material on the remaining natural nail.
- Place the prosthetic nail at a steep angle on the proximal nail wall and gently push it down in the direction of the toe tip.
- Prior to hardening, remove excess material with a spatula.
- Hold the prosthetic nail in place with your fingers until it has completely adhered.
- Apply tamponade.
- The prosthetic nail is re-usable once all the bonding material has been removed with a grinding tool.

6.4 Unguisan® nail plate prostheses

Materials

For a plate prosthesis, use a pre-shaped nail plate made of transparent cold-mouldable plastic material.

Unguisan is a two-component synthetic resin consisting of powder and hardener liquid. Immediately after those two components are combined, a chemical cross-linking process (polymerization) occurs lasting a few minutes. During this time, the material can be shaped into the desired form. The result is an artificial nail that closely resembles a natural nail in colour, shape and texture and bonds solidly and gently to the natural nail.

Work materials (image 6.19)

- artificial nail plate made of transparent plastic
- orthonyxia round nose pliers
- Unguisan powder and hardener liquid
- cutting tool
- measurement spoon
- spatula

Indications

- loss of nail caused by trauma
- onychorrhexis
- onychoschizia
- onychogryposis
- chronic nail injuries
- temporary deformity
- cosmetic reasons

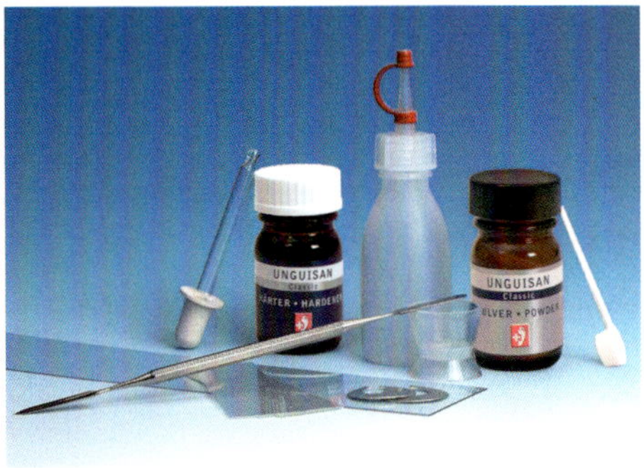

Image 6.19 Work materials

Contraindications
- open wound
- nail bed injuries
- nail or skin mycoses

Instructions
- Remove loose or damaged nail parts and hornifications.
- Ensure that the remaining natural nail and the nail bed are dry, grease-free and clean.
- Apply dry tamponades and adhesive film where needed to provide adequate level compensation for the artificial nail.
- Use a pre-shaped nail plate made of transparent cold-mouldable plastic material and shape it with hand tools (e.g., orthonyxia round-nose pliers) and grinding tools to fit the original nail organ. Combine and blend Unguisan powder and hardener liquid (approximately 20 drops hardener per white measuring spoon of powder). Apply the mixture with a spatula once it has a pasty consistency that will adhere the artificial nail plate to the remaining natural nail. The evenly distributed material and Unguisan's unique colour create a natural-looking artificial nail.

The most significant advantage of a plate prosthesis is its effect on the entire nail organ. The applied pressure during the hardening process remains constant, thereby pushing upward pointing toe tips or pronounced nail walls allowing the natural nail to grow without being obstructed.

Depending on the individual situation, a nail prosthesis can be worn up to three months, thereby achieving long-term therapy results, which also highlights the economic benefit of this method. The patient is comfortable and is not hindered in his daily activities. The artificial nail grows with the natural nail and can be shortened with a diamond file.

Part of the natural nail must be present to ensure proper adhesion of the artificial nail.

Unguisan processing issues

If Unguisan does not completely harden, but "crystallizes" instead, there can be various causes for this:

1. The hardener liquid is compromised in some way, e.g., by incorrect storage, using expired materials or the presence of dirt.
2. The mixing ratio is incorrect.
3. The mixture was not blended long enough.
4. The mixed quantity is too small (the desired homogeneity of the compound has not been achieved).

If the first cause can be eliminated, we recommend the following approach:

Take at least two measuring spoons of the powder. Slowly add the liquid until the mixture has the consistency of fresh honey. The consistency of the mixture should be slightly more liquid and under no circumstances less liquid. Giving an exact recommendation on how many drops should be added to one spoon is difficult since the drop size might vary for each pipette and other factors such as temperature, air moisture, etc., must be taken into consideration.

Blend powder and liquid thoroughly until a homogenous mixture has been achieved. Definitely keep blending until the hardening process starts to set in. The mixture becomes pasty and loses its shine looking more opaque. Only now is the mixture ready to be poured, leaving enough time to prepare the nail plate.

The following illustrates a few application examples (images 6.20 to 6.23).

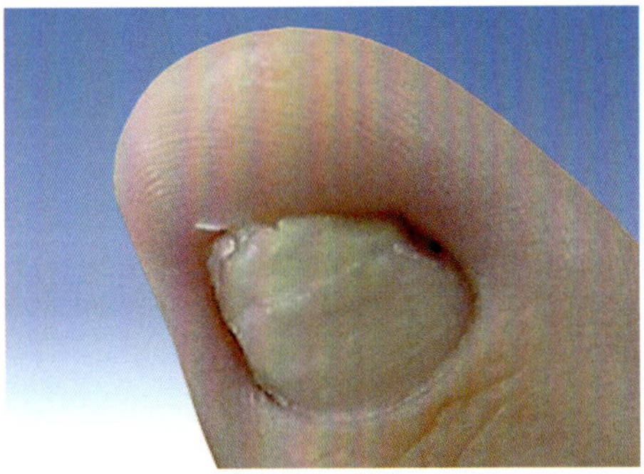

Image 6.20 Plate prosthesis before

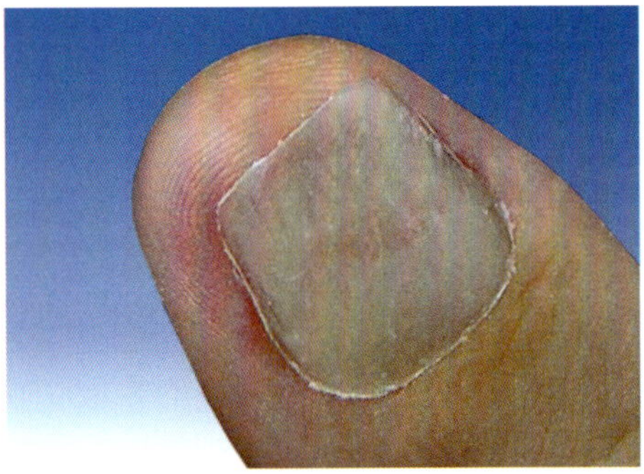

Image 6.21 Plate prosthesis after

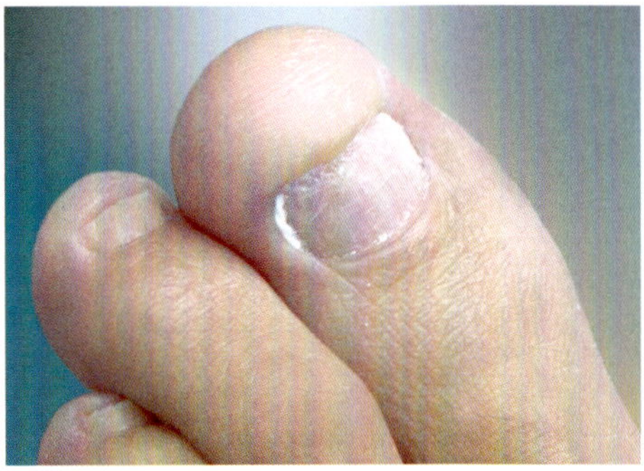

Image 6.22 Casting prosthesis before

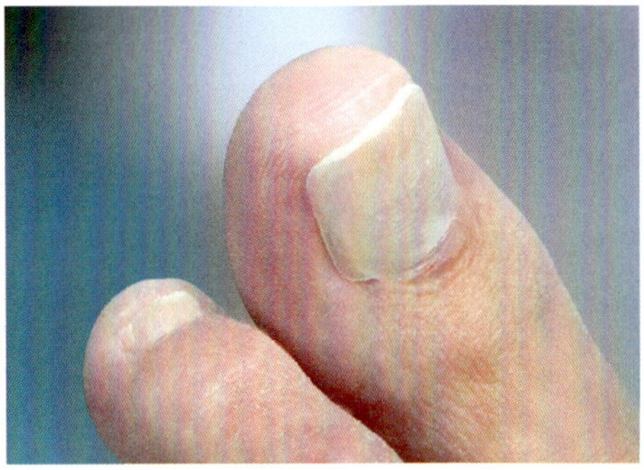

Image 6.23 Casting prosthesis after

6.5 Impro System (Erkodent)

Materials

Thermoplastic polyethylene terephthalate (pet)-foil and synthetic material (powder and liquid).

Work materials (image 6.24)

- impression material and Kneton hardener (condensation-cured silicone)
- impression tray
- impression spoon
- Erko super hard plaster
- mixing bowl
- blocking out plaster
- Onycholit liquid
- Onycholit powder, clear and pink
- scissors
- form pot
- Erkodur foils
- spirit lamp
- foil holder
- degreasing agent

Indications

- nail plate replacement
- partial replacement of the nail plate
- correcting an upward pointing toe tip
- correcting a nail bed too narrowly formed distally

Contraindications

- nail bed injury
- nail bed infection
- granulation tissue
- eczema in the nail bed area

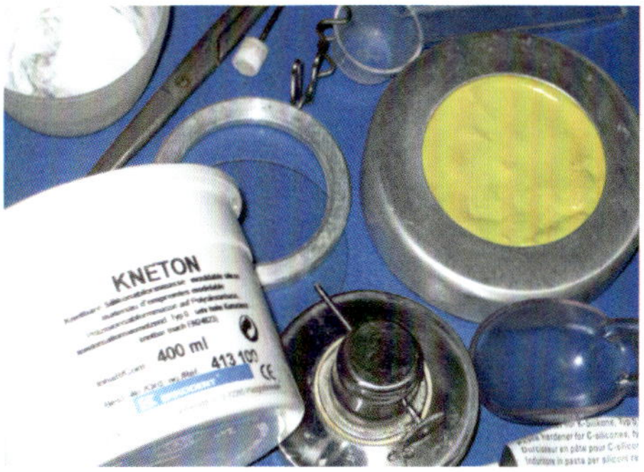

Image 6.24 Work materials

- onychomycosis
- complete nail loss, can have different causes

Instructions (images 6.25 to 6.45)

Blend the Kneton impression material with hardener paste, according to the instructions, until the material displays uniform colouring. The blending process should take a maximum of 30 seconds.

Insert the mixture into the Eckle impression spoon and flatten it.

Place the spoon on the toe and press down applying sufficient pressure. Remove the spoon after approximately three to four minutes and cut excess overhanging material from the spoon.

Pour Erko super hard plaster into the Kneton mould.

Remove the plaster model once the plaster is completely hard and cut away any excess mould material.

The new nail shape or missing nail parts are contoured and built up with Infra material. Apply the blocking out plaster material with a spatula. Smooth the surface with a moist brush or, after the material has hardened, use fine sandpaper to give the nail its final shape. Start at the remaining nail fold and grind off the plaster in a slightly slanted inwards growth direction of about two to three millimetres deep. Also use a grinding tool to remove the possibly upward pointing toe tip.

Insert the Erkodur foil in the foil holder and carefully warm both sides over a spirit lamp.

Test the softness of the foil with a blunt instrument and, if it leaves indents, the foil is ready for deep-drawing.

Place the foil holder on the form pot and press the prepared plaster model downwards at an angle through the pre-heated foil into the form pot. Remove the plaster model after a few seconds. Allow foil holder and foil to cool down before removal.

Compress the yellow material in the form pot to create a smooth surface.

Cut out a rough shape of the nail plate with scissors. The accurate fit will be determined on the patient.

Smooth the edges of the artificial nail plate with a file or a sanding wheel and sand the inside of the nail creating a rough surface.

Degrease the artificial nail plate, remaining natural nail and nail bed.

Mix Onycholit until it displays the desired colour (pink, clear) and has a viscous consistency.

Apply Onycholit to the artificial nail plate and on the remaining natural nail or nail bed.

Place the artificial nail plate and only press down on the area of the remaining natural nail. Pull the upward pointing toe tip downwards with the other hand, thereby using the artificial nail plate as a corrective tool. Remove the soft excess with a spatula. Alternatively, a cyanoacrylate adhesive (instant adhesive) can be used to secure the nail, but it must only be applied to the healthy part of the natural nail. This facilitates the evaluation and observation of the growing nail.

Secure the artificial nail plate with an adhesive strip and use a grinding tool to give the nail its final shape.

Finish by applying cream to the nail plate.

The nail plate must be cut every four to six weeks, depending on the individual growth rate, to prevent the plate from lifting.

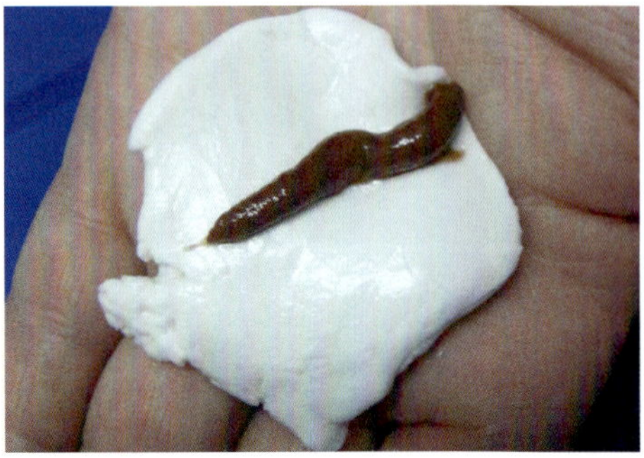

Image 6.26

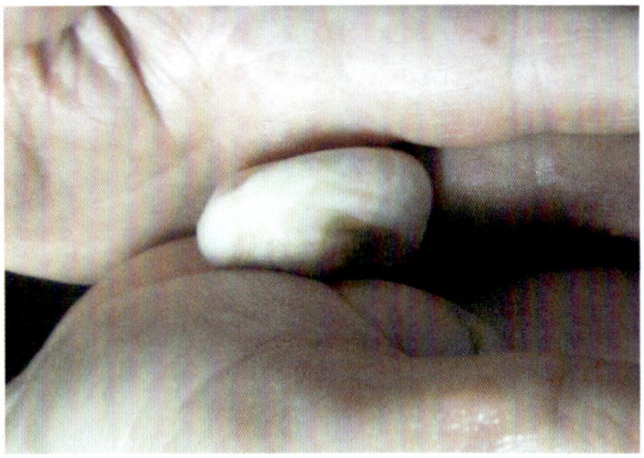

Image 6.27

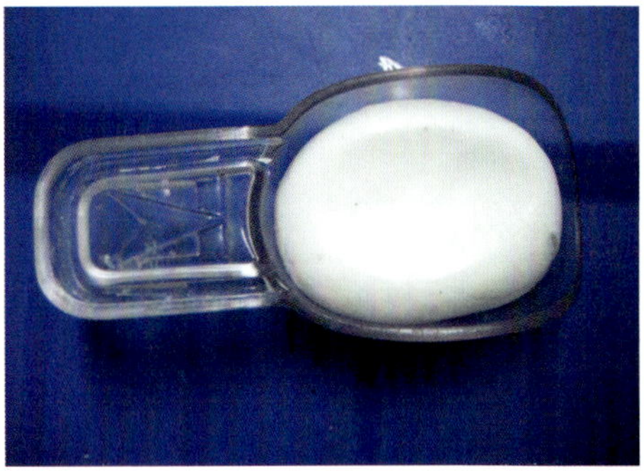

Image 6.28

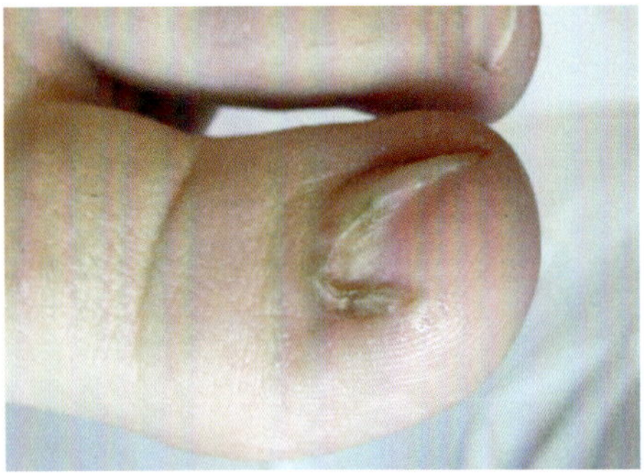

Image 6.25

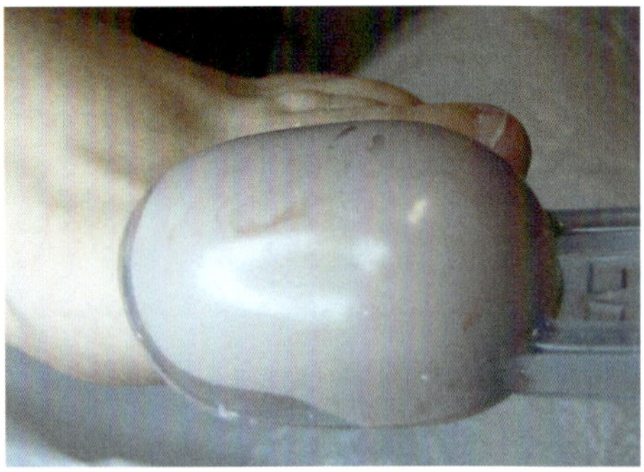

Image 6.29

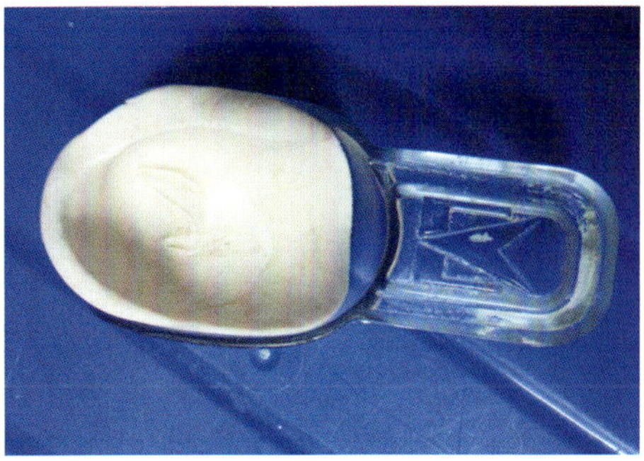

Image 6.30

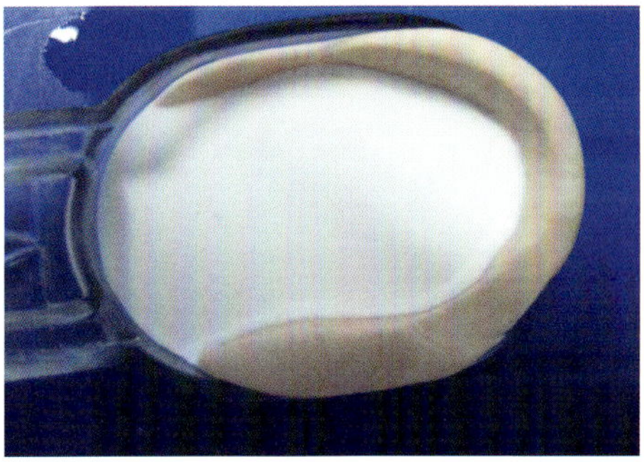

Image 6.31

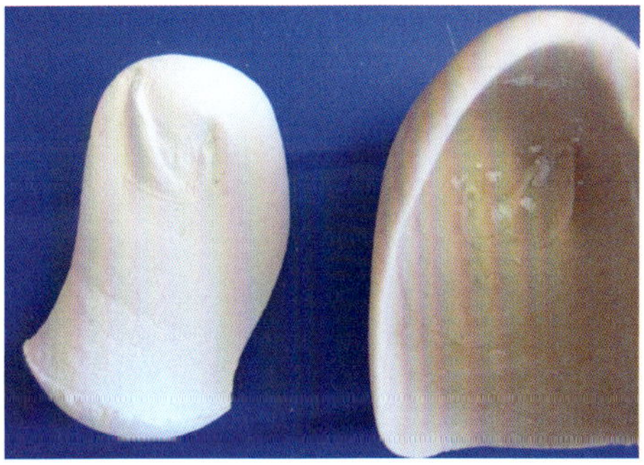

Image 6.32

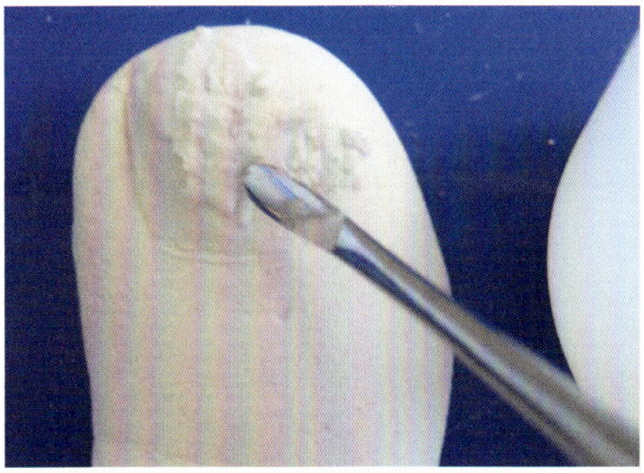

Image 6.33

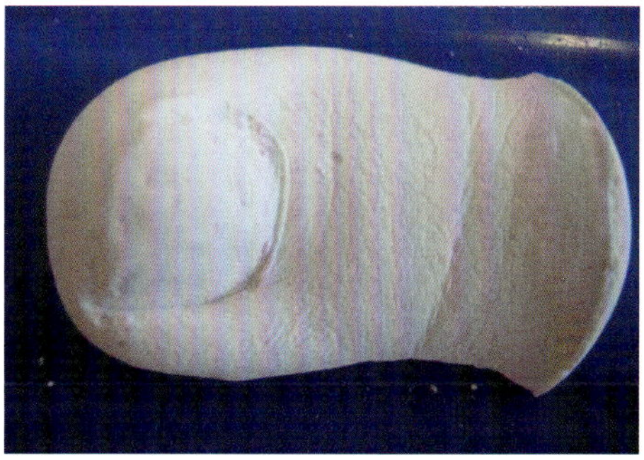

Image 6.34

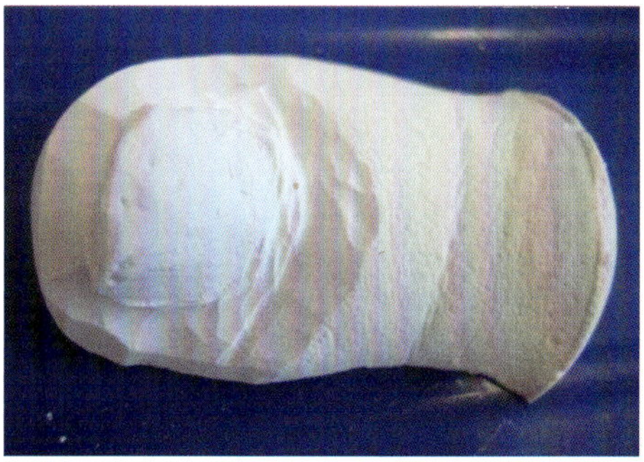

Image 6.35

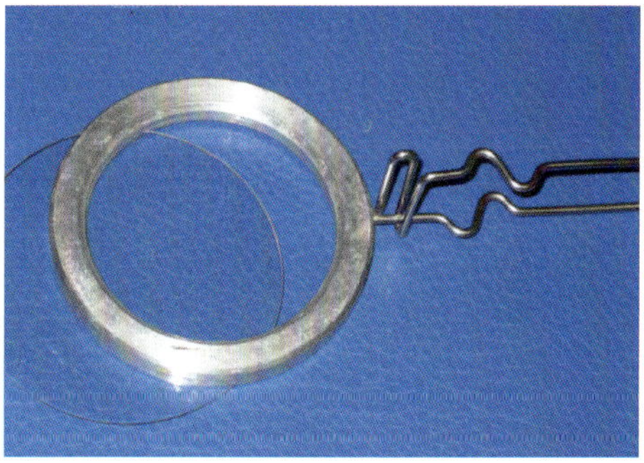

Image 6.36

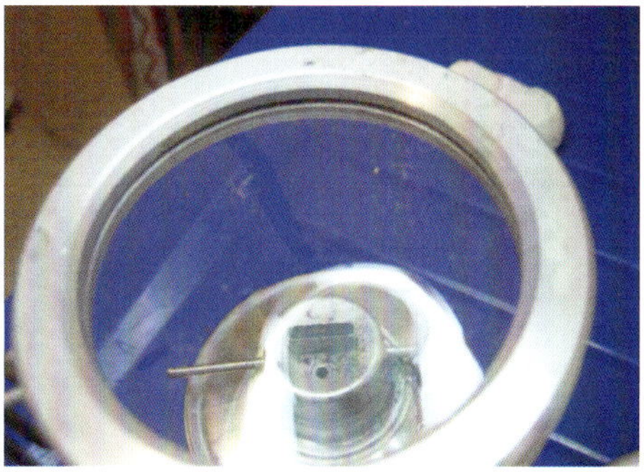

Image 6.37

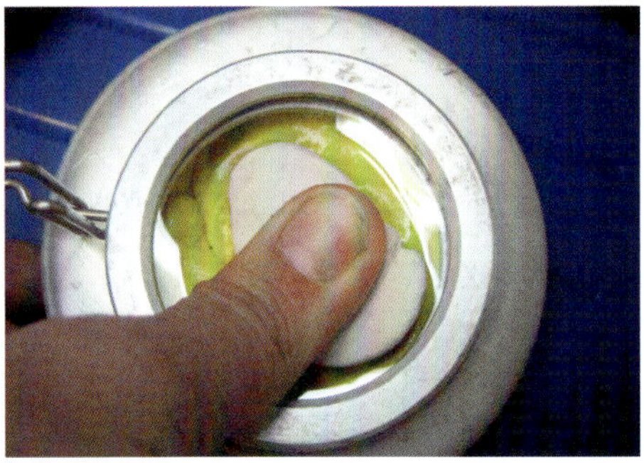

Image 6.38

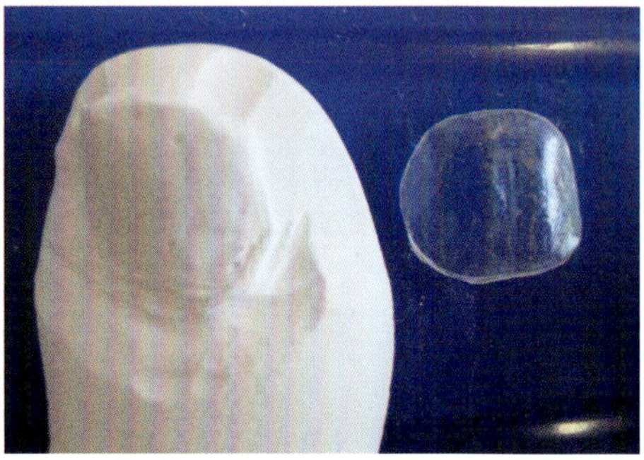

Image 6.42

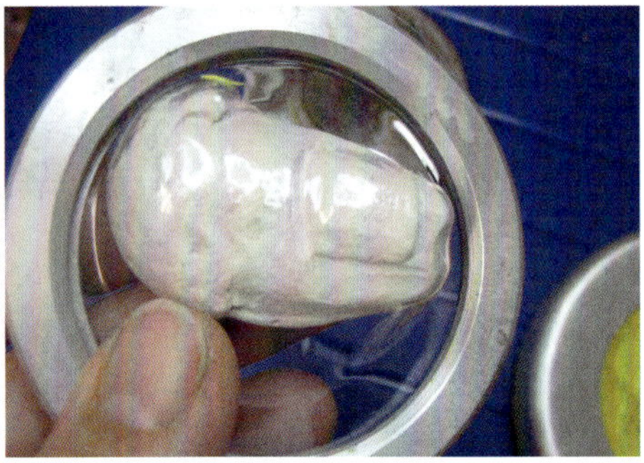

Image 6.39

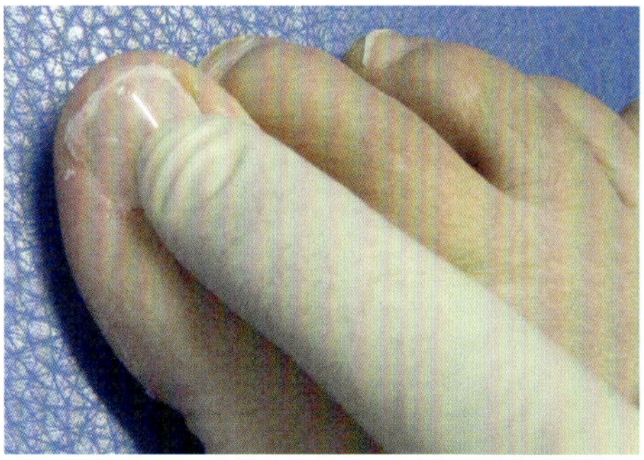

Image 6.43

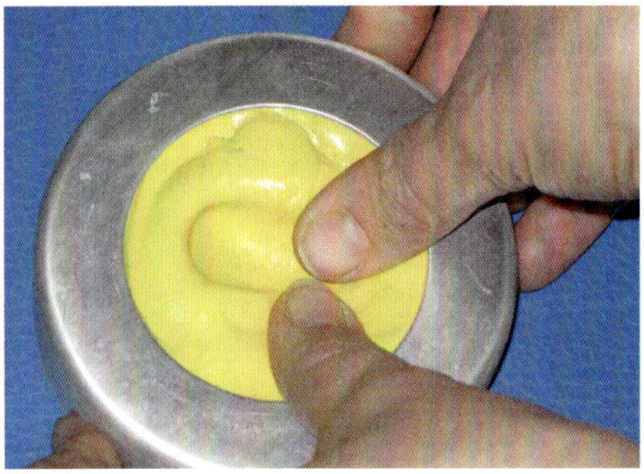

Image 6.40

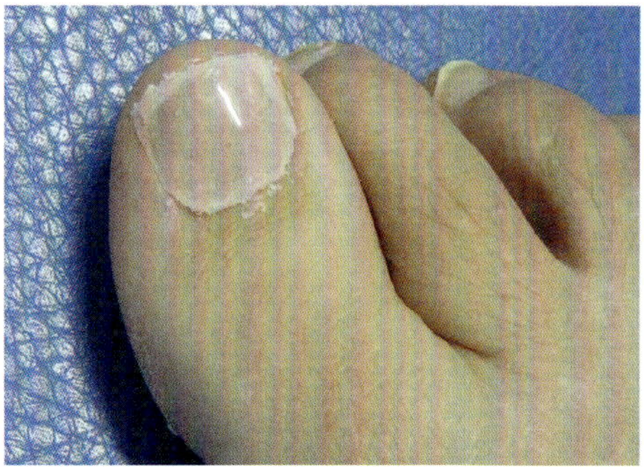

Image 6.44

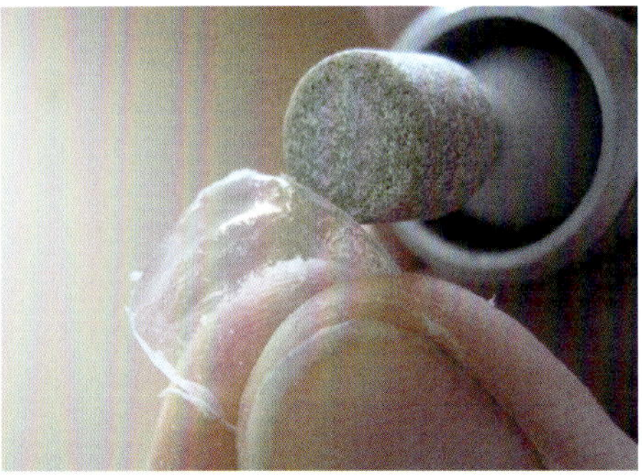

Image 6.41

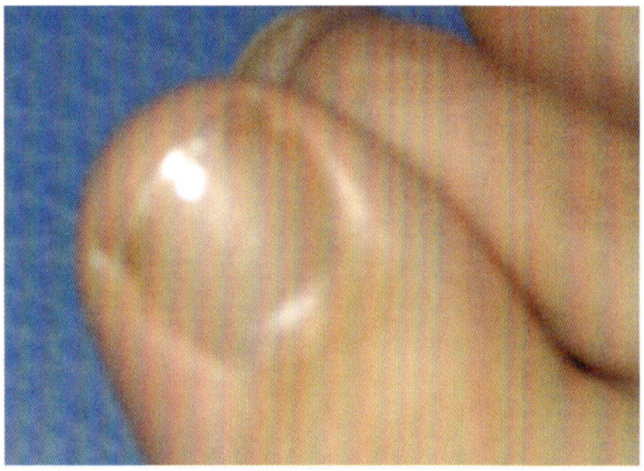

Image 6.45

6.6 BS Nail

Materials
Nail strip made of glass fibre.

Work materials *(image 6.46)*
- BS nail liquid
- BS filler, powder and liquid
- surgical spirit
- nailstrip made of glass fibre
- applicator
- BS nail liquid dry

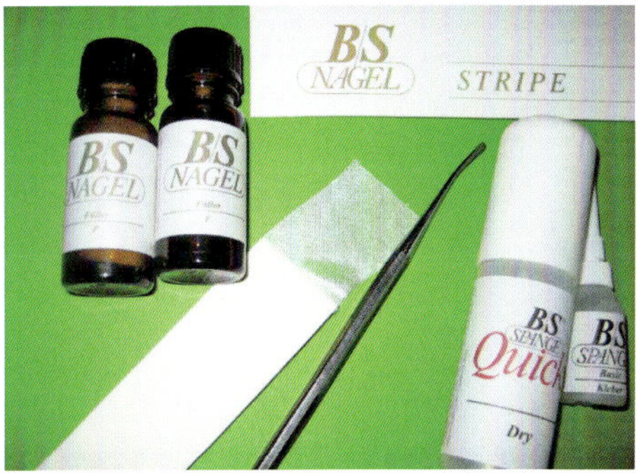

Image 6.46

Indications
- nail plate replacement
- partial replacement of the nail plate
- reinforcing a thin nail plate
- correcting an upward pointing toe tip
- correcting a nail bed too narrowly formed distally

Contraindications
- nail bed injury
- nail bed infection
- granulation tissue
- eczema in the nail bed area
- onychomycosis
- complete nail loss, can have different causes

Instructions

Partially loosened or torn nail
- Degrease nail with surgical spirit or acetone (image 6.47).

Image 6.47

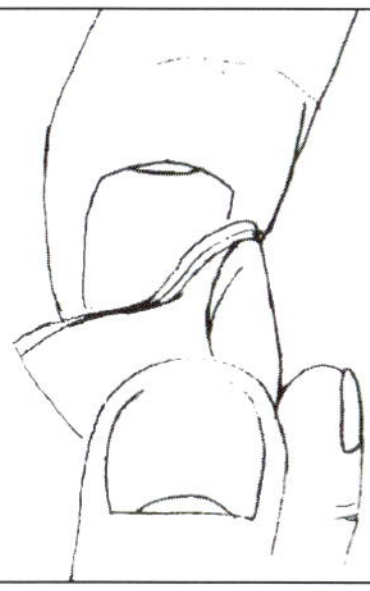

- Once the surgical spirit has evaporated, apply a small amount of nail liquid under the loose nail plate (image 6.48). Wait three seconds.

Image 6.48

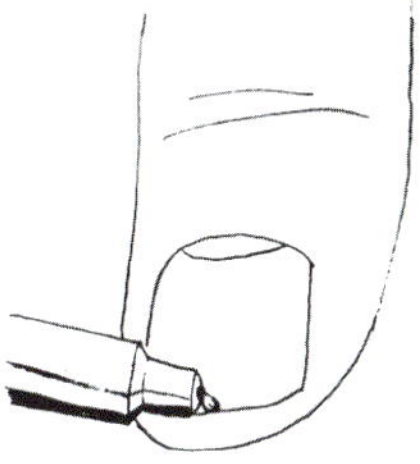

- Cut a self-adhesive BS glass fibre strip and place it on the nail for reinforcement. The strip must fit the width of the nail (images 6.49 to 6.51).

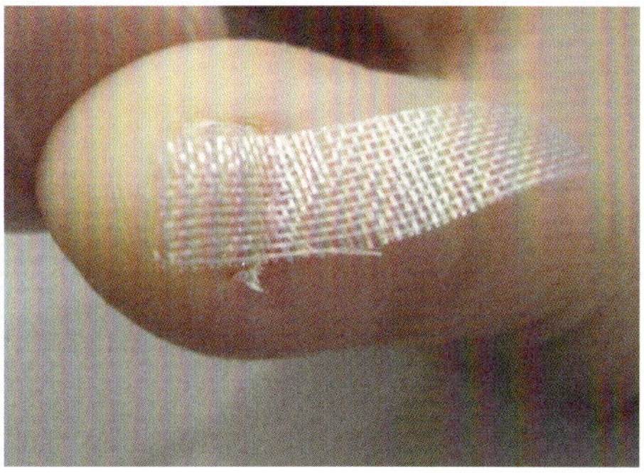

Image 6.49

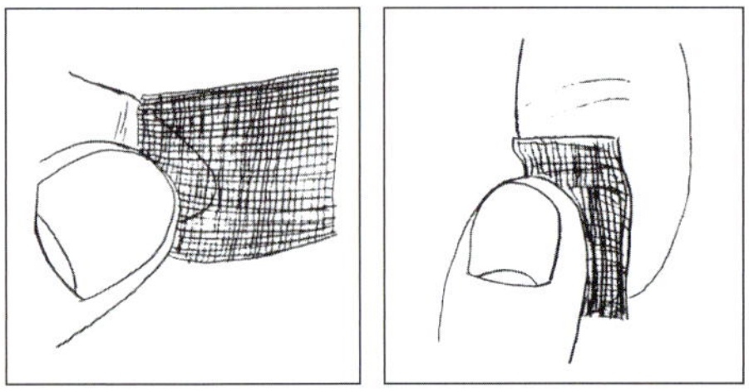

Image 6.50 and 6.51

- Apply a small amount of BS nail liquid (cyanoacrylate) ensuring not to come 1 mm within the cuticle or lateral nail fold since it can cause irritation in those areas (images 6.52 to 6.55).

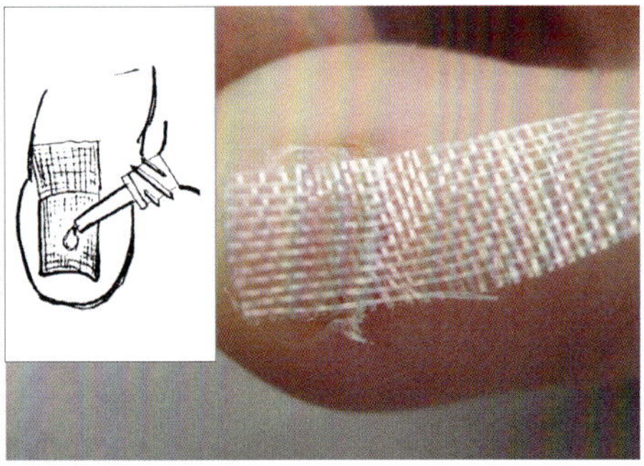

Image 6.52 and 6.53

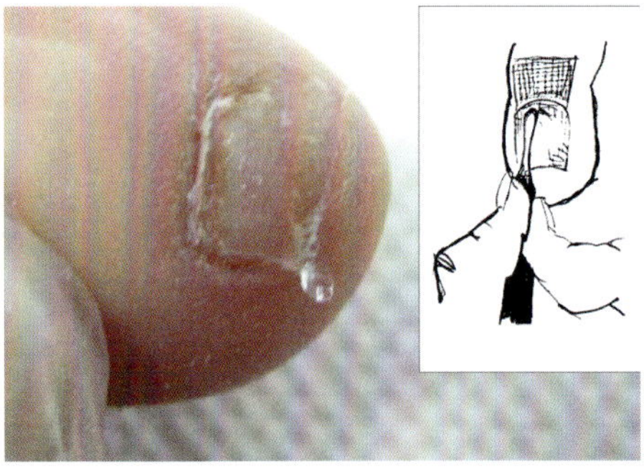

Image 6.54 and 6.55

- Spray BS nail liquid dry (accelerates drying) on the nail. Hold the bottle 10 cm away from the nail while spraying. The artificial nail dries instantly and is ready for further processing. Applying too much nail liquid may cause the nail to get hot after spraying (images 6.56 and 6.57).

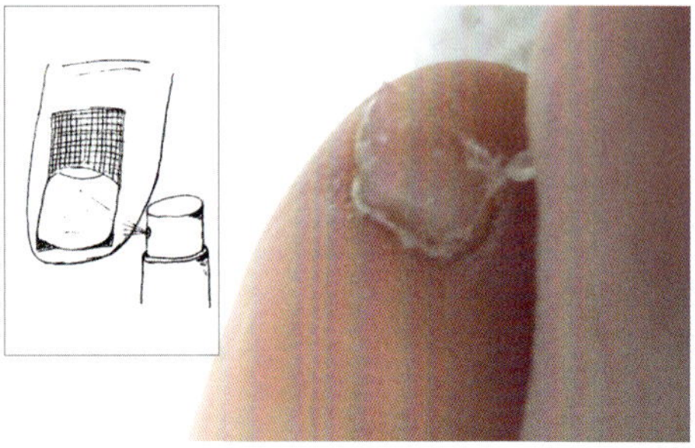

Image 6.56 and 6.57

- Gently pull off the extra glass fibre strip at the nail root and carefully grind off all other glass fibre remnants around the nail with corundum stone (images 6.58 to 6.61).

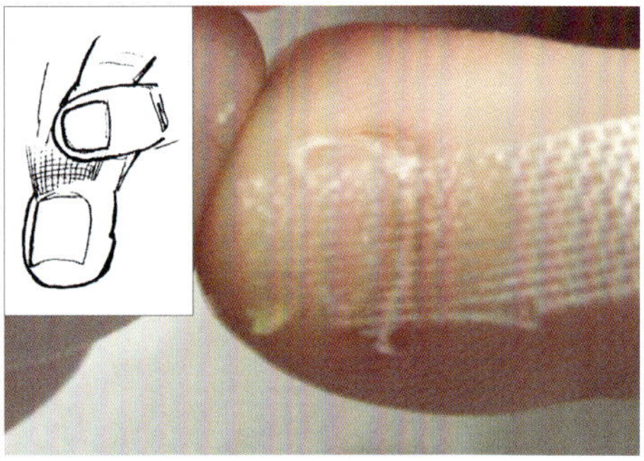

Image 6.58 and 6.59

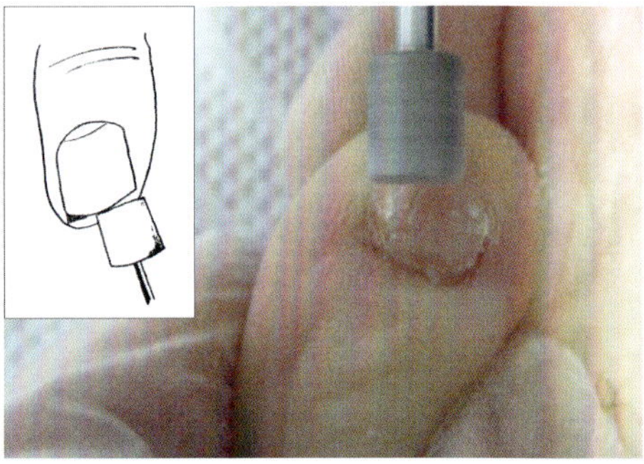

Image 6.60 and 6.61

- Finally, apply nail polish to the nail plate and spray with BS nail liquid dry spray to prevent the nail polish from running into the nail fold. If this happens, remove immediately (images 6.62 to 6.64)!

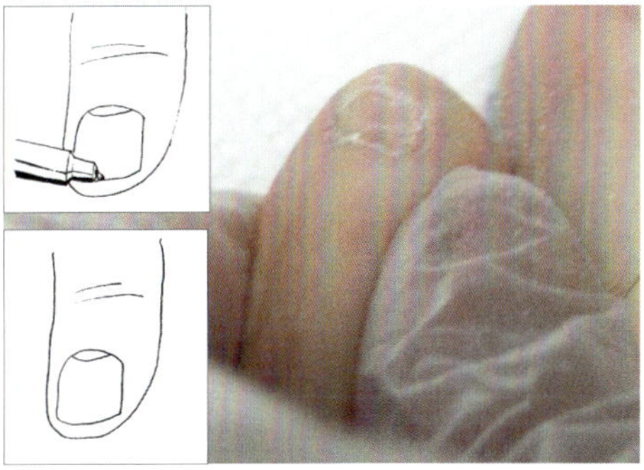

Image 6.62 to 6.64

Replacing a partially missing nail

At least half of the nail should still be there.

- Replace the missing nail part with soft pliable material ensuring that it is flush with the remaining part of the nail (images 6.65 to 6.68).

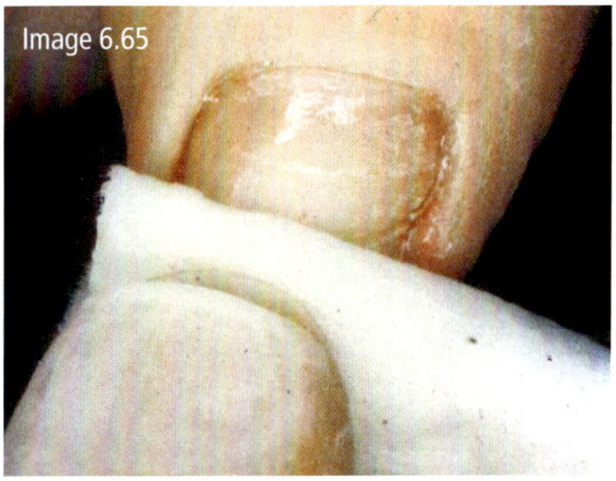

Image 6.65

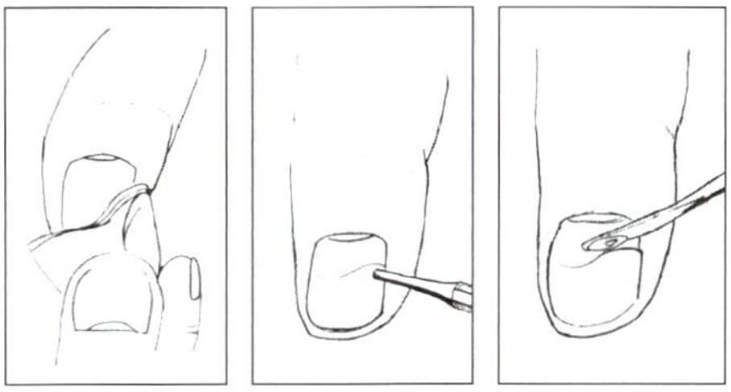

Image 6.66 to 6.68

- After approximately three minutes, the material has hardened. The process is similar to that of the partially loosened nail except that the reinforcement step must be repeated three times (image 6.69).

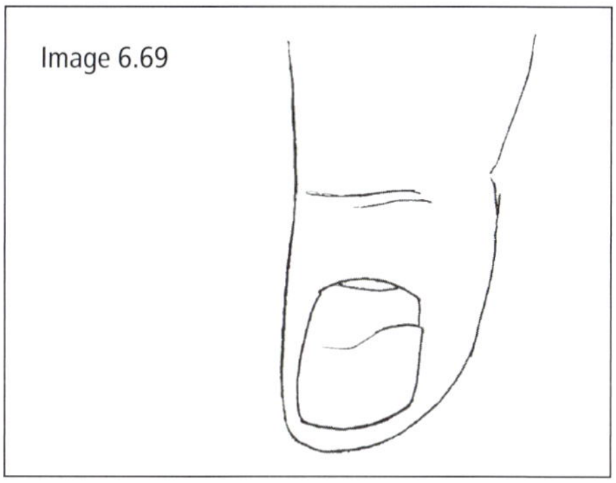

Image 6.69

- Cut a self-adhesive BS glass fibre strip and place it on the nail for reinforcement. The strip must fit the width of the nail (images 6.70 to 6.72).

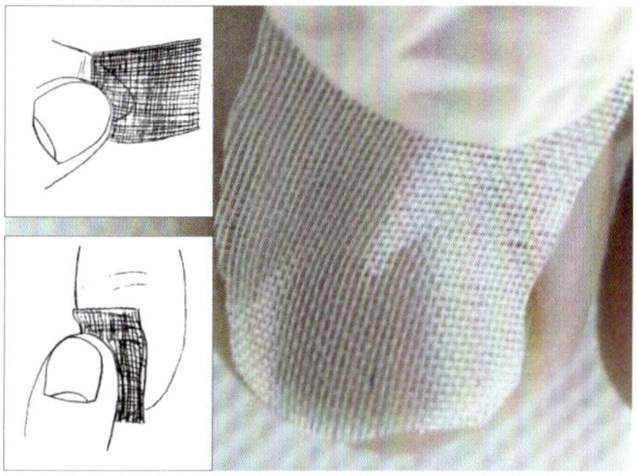

Image 6.70 to 6.72

- Apply a small amount of BS nail liquid (cyanoacrylate) ensuring not to come within 1 mm of the cuticle or lateral nail fold since it can cause irritation in those areas (images 6.73 to 6.76).

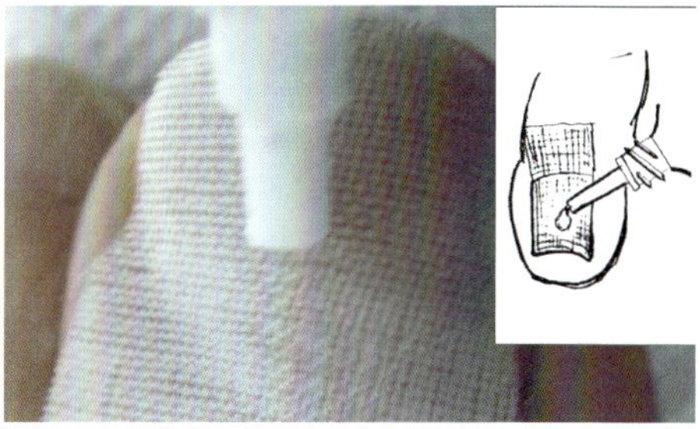

Image 6.73 and 6.74

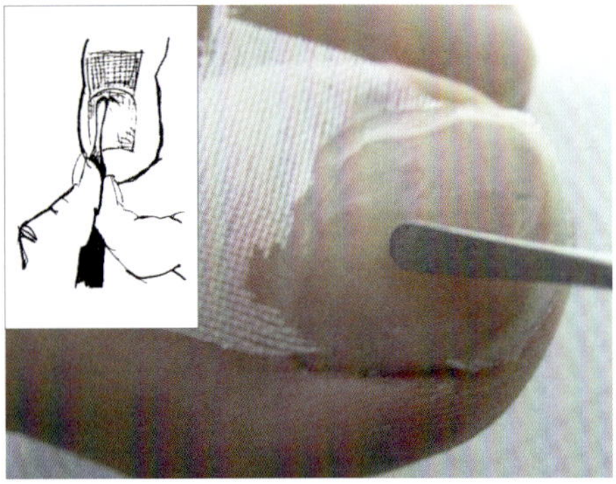

Image 6.75 and 6.76

- Spray BS nail liquid dry (accelerates drying) on the nail. Hold the bottle 10 cm away from the nail while spraying. The artificial nail dries instantly and is ready for further processing. Applying too much nail liquid may cause the nail to get hot after spraying (images 6.77 and 6.78).

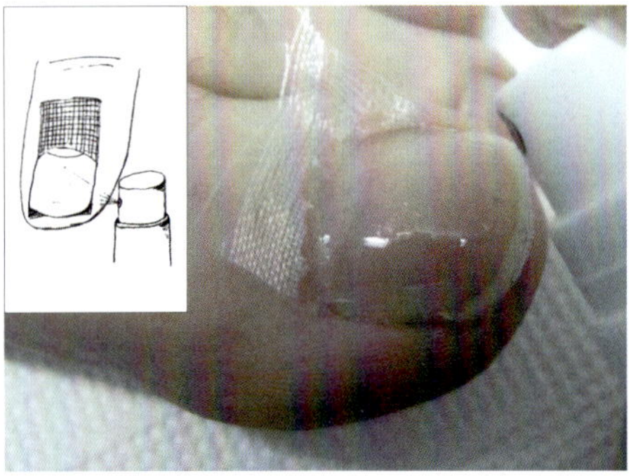

Image 6.77 and 6.78

- Gently pull off the extra glass fibre strip at the nail root and carefully grind off all other glass fibre remnants around the nail with corundum stone (images 6.79 to 6.82).
- Finally, apply nail polish to the nail plate and spray with BS nail liquid dry spray to prevent the nail polish from running into the nail fold. If this happens, remove immediately! (images 6.83 to 6.85).

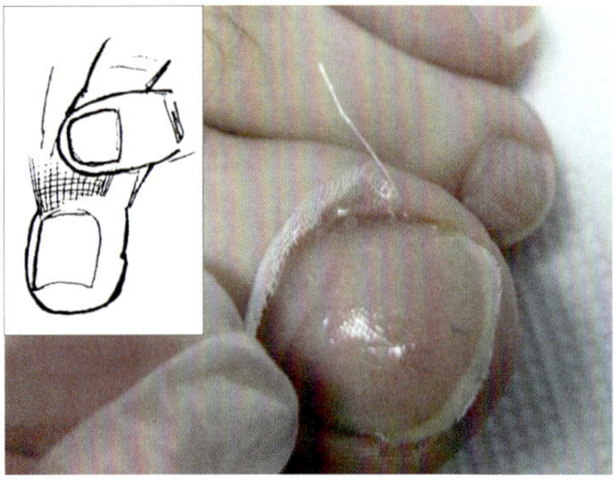

Image 6.79 and 6.80

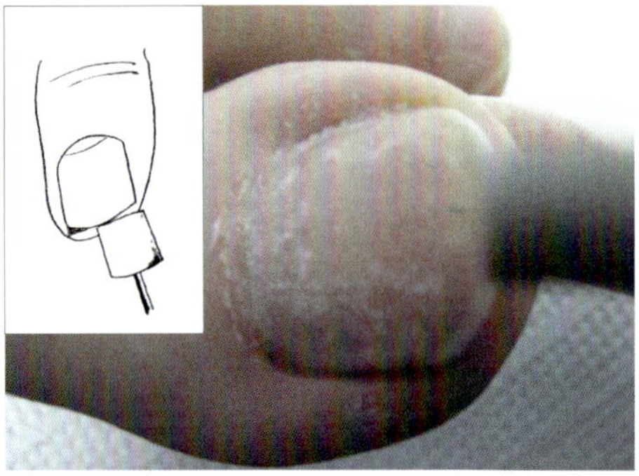

Image 6.81and 6.82

Image 6.83 to 6.85 ▼

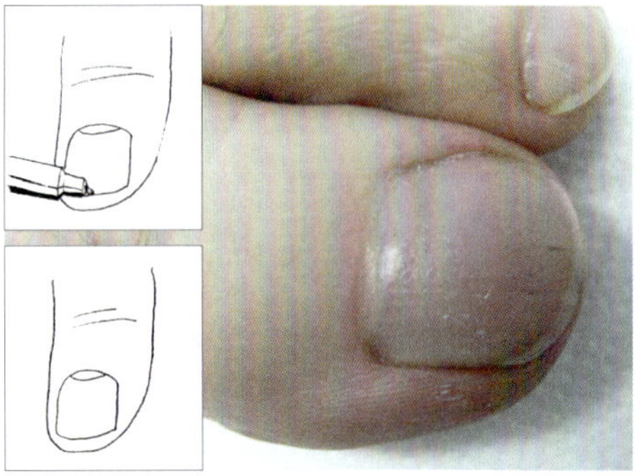

Covering a subungual clavus

- As a prophylactic measure, place a Propolis-impregnated piece of Copoline on the core area of the clavus (images 6.86 and 6.87).
- Blend equal parts of BS filler in a dappen dish (image 6.88).
- Fill the clavus area to the upper edge of the nail to prevent the nail bed from drying out and provide soft padding for the nail bed (image 6.89).

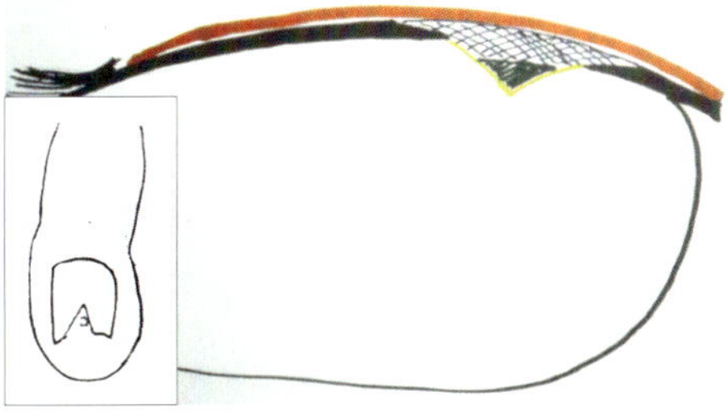

Image 6.86 and 6.87

- Cover the nail with three layers of BS stripe (same method as replacing a partially missing nail) (images 6.91 to 6.92).
- Smooth uneven spots with a corundum stone or diamond bur and seal the nail surface with BS nail polish (images 6.93 to 6.98).

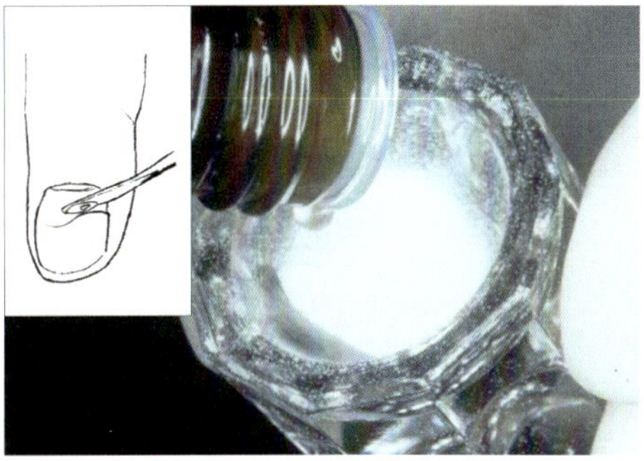

Image 6.88 and 6.89

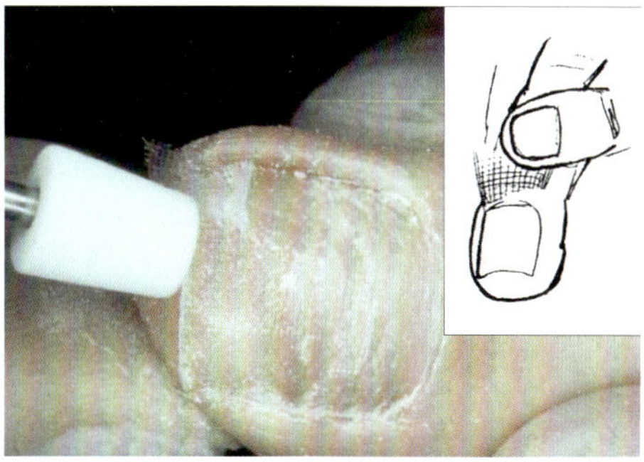

Image 6.93 and 6.94

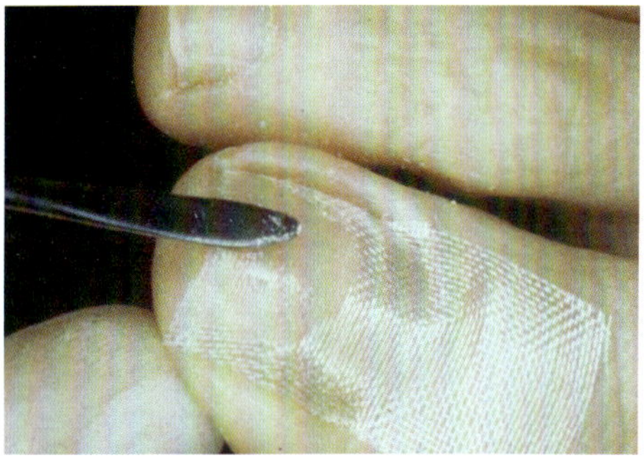

Image 6.90

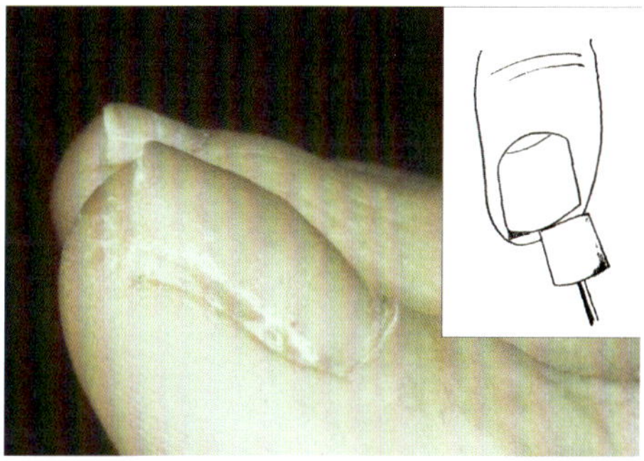

Image 6.95 and 6.96

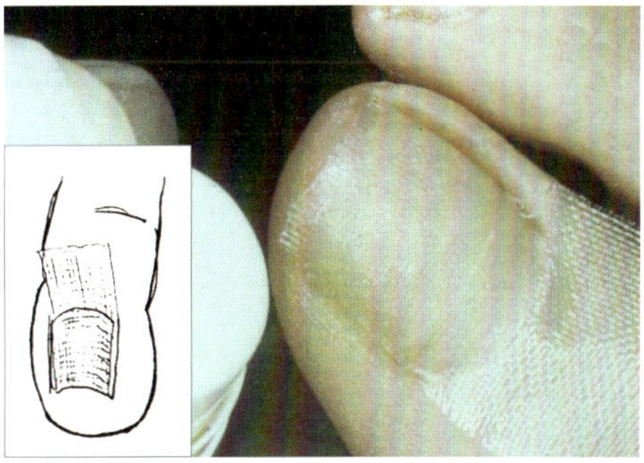

Image 6.91 and 6.92

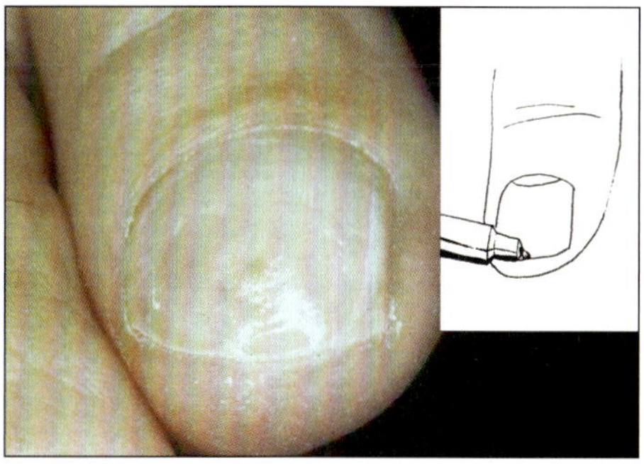

Image 6.97 and 6.98

6.7 Light-curing technique for nail prosthetics

Materials

- Special light-curing materials.
- Work materials
- gel (LCN or Gerlach)
- brush
- cleansing agent
- tamponade

Indications

- nail plate replacement
- partial replacement of the nail plate
- correcting an upward pointing toe tip
- correcting a nail bed too narrowly formed distally
- friction protection (for the tip of the toe)
- nail damage caused by psoriasis, onychorrhexis or onychodystrophy

Contraindications

- nail bed injury
- nail bed infection
- granulation tissue
- eczema in the nail bed area
- onychomycosis
- complete nail loss, can have different causes

Instructions (images 6.99 to 6.103)

Gel is the base material. Apply evenly on the smoothed and degreased nail plate with a small bristle brush. Cure with a 400 nm UV-light for approximately two minutes. If needed, apply several layers of gel. The curing process leaves a sticky film which is easily removed with a cellulose swab. This technique has the advantage of creating a more flexible prosthetic nail option, whereby the artificial nail can be ground and is fracture and tear resistant.

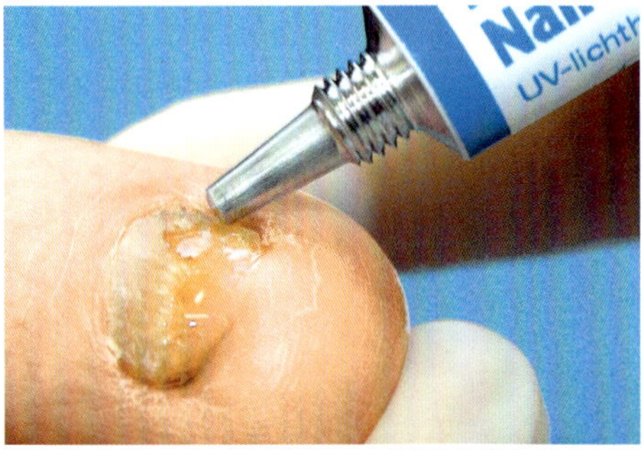

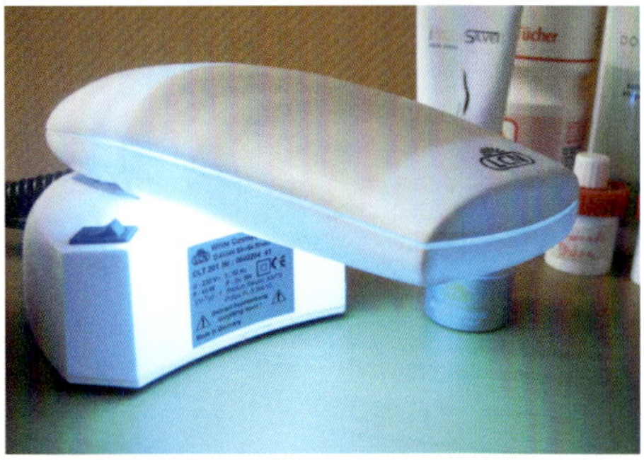

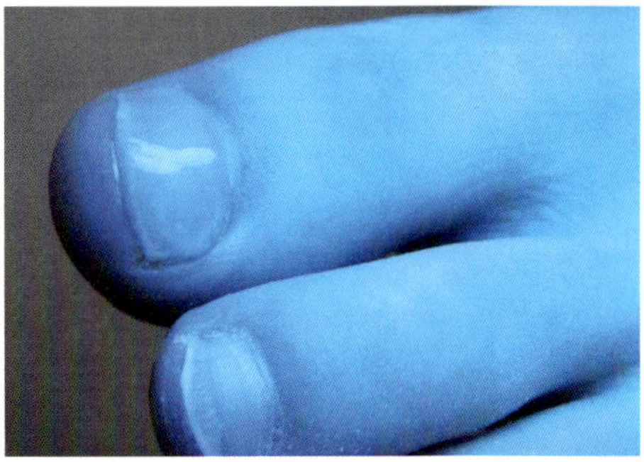

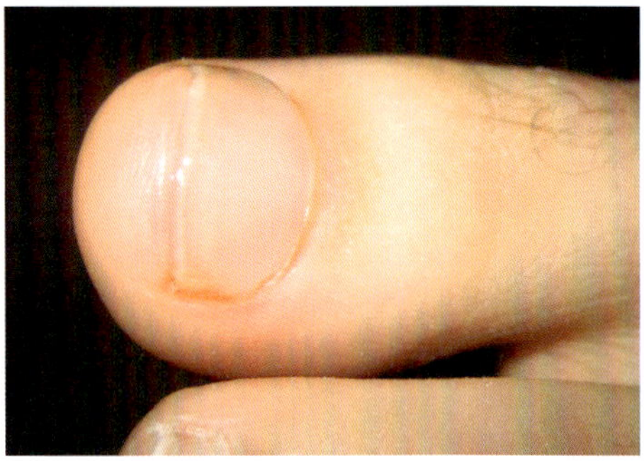

Image 6.100 to 6.103 (top to bottom)

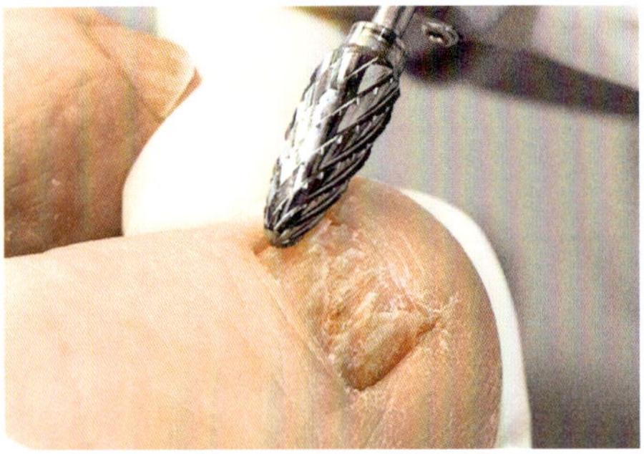

◀ Image 6.99

6.8 Acrylate material

Materials
Acrylate adhesive material and medical fleece.

Acrylate adhesive is the base material. It offers a disinfecting and fungicidal effect. The material is viscous, has a pink tint and comes in tubes. Evaporation of the solvent causes the material to harden.

Work materials
- acrylate adhesive material
- medical fleece such as Copoline
- spatula

Indications
- minor partial nail replacement
- nail damage caused by psoriasis, onychorrhexis or onychodystrophy

Contraindications
- nail bed injury
- nail bed infection
- granulation tissue
- eczema in the nail bed area
- onychomycosis

complete nail loss, can have different • causes

Instructions (images 6.104 to 6.106)
- Degrease and smooth the existing part of the natural nail.
- Apply the material thinly onto the nail and the nail bed directly from the tube, as needed, to complete the nail. Use a spatula to distribute the material evenly.
- Three to four layers are usually sufficient.
- Allow the material to dry for at least two minutes before adding another layer.
- Adding layers of Copoline provides additional reinforcement for the artificial nail.
- Avoid applying the material too thickly since it can form bubbles and then the drying time increases to 30 minutes.
- Once completely hardened, smooth and cut the nail.

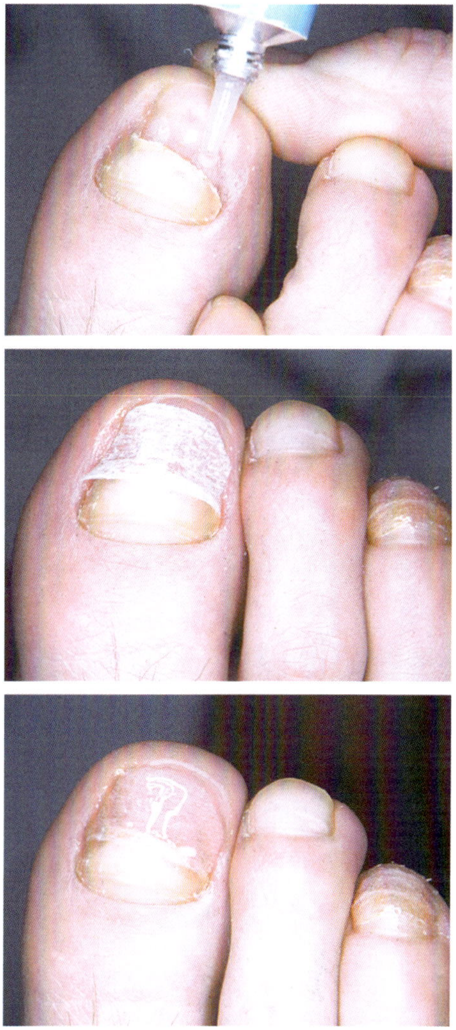

Images 6.104 to 6.106
Steps to create an artificial nail plate with Gehwol nail repair gel (Gerlach)
Source: Klaus Grünewald, Theorie der medizinischen Fußbehandlung – tome 2, 3rd edition 2016. Verlag Neuer Merkur

6.9 Unguisan® technique

Materials

Acetate silk tape and cyanoacrylate adhesive.

Work materials

- acetate silk tape
- cyanoacrylate adhesive
- scissors

Indications

Partial replacement of a nail plate.

Contraindications

- nail bed injury
- nail bed infection
- granulation tissue
- eczema in the nail bed area
- onychomycosis
- complete nail loss, can have different causes

Instructions (images 6.107 to 6.109)

- Apply tamponade before anything else!
- Slightly roughen, degrease and dry the nail surface.
- Cut a piece of acetate silk tape slightly larger than the part that needs to be replaced and place on the damaged area.
- Cut a second wider piece of acetate silk tape and place over the first piece.
- Carefully distribute the adhesive on the entire acetate silk surface.
- The silk material becomes transparent resembling a natural nail.
- The prosthesis can be sanded and shaped with nail tongs or corner nippers.

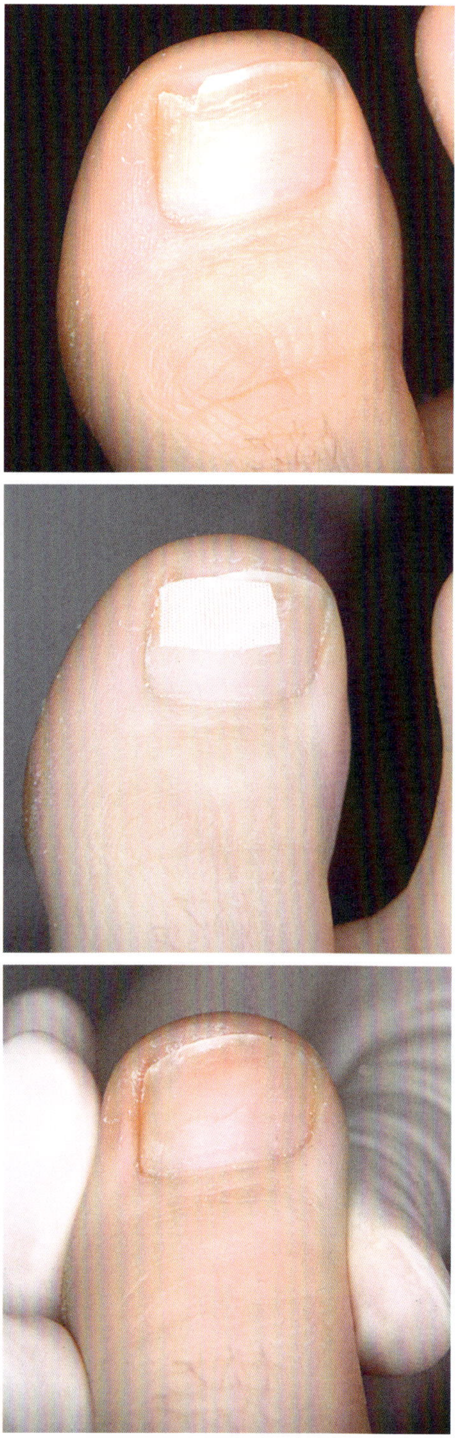

Images 6.107 to 6.109 Unguisan technique

Source: Klaus Grünewald, Theorie der medizinischen Fußbehandlung – tome 2, 3rd edition 2016, Verlag Neuer Merkur

6.10 Brush application for synthetic materials

Materials

Primer and synthetic material (powder and liquid).

Work materials

- primer
- synthetic material
- brush
- two dappen dishes

Indications

- minor partial nail replacement
- nail damage caused by psoriasis, onychorrhexis or onychodystrophy

Contraindications

- nail bed injury
- nail bed infection
- granulation tissue
- eczema in the nail bed area
- onychomycosis
- complete nail loss, can have different causes

Instructions

- Degrease and sand the nail plate. Apply a thin layer of primer.
- To apply the synthetic material, first dip a fine brush into the liquid and then into the powder.
- The powder combined with the moisture on the brush becomes pasty during the brush application and hardens. Clean the brush thoroughly afterwards. Once the material has completely hardened, sand and shape the nail as usual.

Tamponades and taping

7

List of medicinal products in this book with German brand names – ingredients and possible brand names outside Germany

Chapter 7.1

- Octenisept – antiseptic, containing Octenidine dihydrochloride and Phenoxyethanol
- Propolis – bee glue

Chapter 7.2

- Betaisodona wound gauze – Betaisodona contains povidone iodine
- Nebacetin – in Germany no longer available; “triple antibiotic ointment,” international with a common brand name Neosporin
- Vindex compresses – impregnated with Peruvian balsam, alkaline Bismuth nitrate and Bismuth subgallate
- Dolerma – nail fold oil with wheat germ oil, water, lanolin, alcohol, menthol, citronella oil, camphor, perfume, xanthan gum

7 Tamponades and taping

7.1 Copoline

Material
- Copoline
- ready-to-use single-layer gauze material

Work materials (image 7.1)
- excavator and probe
- Copoline
- disinfectant

Indications
- injuries and infection in the nail fold are
- painful callus skin

Contraindications
Can cause infection if left for more than three days.

Insertion (images 7.2 to 7.5)
Cut a correctly sized piece of Copoline and moisten with Octenisept, Propolis or Dolerma. Place the tamponade flat on the nail plate and gently push it under the lateral free nail margin.

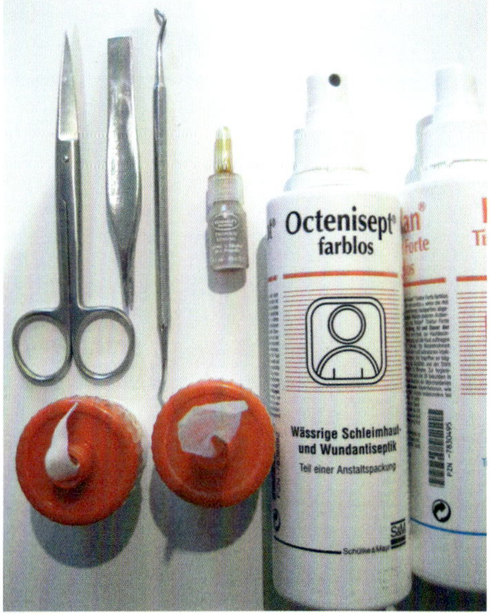

Image 7.1

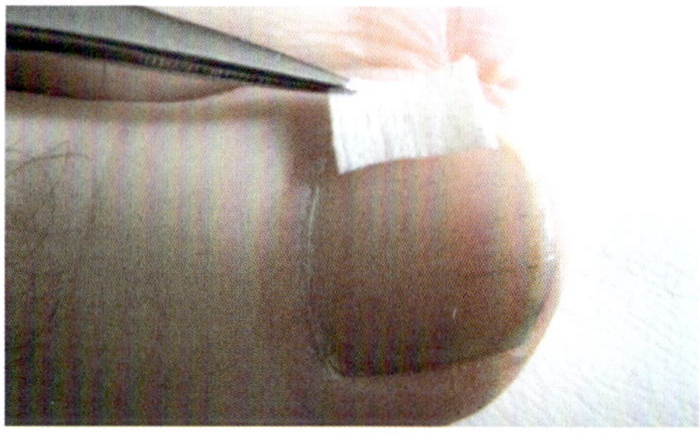

Image 7.2

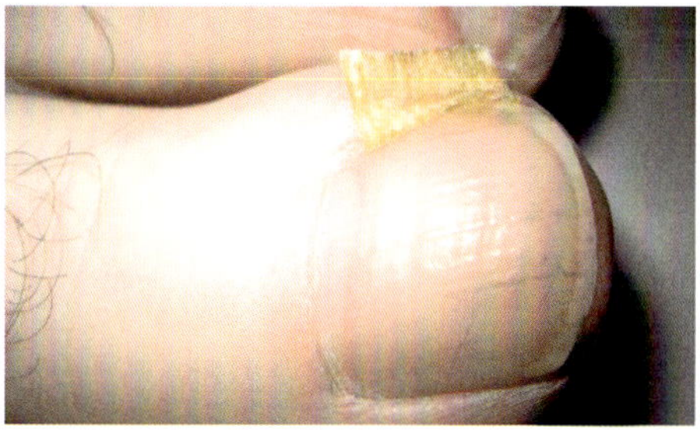

Image 7.3

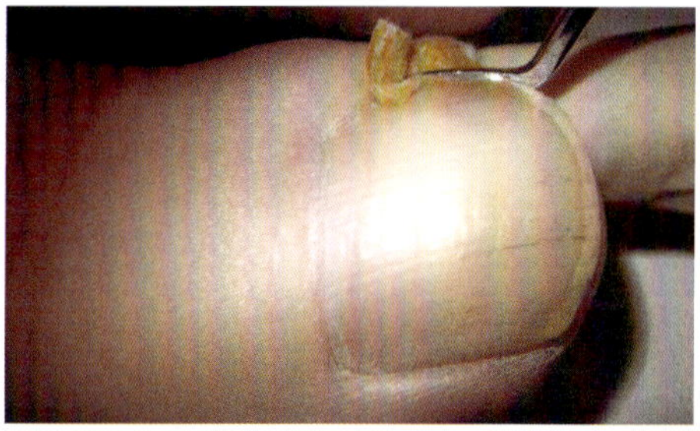

Image 7.4

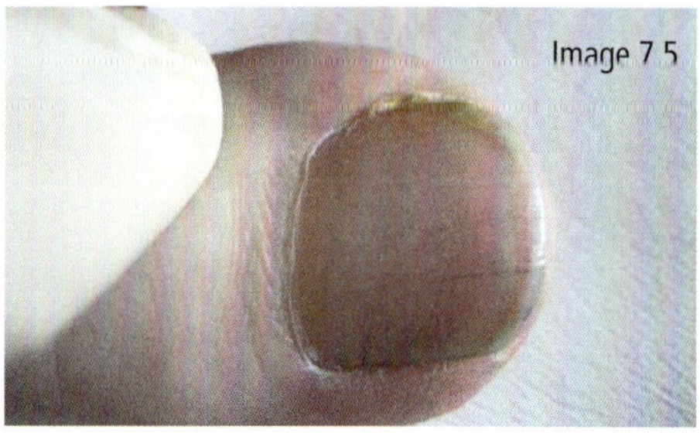

Image 7.5

Application time
One to three days.

7.2 Copoline with medicated gauze and compresses

Material

Ready-to-use, single-layer gauze material on which disinfecting ointments can be applied. The advantage of these tamponades is that they are perfectly hygienic and ready to use.

- Medicated wound gauzes:
- Betaisodona wound gauze
- Nebacetin gauze (only available on prescription)
- Vindex compresses

Work materials

- Copoline with active medication
- Sterile/disinfected forceps
- Sterile/disinfected excavator or probe

Indications

- nail fold injuries
- painful callus skin

Contraindications

Can cause infection or allergic reaction if left for more than three days.

Application

The gauze is protected by two layers of foil and can be cut to the desired size. To expose the gauze pad, rub the two pieces of foil against each other with your fingers. Remove the medicated gauze pad with sterile and disinfected forceps and gently insert it into the nail fold with a sterile instrument.

Application time

One to three days.

7.3 Ligasano tamponade

Material

Ligasano white sterile is a therapeutic polyurethane foam dressing for wound treatment, known for its fast-remittent compressional stress and reliable absorbency. Its surface structure triggers a mechanical stimulus in wounds and on the skin, encouraging blood circulation. This promotes exudation and, therefore, the cleansing of contaminated or infected wounds and facilitates granulation and epithelization of "clean wounds". The material does not contain additional active substances, is completely hypoallergenic and ensures efficient dressing change without disturbing wound healing.

Work materials

- excavator or tamponade probe
- Ligasano white sterile (images 7.6 to 7.8)
- scissors
- disinfectant

Indications

- contaminated or infected wounds
- problematic wounds in their cleaning, granulation and epithelization phase
- chronic wounds, burns, abrasions, for postoperative dressings, meshgraft covers, and for activating stagnating wounds

Contraindications

- None.

Complications

None with proper application. Does not adhere to the wound! In rare cases, Ligasano white must be slightly moistened during application.

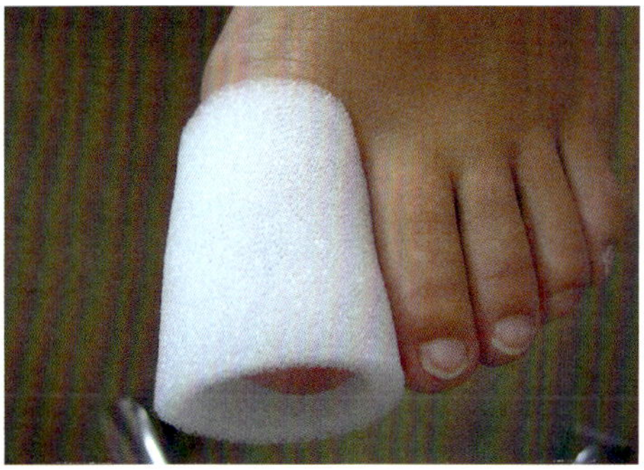

Image 7.6

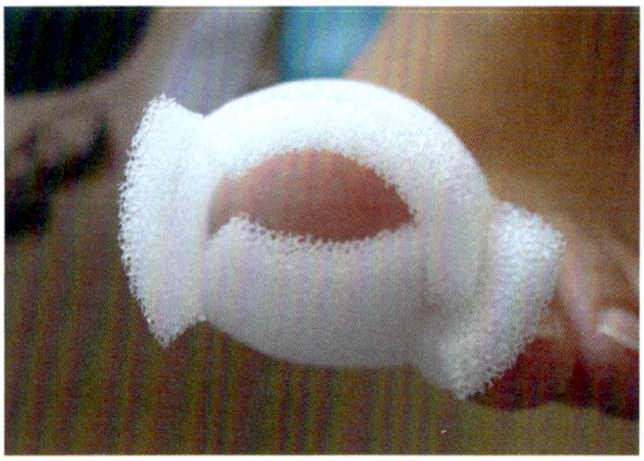

Image 7.7

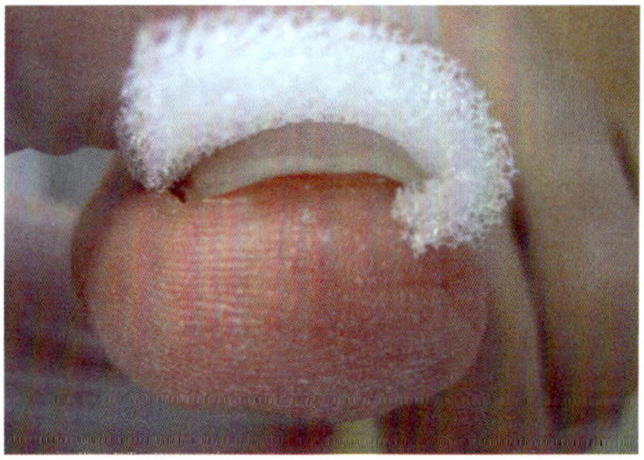

Image 7.8

Application

- Cut a correctly-size piece of Ligasano.
- Apply Prontoman gel, Propolis or Octenisept gel to the nail fold.
- Place the tamponade flat over the nail fold and gently insert it into the nail fold and under the lateral free nail margin with the excavator.

Application time

The tamponade must stay on the wound one to three days (images 7.9 to 7.12).

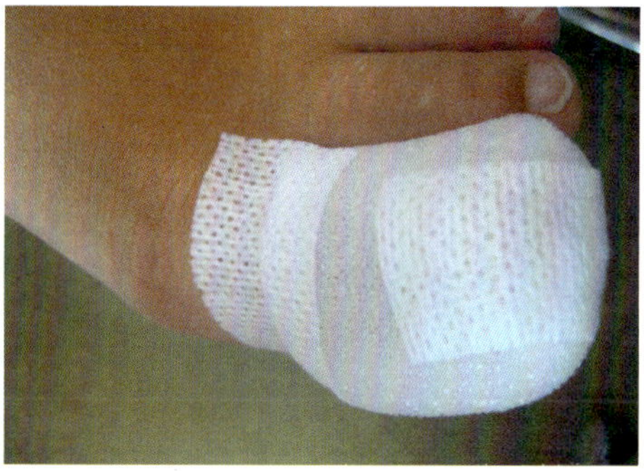

Image 7.9

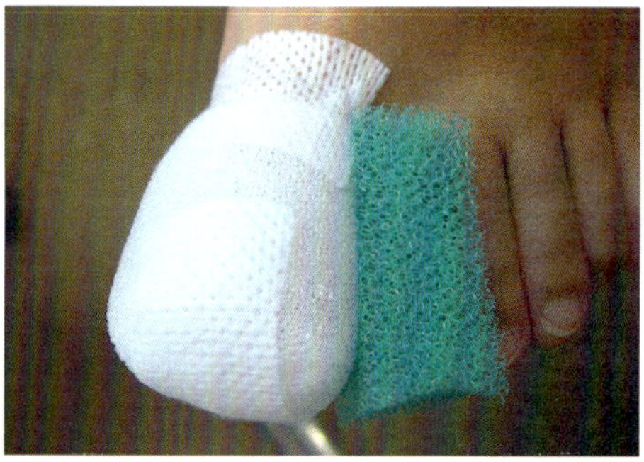

Image 7.10

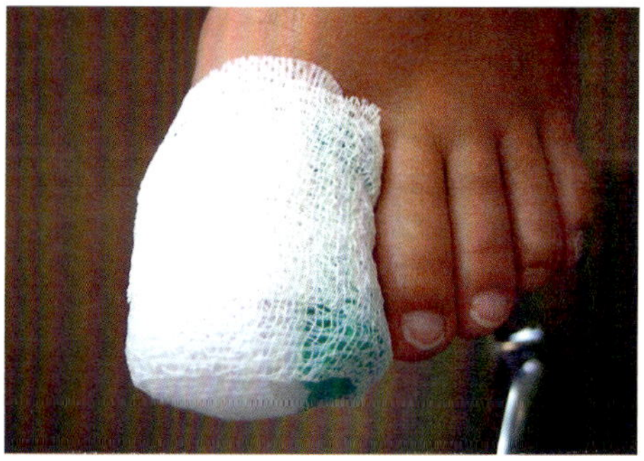

Image 7.11

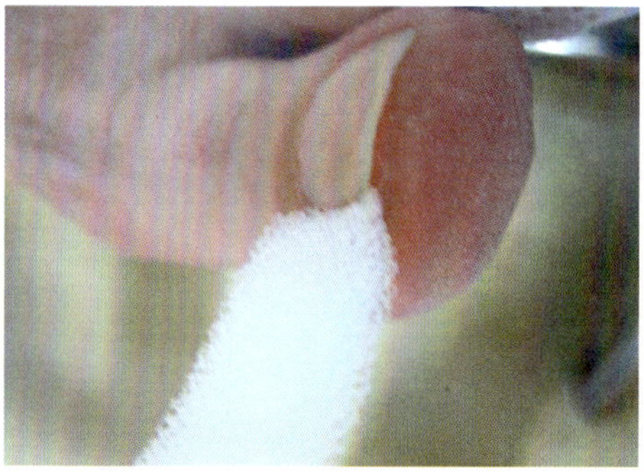

Image 7.12

7.4 Smig

Material (image 7.13)
Smig is a pliable synthetic material that is usually used as an adhesive cushion liner for dentures. It consists of a combination of PBMA, polypropylenglycol monolaurate and food colouring.

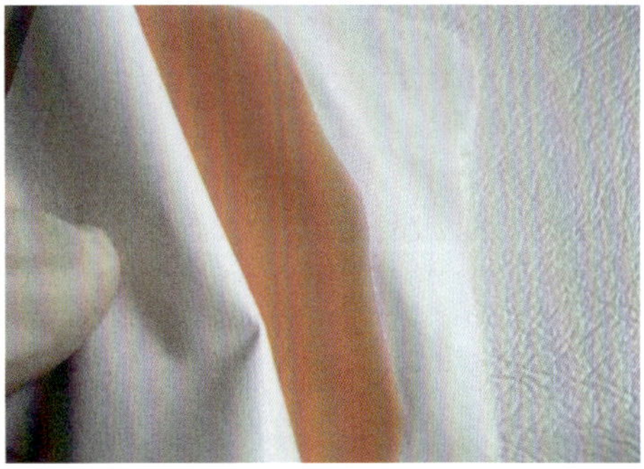

Image 7.13

Work materials
- Smig scissors
- dappen dish
- forceps
- excavator
- narrow metal spatula or nail blade

Indications
- protects the nail fold from friction
- protects the nail during treatment with nail correction braces
- painful callus

Contraindications
Nail fold infections.

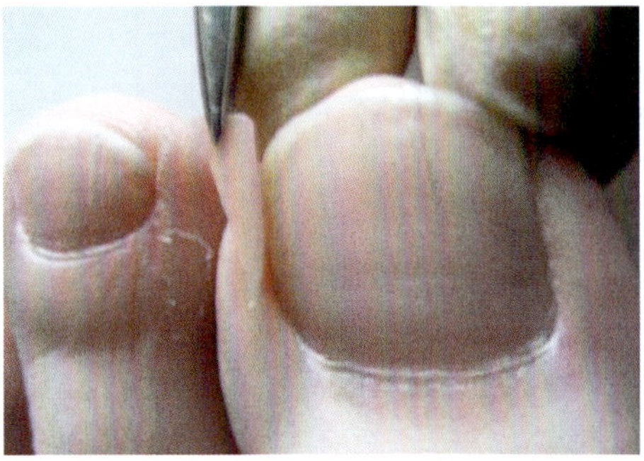

Image 7.14

Application (images 7.14 and 7.15)
Cut a small wedge out of the Smig sheet making sure that its length and width conform to the size of the nail fold. Apply some acetone solvent to the Smig wedge. Then gently insert the wedge into the nail fold with a spatula or an excavator, making sure not to push it in too deeply since that causes irritation. Once the solvent has completely evaporated, it is a pliable, soft tamponade.

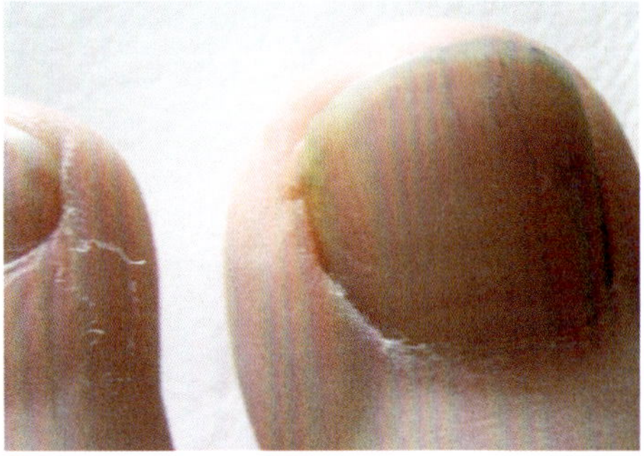

Image 7.15

Application time
The Smig wedge stays in the nail fold for four weeks. If there is no sign of irritation, it can even stay up to eight weeks.

7.5 Gutta-percha compound in sheet form

Material

Gutta-percha (Malayan getah "rubber", percha "tree") is the dried-up sap of the tropical gutta-percha tree.

It chemically resembles caoutchouc.

Work materials

- gutta-percha compound
- scissors
- dappen dish
- forceps
- chloroform
- excavator
- narrow metal spatula or nail blade

Indications

- protects the nail fold from friction
- protects the nail during treatment with nail correction braces
- painful callus

Contraindications

Nail fold infections.

Application

- Cut a small wedge out of the gutta-percha sheet making sure that its length and width fit the nail fold correctly.
- Immerse the gutta-percha wedge for 12 seconds in chloroform to soften it and immediately insert it into the nail fold. Periodic application of chloroform to the wedge with a small spatula or nail blade is recommended.
- After the solvent has evaporated, the body temperature causes the gutta-percha to stay somewhat pliable and it is, therefore, suitable for the preliminary correction of rolled nails.
- Leave the gutta-percha wedge in the nail fold until the next treatment appointment, provided there is no sign of irritation. To prevent irritation, always smooth out gutta-percha in the nail fold area.

Application time

The gutta-percha wedge stays in the nail fold for four weeks. If there is no sign of irritation, it can even stay up to eight weeks.

7.6 Orthoses silicones

Material
- silicone, e.g., Bland-Rosé (distribution: Bernd Stolz Company)
- Erkoton HE (Erkodent)
- Soft Pipe (Süda)
- Peclavus orthosis soft (Ruck)

Work materials
- silicone
- mixing pad
- spatula

Indications
- protects the nail fold from friction
- protects the nail during treatment with nail correction braces
- painful callus

Contraindications
Nail fold irritation and infection.

Application (images 7.16 to 7.20)
Mix the silicone according to the manufacturer's recommendation and carefully work it into the nail fold and under the free nail margin with a spatula.

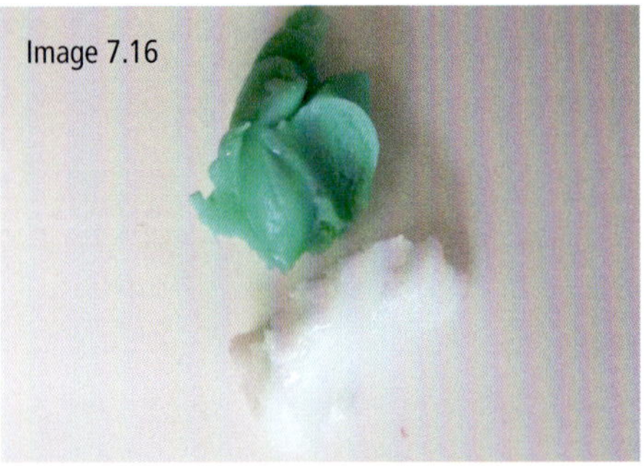
Image 7.16

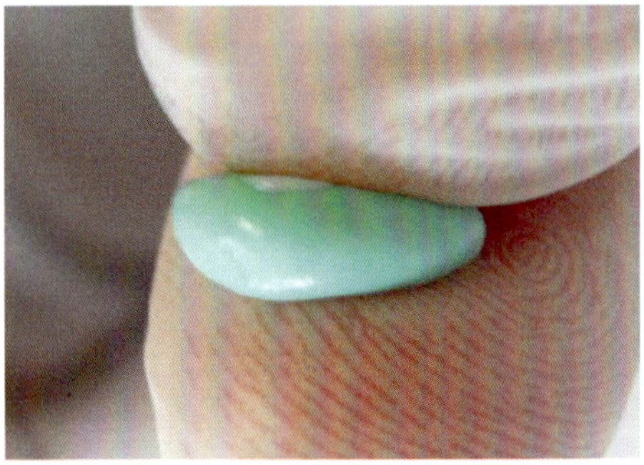
Image 7.17

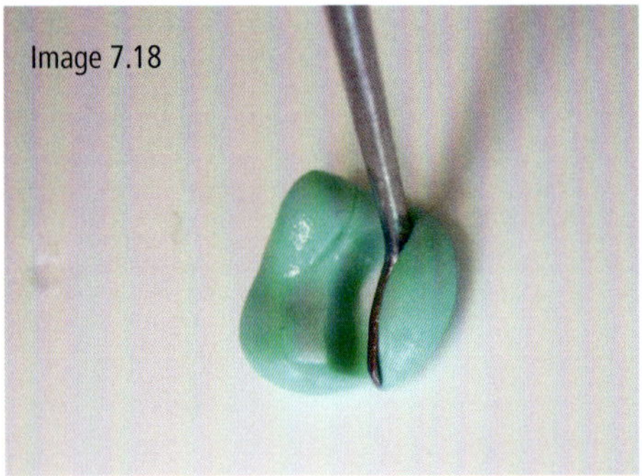
Image 7.18

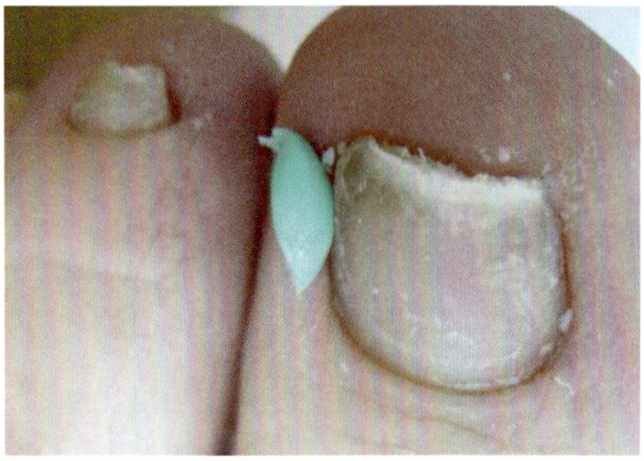
Image 7.19

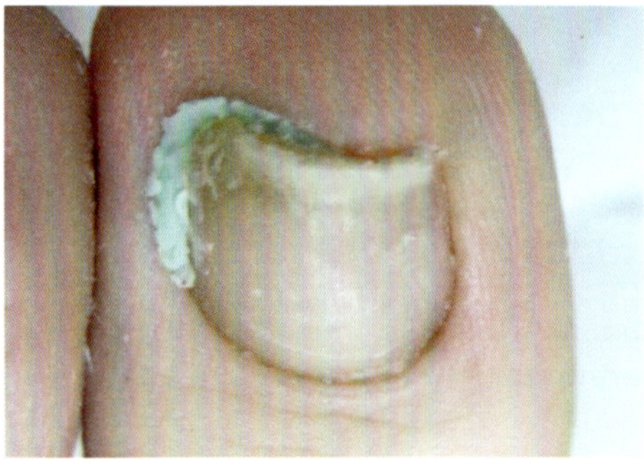
Image 7.20

Application time
If there is no sign of irritation, an orthosis tamponade can be left in the nail fold for four to even eight weeks. After four weeks, the tamponade must be repositioned.

7.7 Sulci protectors

Material (image 7.21)

Sulci protectors are small plastic tubes with a longitudinal slit and come in different sizes.

Work materials

- sulci protector
- forceps
- applicator
- scissors
- spatula
- Gerlach nail compound
- Unguisan or instant adhesive

Indications

- protects the nail fold from friction
- protects the nail during treatment with nail correction braces
- painful callu

Contraindications

Nail fold irritation and infection.

Application (images 7.22 to 7.26)

Cut the sulci protector tube to fit the length of the lateral free nail margin. Use forceps or a special injector (Greppmayr) to slide the tube onto the lateral free nail margin from distal to proximal.

Round the tip of the tube off prior to sliding it onto the lateral free nail margin.

The visible tube part on the nail plate must be secured with Gehwol nail compound (Gerlach), Unguisan (Greppmayr) or instant adhesive.

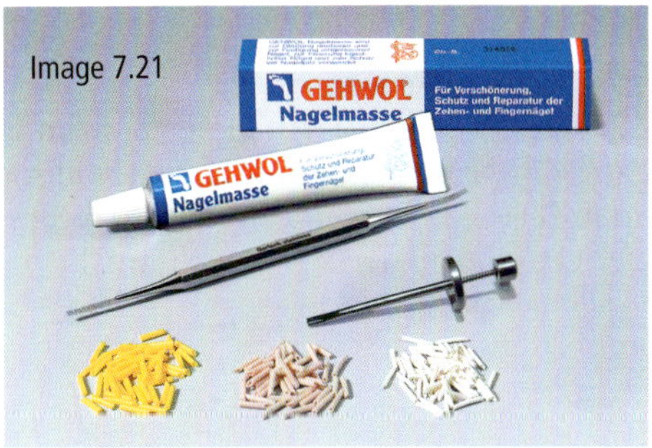

Image 7.21

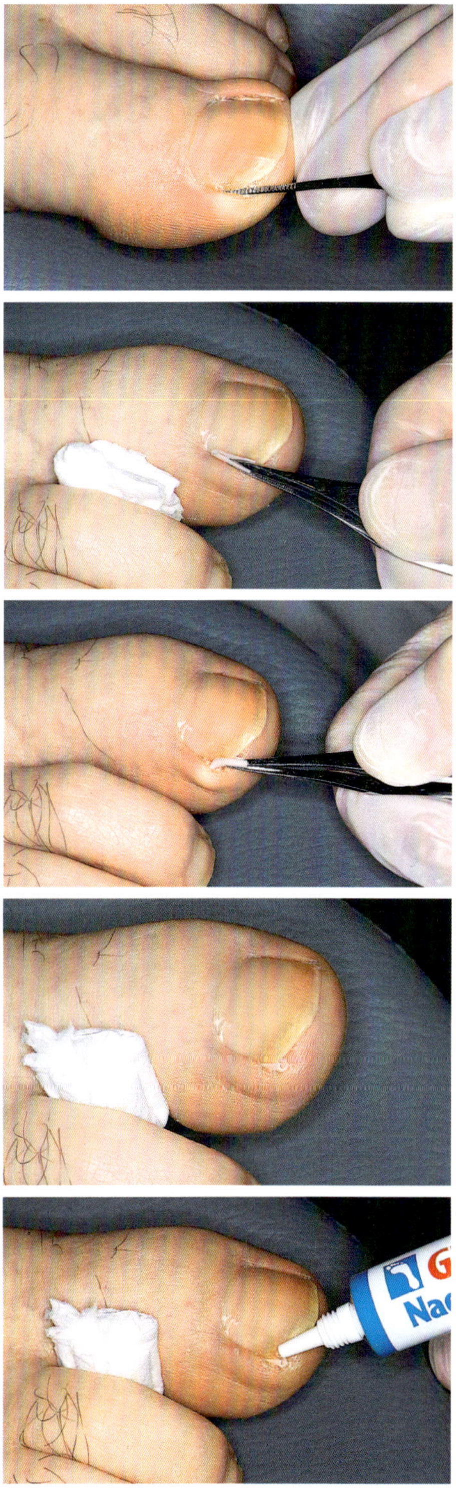
Image 7.22 to 7.26

Source: Gerlach

Application time

If there is no sign of irritation, a sulci protector can be left in the nail fold for four to even eight weeks. After four weeks, it must be repositioned.

7.8 Products with superior packing characteristics

Prontoman gel (image 7.27)

Active substance: PHMB.

Image 7.27

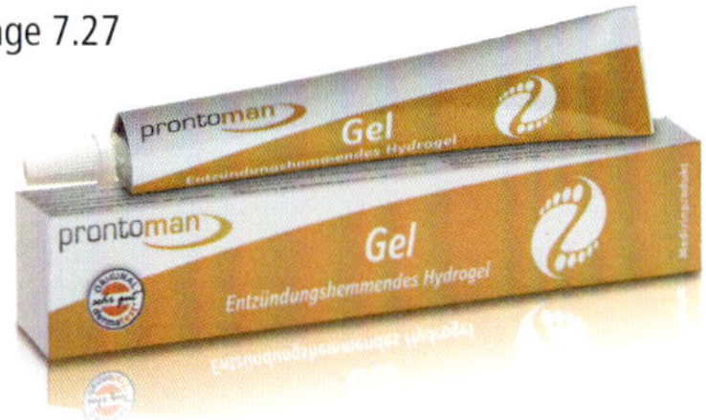

The gel prevents pathogens from entering through minor fissures or injuries in the nail bed. It seals the injury site and promotes healing. Using it with tamponades or braces has also been proven successful. Patients who suffer from unguis incarnatus can apply the gel twice daily at home on the affected area. This prevents infection and promotes the healing process.

Prontoman spray (image 7.28)

Active substance: PHMB.

Prior to treatment, the feet must be sprayed with Prontoman spray to eliminate germs. To soften callus skin, the affected area should be sprayed repeatedly. After approximately two minutes, the dead skin cells turn white and start to loosen. Compared to other chemical callus softeners, this process is purely physical. It does not affect healthy skin. The risk of an injury is minimized since the loosening dead skin cells are gently removed with an excavator without causing trauma to the skin.

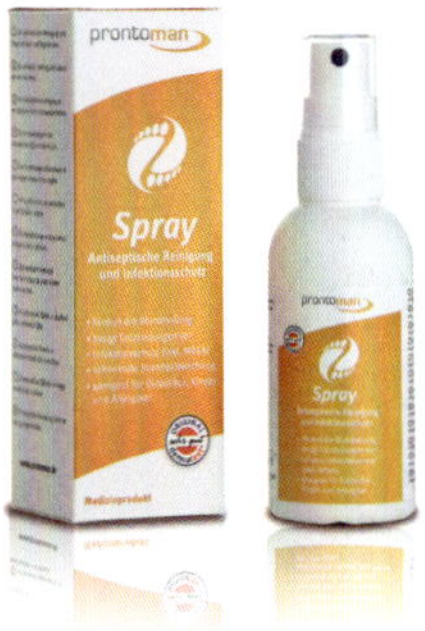

Image 7.28

After a longer exposure time, thick callus skin in the heel or ball area is also easily removable. Applying cotton pads or compresses moistened with Prontoman spray to the affected areas and covering it with plastic wrap for 10 to 12 minutes has also been proven to be effective.

Propolis solvent (image 7.29)

Active substance: Natural keratolytic

Indications

- skin care
- softening of callus skin
- fixing and preserving of tamponades or impregnation of dressings
- skin care after tattoos, permanent make-up and piercings
- sealing of minor skin abrasions
- acne skin care
- animal care

Mode of action

Propolis solvent has a resin base and is, therefore, not water soluble. It does not penetrate deep skin layers but rather covers the outer layer of the skin with a protective film. It mechanically softens excess callus skin, thereby, facilitating its removal.

The solvent's dry ingredient promotes skin elasticity and smoothness and the contained bioflavonoids inhibit the multiplication of microorganisms.

Application

Start by applying Propolis to the skin selectively and then distribute it evenly on

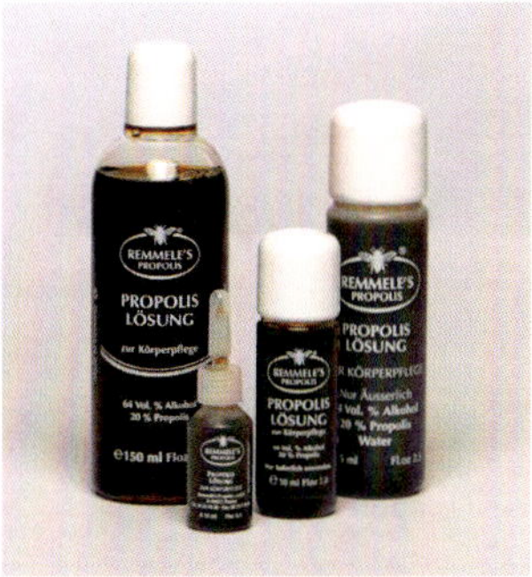

Image 7.29

the affected area. The natural product's properties might cause some discolouration. This will disappear once the solvent has dried. Be careful not to rub the solvent into your eyes!

octenisept® spray (image 7.30)

- broad spectrum of antiseptic efficacy
- fast onset of action from the first minute
- good skin and mucous membrane tolerance
- suitable for infants and premature babies
- painless application
- colourless

Composition

100 g solvent contains:

- Medically active ingredients:
  - 0.1 g Octenidine dihydrochloride
  - 2.0 g 2-Phenoxyethanol (Ph.Eur.)
- Other ingredients:
  - (3-amidopropyl cocoate) dimethylammonium acetate
  - Sodium D-gluconate
  - Glycerol 85 %
  - Sodium chloride
  - Sodium hydroxide
  - Purified water

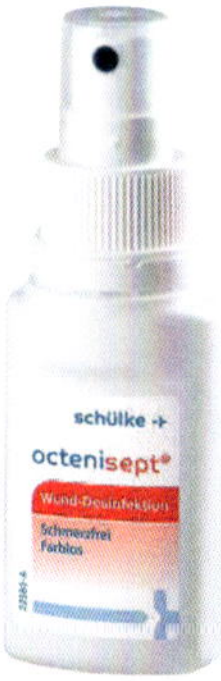

Image 7.30

Applications

Wound treatment:

Antiseptic treatment of traumatic, acute, chronic, surgical and burn wounds.

Mucous membrane antiseptic:

As an antimicrobial whole-body wash for MRSA-populated patients.

Microbiological efficacy against:

- bacteria, including chlamydia trachomatis and mycoplasma
- fungi and yeast
- protozoa (trichomonads)
- viruses (herpes simplex, HBV, HCV and HIV)

Instructions

The skin and mucous membrane areas must be evenly and thoroughly moistened with the antiseptic in preparation for the following application methods.

Swab method: Wipe areas under aseptic conditions with impregnated swabs. This is the preferred method of application due to the anatomic and physiological conditions of the mucous membrane.

Spray method: octenisept® can be sprayed directly on skin and mucous membrane areas.

Special instructions

- To prevent tissue injury, the product must not be injected or applied to tissue with pressure. Adequate drainage from wound cavities must be provided (e.g., for flexible drain tube).
- Do not swallow octenisept® or allow it to enter the blood stream, e.g., by accidental injection.
- Do not mix octenisept® with other compounds and do not use it in combination with PVP-iodine based antiseptics since it can cause brown to violet skin discolouration.
- Dressings and incision foils can be applied once octenisept® has dried off completely.

- In rare cases octenisept® may cause a slight burning sensation.
- The spray can be warmed up to body temperature.
- Do not use beyond the expiry date.
- Once the container has been opened it should not be used for more than three years and not beyond the expiry date.
- Keep out of the reach of children.

octenisept® gel (image 7.31)

Non-irritating, non-sensitising, pain-free, without tissue toxicity, no impairment of granulation or epithelialisation.

Composition
Aqua purificata, Propylene Glycol, Hydroxyethylcellulose, Octenidine HCl.

Applications
octenisept® gel is applied to acute skin injuries, such as grazes, cuts and minor burns (e.g., sunburn). For optimal healing, the wounds should be supplied with enough moisture. The healing process requires skin cells to divide and migrate which a moist environment promotes. In addition, the wound must be protected from infection.

The special formula in octenisept® gel supplies the wound with moisture and forms a protective barrier against bacteria. This protective layer prevents pathogens from entering the wound as they have already been inactivated in the gel, therefore, preventing inflammation and infection while promoting and accelerating natural wound healing.

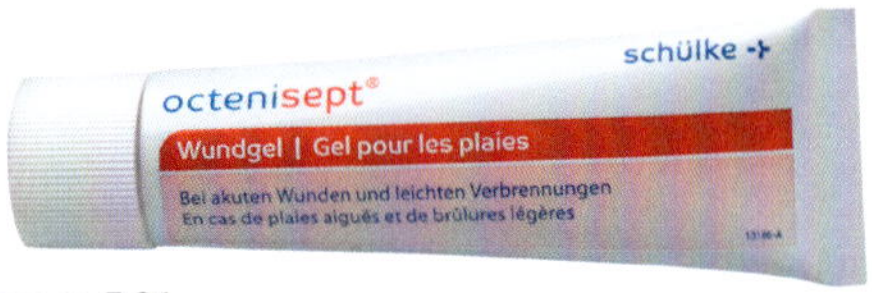

Image 7.31

Instructions
Disinfect the wound immediately after the injury occurs with octenisept® wound disinfectant. Apply a thin gel layer on the wound and, if required, cover the wound with dressing or plaster. Apply the gel one to two times daily until the wound has healed completely. The tip of the gel tube must not touch the wound or other surfaces due to hygienic reasons.

Spirularin Nail Serum/ Spirularin VS (image 7.32)

This new and exceptional serum consists of special microalgae substances derived from the arthrospira species. These substances are extracted through a patented preparation process and protect effectively against fungi and bacteria invasion while promoting the skin's regeneration process. Arthrospira algae have been around for 3.6 billion years and are, therefore, one of the oldest life form on earth. Enzymes of the artificially stressed microalgae extract destroy fungi by attacking its chitin structures. These enzymes do not cause undesirable side effects since human skin and nails do not contain chitin structures and also protect against bacteria, such as Staphylococcus areus.

Polysaccharide-calcium-spirulan is an active component in the treatment of warts. It effectively inhibits the absorption, penetration and replication of viruses. Regenerative skin tissue under the warts is protected from HPV viruses gradually replacing wart tissue. The treatment is pain-free and does not cause skin injuries. There is no restriction on use for diabetics or during pregnancy and breastfeeding. The alga consists of 240 ingredients and has a high bioavailability. It stimulates the metabolism and supplies the skin with essential vitamins, minerals, micronutrients and antioxidants.

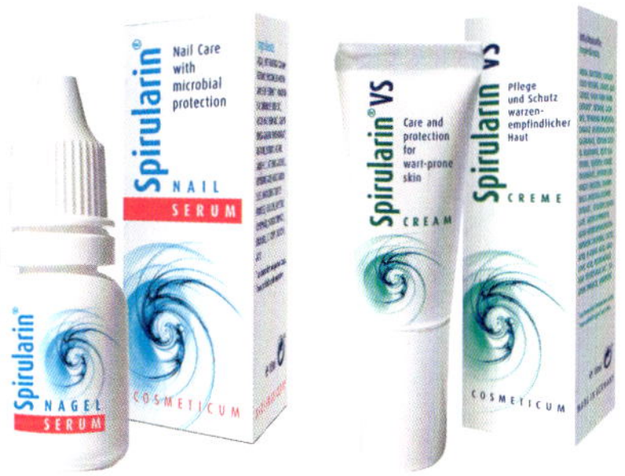

Image 7.32

Spirularin Nail Serum

Active substances and their healing effects:

- Arthrospira micro algae extract (high concentration):
  - anti-microbial (bacterial) protection +++
  - anti-inflammatory effect
  - cell regeneration + 26 %
- Hamamelis extract:
  - astringent effect
- Nail care oils:
  - jojoba oil
  - coconut oil
- Liquorice root extract:
  - sensitivity reduction

Spirularin VS Fluid

Active substances and their healing effects:

- Arthrospira micro algae extract (high concentration):
  - inhibits virus activity
  - cell regeneration + 26 %
  - anti-microbial
- Willow bark extract:
  - anti-bacterial
  - keratolytic effect
- Hamamelis extract:
  - toning effect
  - astringent effect
- Liquorice root extract:
  - anti-microbial
  - skin sensitivity

Inhibitory effect of the active microalgae extracts spiralin on various pathogenic organisms:

Bacteria	
Staphylococcus lentus	+++
Bacillus subtilis	+++
E.coli K12	++
Staphylococcus epidermidis	++
Pseudomonas aeruginosa	++
Propionibacterium acnes	+++
Fungi/yeasts	
Candida glabrata	+++
Candida albicans	+++
Dermatophytes	
Trichophyton rubrum	+++
Trichophyton mentagrophytes	+++
Microsporum canis	+++

\+ = > 30%
++ = > 50%
+++ = > 80%

Prof. Imhoff, Institute MicrobiMaris, API center at the Kiel University

7.9 Taping and nail diseases

Taping is a therapeutic method designed to treat painful muscles, tendons and the skeletal apparatus. The colourful tapes are applied on the muscle and are especially effective for acute symptoms, pain prevention and chronic pain. During the treatment, flexible cotton-based adhesive tapes are applied directly to the skin where they stay for a period ranging from a few days to two weeks. These tapes can be easily removed and are hypoallergenic. They are extremely stretchable, water-resistant and air and moisture permeable.

Mode of action

The taping technique is simple yet very effective. It supports the body's natural healing process by stimulating different skin receptors. The wave-like tape microscopically lifts the skin, promoting blood and lymph circulation, thereby allowing for a decrease in inflammation and pain. In addition, properly applied tapes function as muscle support and improve proprioception.

Taping effects the following areas in the body:

- muscle attachments and muscles
- joint function
- pain receptors
- skin sensors
- fascias
- circulatory system
- meridians and acupuncture points
- scar tissue
- visceral system

Treatment abilities

- augmentation (joint support)
- proprioception (improves physical perception)
- compression (prevents swelling)
- fixation (immobilization)

General taping instructions

Preparation

Prior to applying the tape, the skin must be clean, dry, oil-free and display no sign of skin injury. The area should be shaved to ensure proper adhesion. The patient must be advised not to take baths with oily additives or apply cream to the feet 24 hours before the appointment. It is also not recommended to take a foot bath just before applying the tape. To ensure proper tape adhesion, the skin must be warm which is easily achieved with an infrared light or a cherry stone pillow.

Range of indications in podiatry

- hip joint pain
- knee joint pain
- ankle joint pain or arthrosis
- calcaneal spur
- flat foot
- splay foot
- Hallux valgus
- Hallus rigidus
- hammer and claw toes
- fibromyalgia
- rheumatic diseases
- neuropathic pain
- polyneuropathy
- distorsions
- torn ligament
- overstraining
- sulcus irritation

Contraindications

- open wounds
- acute or chronic skin diseases (e.g., mycotic infections, erythema, erysipelas).
- allergies (allergy test)
- neurodermatitis (possibly tolerable)
- eczema
- thrombosis area
- areas with severe swelling
- large hematoma
- malign tumors
- vascular pathologies (e.g., recent thrombosis and thrombophlebitis)
- medication (e.g., cortisone, antidepressants (sensitive skin))

- radiation, chemotherapy
- severe osteoporosis (caution)

Side effects
- skin irritations
- compartment syndrome
- circulatory problems
- decreasing stabilizing effect
- uncomfortable pinching and constricting of skin (caused by overstretching the tape)
- sore muscles

Application technique
I use hallus-valgus-tape, hallus-rigidus-tape, hammer-and-claw toe-tape (image 7.33) and splay-and-flat foot-tape on patients with nail deformities. For infections in the sulcus, I apply an I-tape.

Step-by-step taping instructions for treating infections in the sulcus area (nail fold)
(See images 7.34 to 7.37)

1. Preparation and measurements
   Measure the tape from the edge of the nail fold to the center of the apex. Then cut the I-tape to fit the width of the nail fold and round off the tape's corners to prevent sharp edges from loosening during friction.
2. To ensure proper adhesion, the patient must be advised not to take baths with oil additives or apply cream to their feet 24 hours prior to the appointment. In addition, clean the skin with a skin disinfectant. Warm feet optimize adherence since the tape's acrylate adhesive bonds faster to warm skin. I recommend the use of an infrared light.
3. Tape application
   Apply the base of the tape below the nail fold. Ensure that the tape does not touch the infected area.
4. Pull the remaining part of the tape firmly towards the plantar area of the toe and rub it down to ensure proper adhesion.

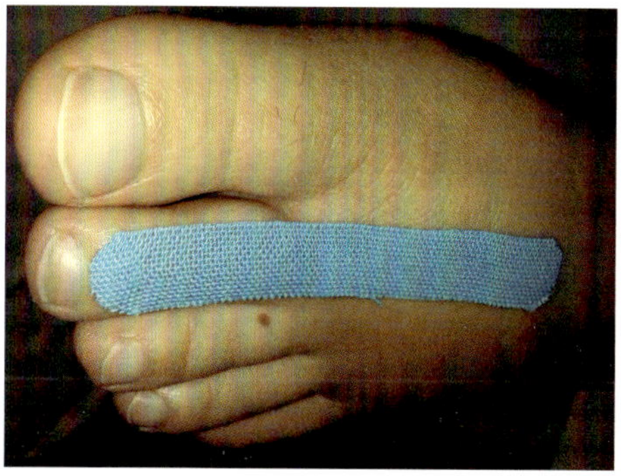

Image 7.33 Tape for hammer toe

5. Advise the patient to wear socks at night.

Training required
Taping is a form of therapy that, if properly applied, promotes healing and provides relief in various parts of the body. The application of different tapes is a technique that definitely requires profound training.

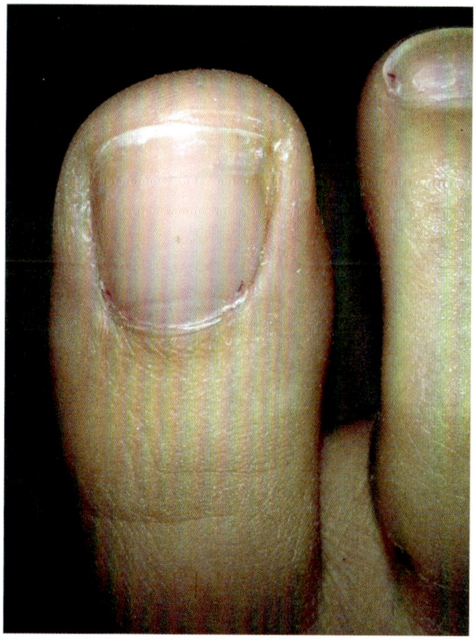

Image 7.34 Sulcus before taping

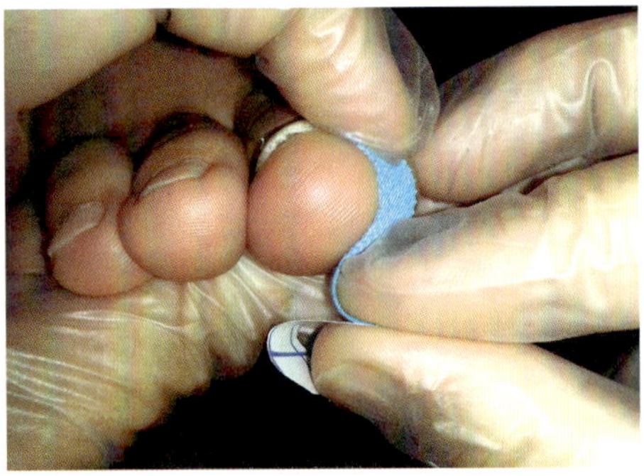

Image 7.35 Applying the tape

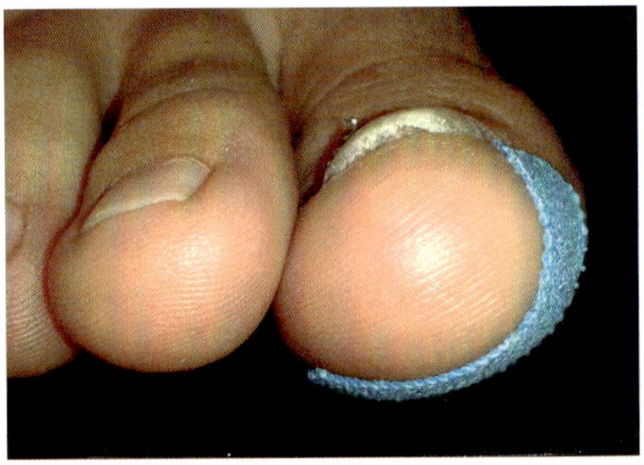

Image 7.36 Applied tape

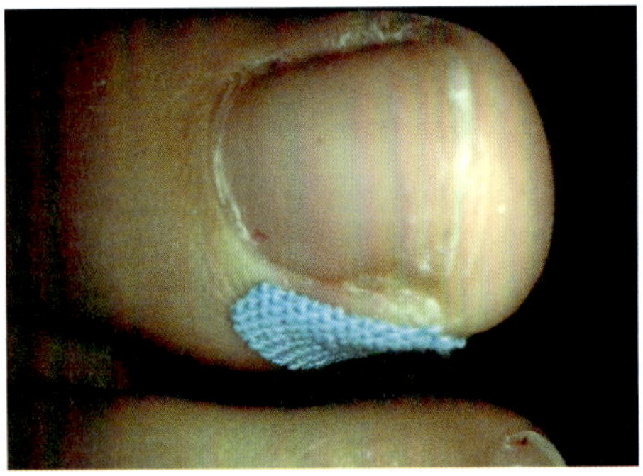

Image 7.37 Sulcus with tape

8

Instruments for the treatment of nails

8 Instruments for the treatment of nails

Overview

Manual instruments (images 8.1 to 8.3)
- double-ended instrument/probe/excavator
- head nipper
- corner nipper
- corner file
- cuticle nipper/scissors/forceps
- scalpel holder #3
- scalpel blades #15
- medi-blades 2
- nail elevator
- forceps

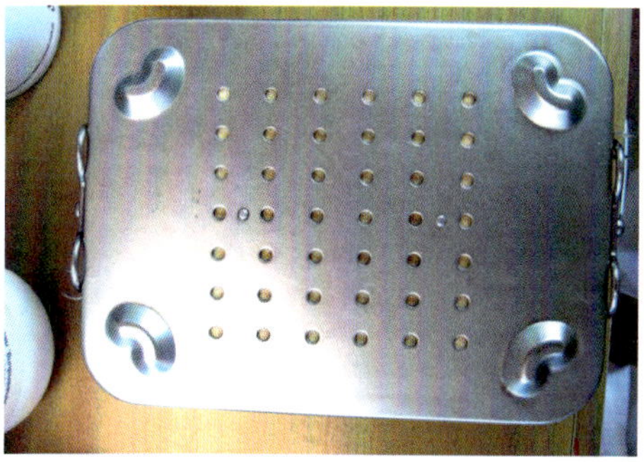

Image 8.1

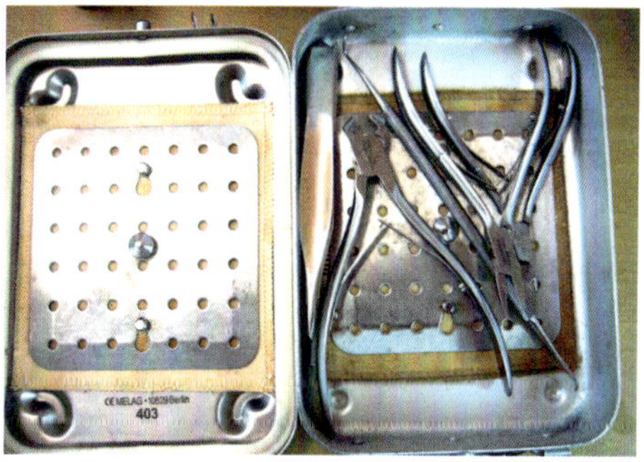

Image 8.2

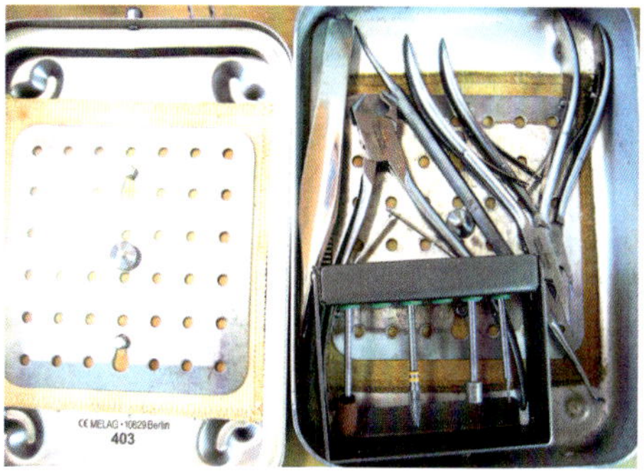

Image 8.3

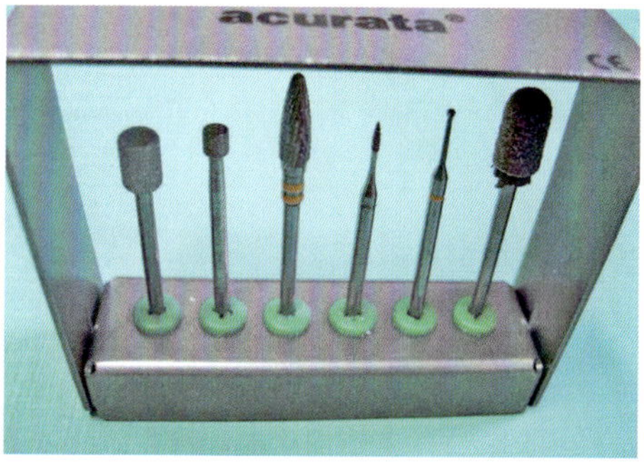

Image 8.4

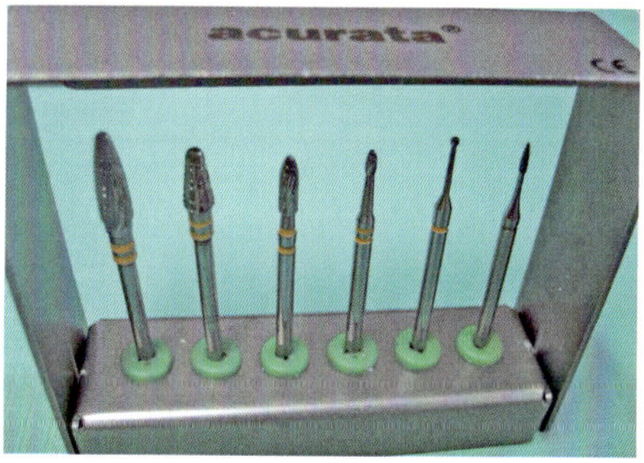

Image 8.5

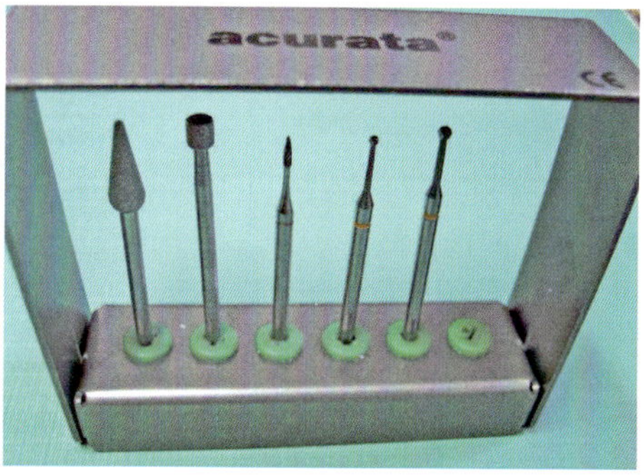

Image 8.6

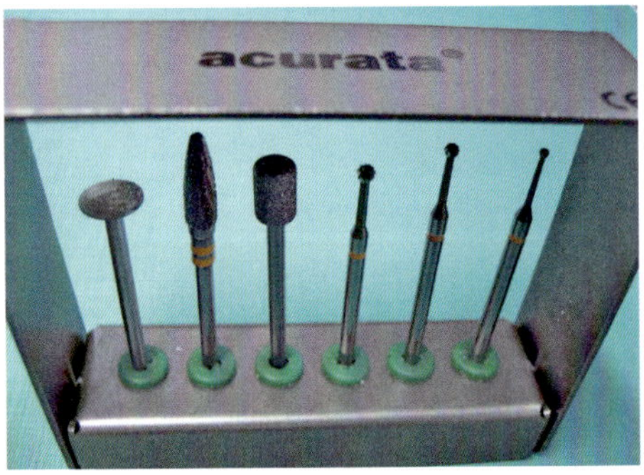

Image 8.7

Image 8.8

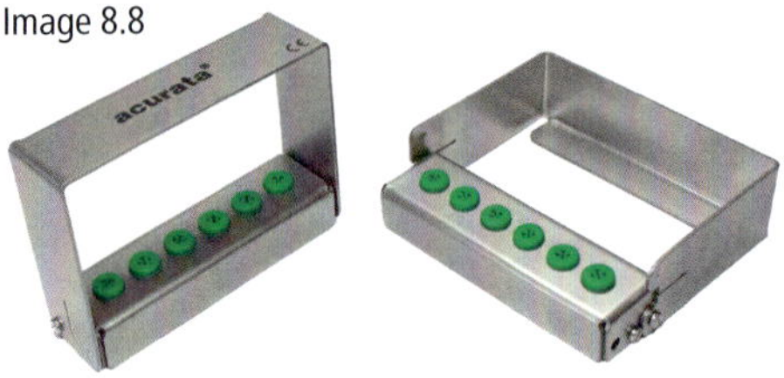

Rotating instruments (images 8.4 to 8.8)

- cutter set for regular nail treatment (image 8.4)
- cutter set for mycotic nail removal (image 8.5)
- cutter set for unguis convolutus or incarnatus (image 8.6)
- cutter set for the preparation and removal of grypotic nails (image 8.7)

Hygiene and care

The sterilization cassette must be closed accurately to guarantee proper instrument sterilization. First the instruments are disinfected in an instrument bath followed by thorough rinsing under running, preferably distilled, water. It is crucial that the instruments are completely dry even in the hinge area before placing them in the autoclave or dry heat sterilizer. Improper maintenance can cause corrosion that permanently damages the expensive stainless steel instruments, rendering them unusable in order to prevent bending, fracturing or other damages. Double-ended instruments are especially prone to bending if incorrectly placed. Be sure to use an approved disinfectant.

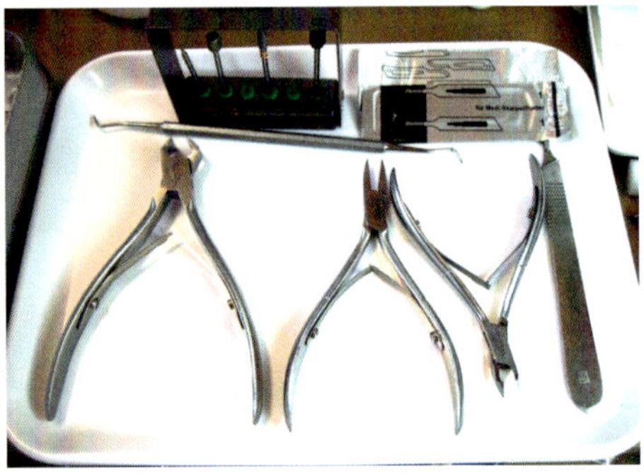

Image 8.9 Set of instruments including cutters

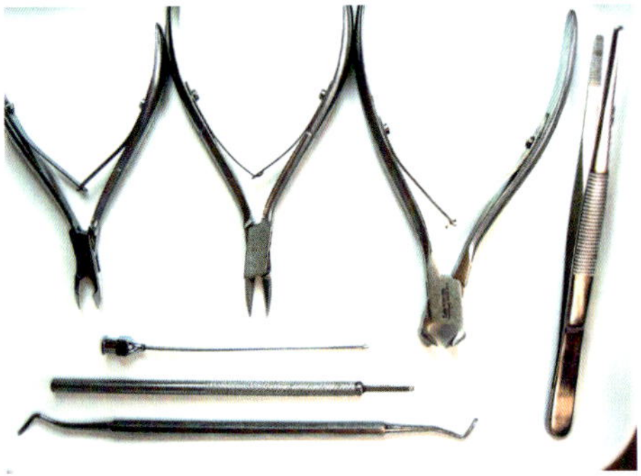

Image 8.10 Treatment set with nail elevator and cannula

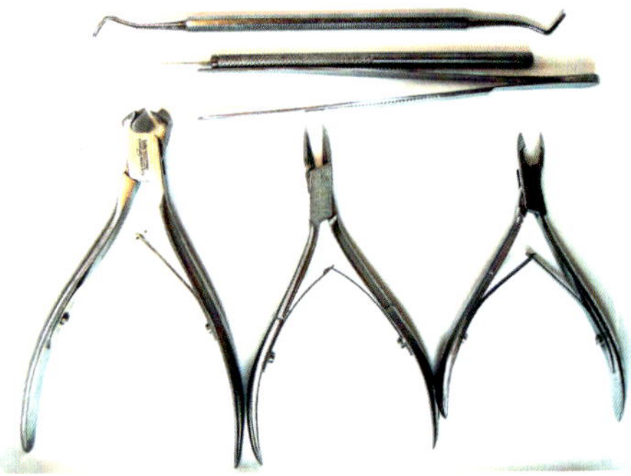

Image 8.11 Instrument set with nail elevator for the treatment of unguis incarnatus

8.1 Different instruments and their applications

The head nipper, with its strong, short cutting edge, is especially suitable for cutting hard, thick nails (image 8.12).

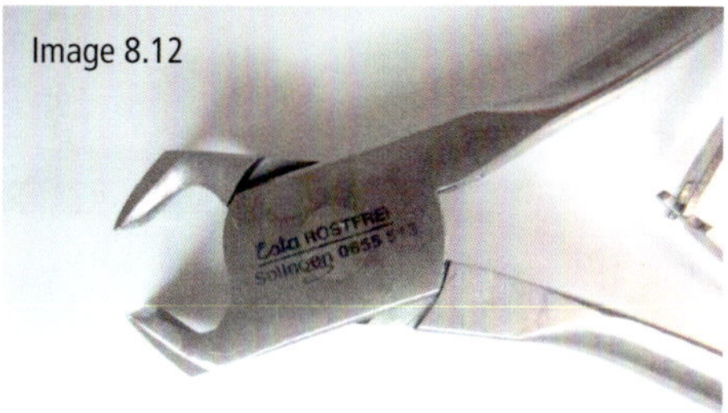
Image 8.12

The corner nipper removes ingrown toenails in the nail fold (unguis incarnatus). Not to be used on hard nails (image 8.13)!

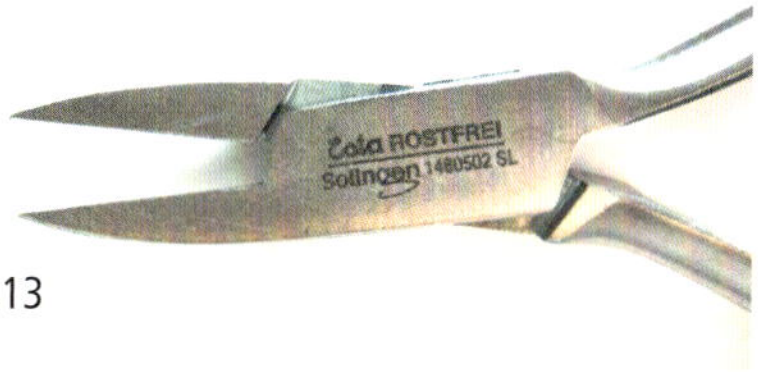
Image 8.13

The cuticle nipper removes cornification in the nail fold and trims cracked skin (rhagades) (image 8.14).

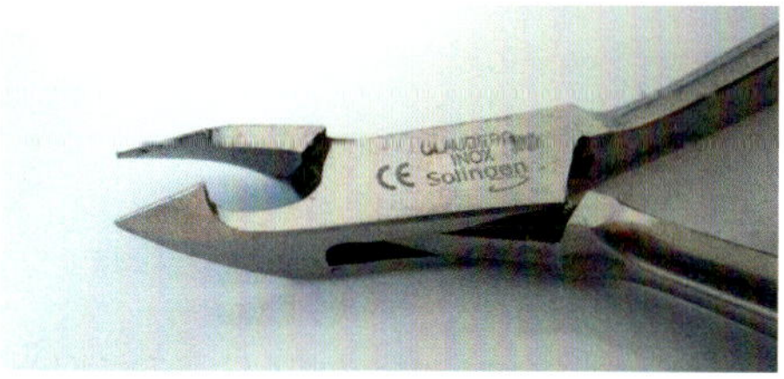
Image 8.14

The scalpel holder # 3 is suitable for the use with interchangeable blades # 15 and/or # 10 (image 8.15).

The corner spoon serves as an examination tool for the nail fold area (image 8.16).

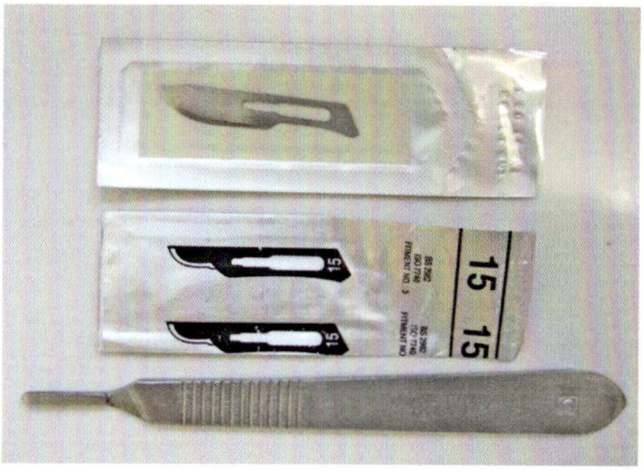

Image 8.15

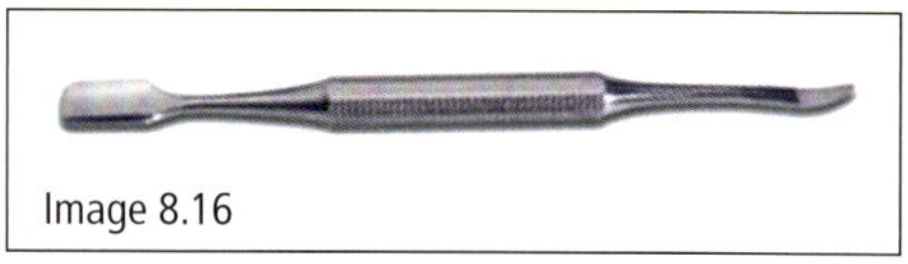
Image 8.16

The tamponade or cotton carrier facilitates the application of various tamponades, such as Copoline, Ligasano, gauze, etc. (image 8.17).

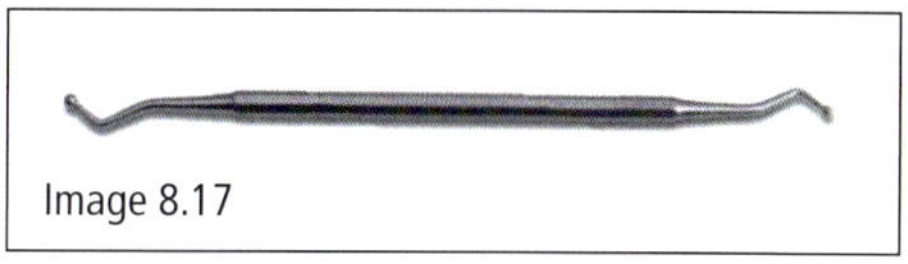
Image 8.17

The metal spatula is suitable for ointment application in the nail fold and for mixing prosthetic nail compounds (image 8.18).

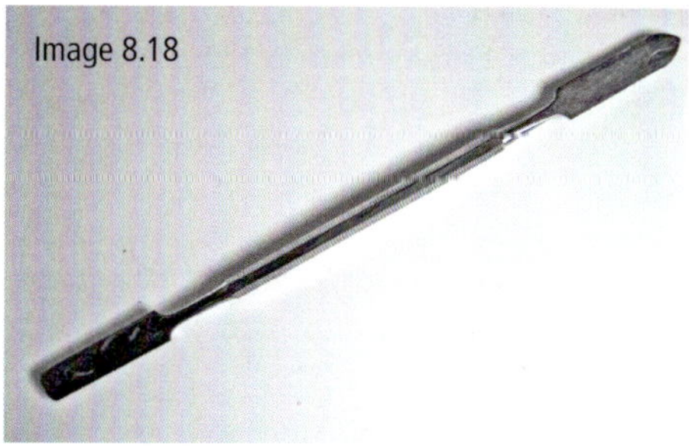
Image 8.18

Forceps, also known as splinter removal forceps, remove cornification in the nail fold area (image 8.19).

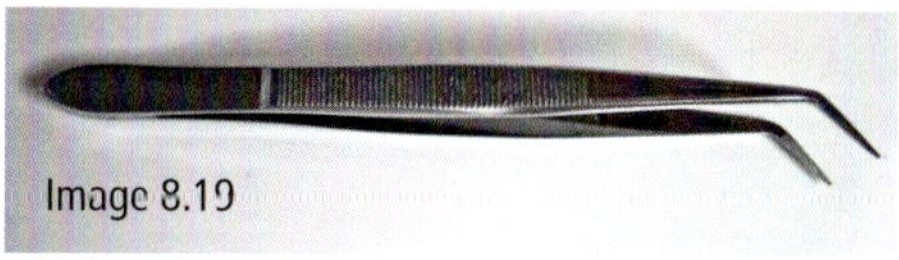
Image 8.19

The excavator is a double-ended instrument used for examining, cleaning and packing the nail fold (image 8.20).

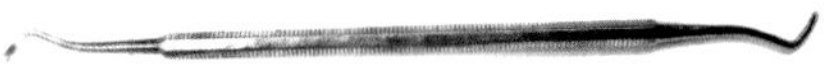

Image 8.20

8.2 Foot treatment: Preparation and procedure

Workspace preparation

All surfaces and the immediate surroundings must be cleaned with an approved surface disinfectant.

Instrument handling

Remove the disinfected and sterilized instruments and cutters from the sterilization cassette or the heat-sealed plastic foil. Covering the instruments with Ruck instrument protection caps or placing gauze over the tips prior to heat sealing will prevent the tips from piercing through the foil.

Disinfection of the patient's feet

Spray the patient's feet with an approved skin disinfectant or thoroughly wipe them with a disinfectant cloth. Advantage: Examining the space between the toes while cleaning. Disadvantage: The disinfectant is not evenly distributed on the skin which might jeopardize proper disinfection. Now the patient's feet can be touched (skin contact).

Examining the feet

Thoroughly examine the patient's feet including the space between the toes. Watch for signs of interdigital mycoses and apply antimycotics as a prophylactic measure (see mycoses). A proper foot examination also includes checking for nail abnormalities and foot static issues (anamnesis report).

Cuticle softener

Spray-on Prontoman spray or a similar product and allow it to work for two minutes. If required, insert a tamponade impregnated with spray into the nail fold. Do not spray regular cuticle softeners on diabetic patients unless it is directly and carefully applied to the cuticle area.

CAUTION!

Cuticle softeners are highly alkaline (pH level 11–12).

It is important to hold the instruments steadily and securely in your hand while resting the same hand on the patient for additional support.

The nail

Prior to cutting the nail, the free margin must be examined with the excavator/double-ended instrument, tamponade applicator or probe. If the excavator moves easily around the sulcus (nail fold) area and front corners of the nail, the nail corners are not ingrown (images 8.21 and 8.22).

Carefully clean the nail fold and the free margin area. The excavator also serves as a retraction tool on the nail wall, allowing a closer look at the nail fold. The probing instruments are also used for tamponade application in the sulcus area.

A healthy, normally grown nail must be treated according to its natural shape:

- Cut the nail to create a rough shape (images 8.23 and 8.24).
- Shape the nail carefully by applying small precise cuts.
- Do not bend the nail plate upwards or downwards and be careful not to cut into neighbouring toes or to cut the nail too short since that might damage the hyponychium.
- Use a **corner nipper** to shape the corners of the nail (images 8.25 and 8.26). Do not cut or round the nail's corners, with the exception of an unguis incarnatus (ingrown toenail), since a nail correction brace will be placed afterwards to remove an ingrown nail fragment or

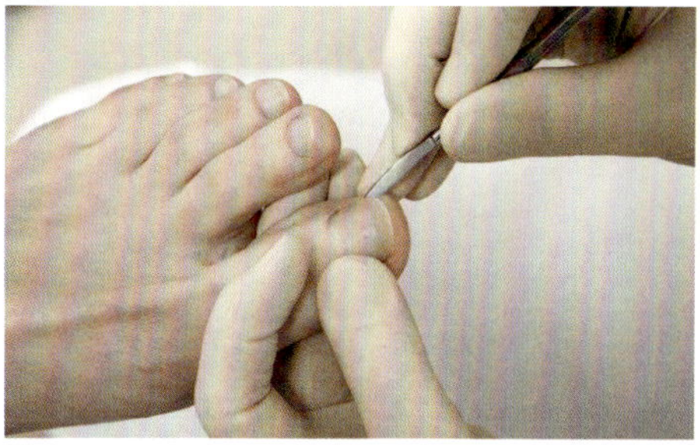

Image 8.21

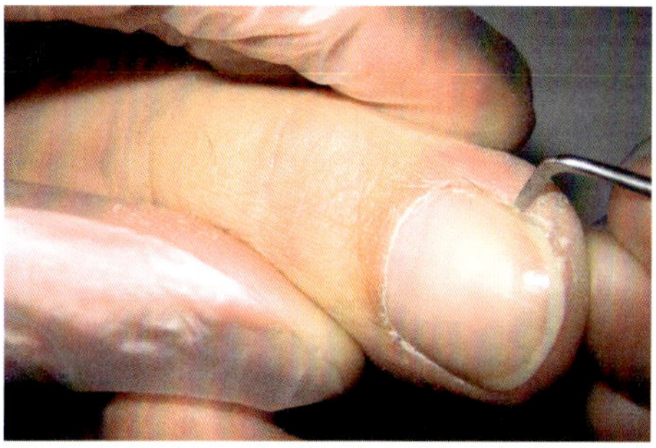

Image 8.22

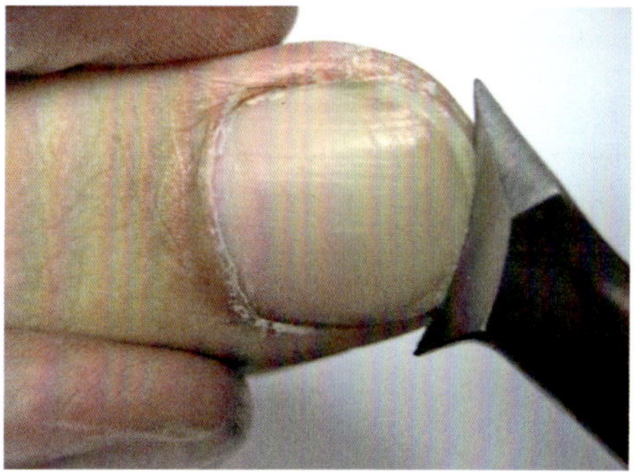

Image 8.23

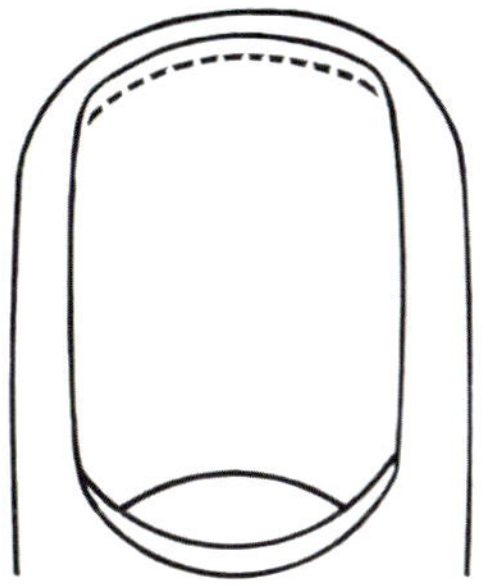

Image 8.24 Correctly cut nail

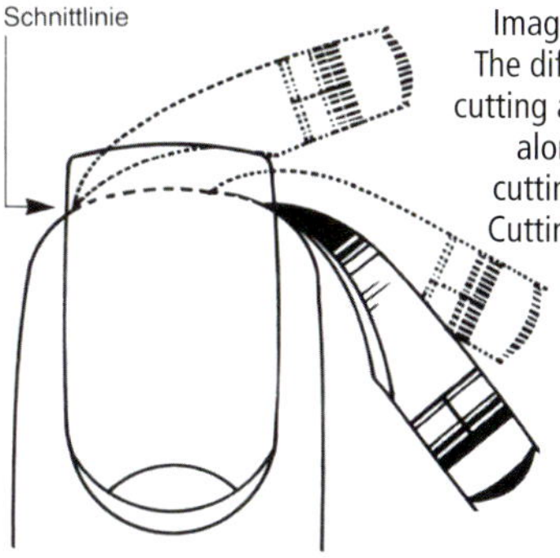

Image 8.25 The different cutting angles along the cutting line Cutting line

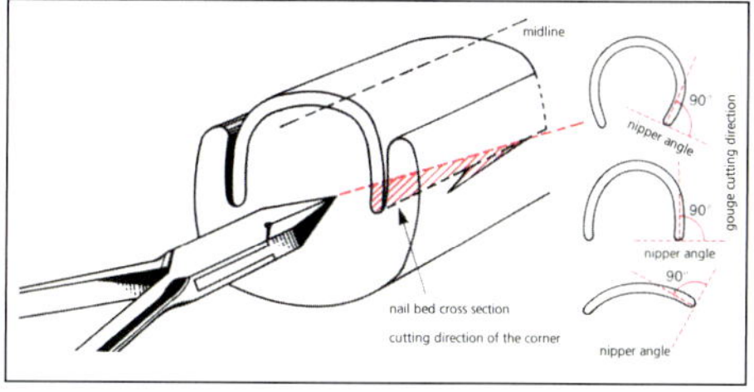

Image 8.26 Cutting direction of the corner nipper

Images 8.24 to 8.26:
Source: Klaus Grünewald: Theorie der medizinischen Fußbehandlung, tome 1, 4th edition 2012, Verlag Neuer Merkur

to straighten the nail's margin (image 8.27).

- If necessary, carefully grind the nail plate to reduce the nail's thickness (image 8.28).
- File or grind the free margin without applying pressure.
- Use a cuticle nipper on the nail fold for removing horny skin particles.
- Lift the skin vertically to the blade and cut, making sure not to damage the underlying skin (cutis).
- Remove callus in the sulcus area with a medi-blade or a scalpel.
- Clean the nail fold with an excavator, corner file, probe or forceps.
- Avoid grinding the nail fold since this can cause micro cuts and injuries.

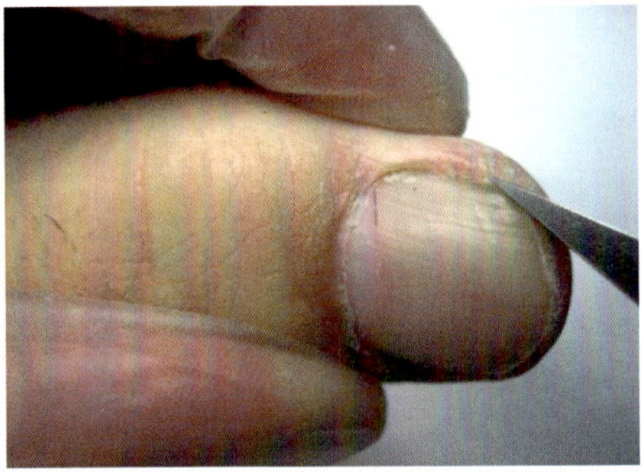

Image 8.27

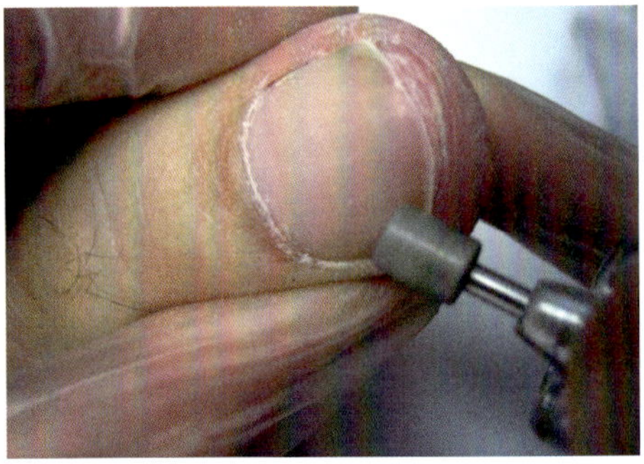

Image 8.28

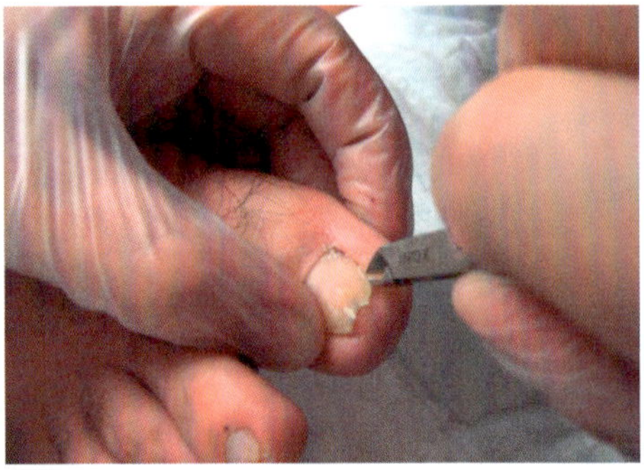

Image 8.29

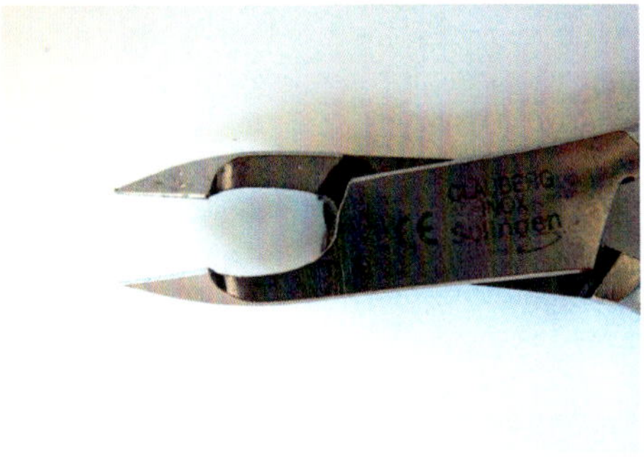

Image 8.30

The cuticle

Gently push back excessive cuticle and use the tip of a cuticle nipper to carefully plug cuticle particles. Hold the instrument at a steep angle for this procedure. Do not remove the cuticle completely in order to prevent micro organism penetration (images 8.29 and 8.30).

CAUTION!

Do not damage the eponychium.

The scalpel

For working on hyperkeratosis, clavus and rhagades, it is recommended to use a size 15 blade. This delicate and small blade works especially well around the nail and in the sulcus area (image 8.31).

Medi blade, gouge and special instruments

These instruments are used for the removal of hard, thick skin on the clavus, in the sulcus area and under the nail (image 8.32). Rotating grinding instruments must be applied with the correct rotation speed and ensure smooth rotation (see rotating instruments 8.3).

Diamond and stainless steel cutting and grinding instruments

Diamond and stainless steel burs come in different shapes and sizes. They perform equally well. Diamond burs are more costly, but last three to four times longer.

After the manual cut, carefully shape the nail with a grinding bur, if necessary.

CAUTION: GRINDING ONLY!

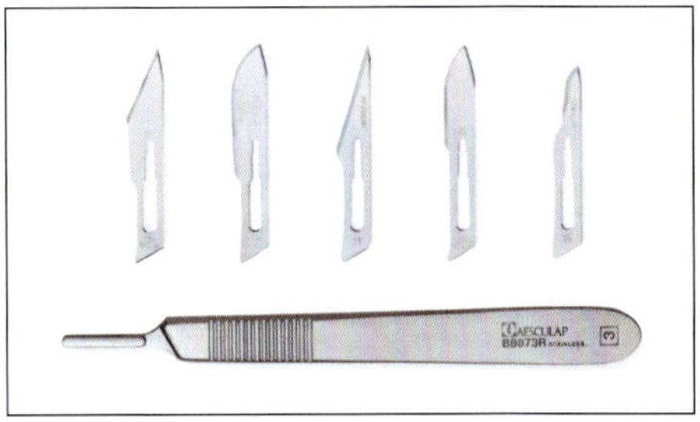

Image 8.31

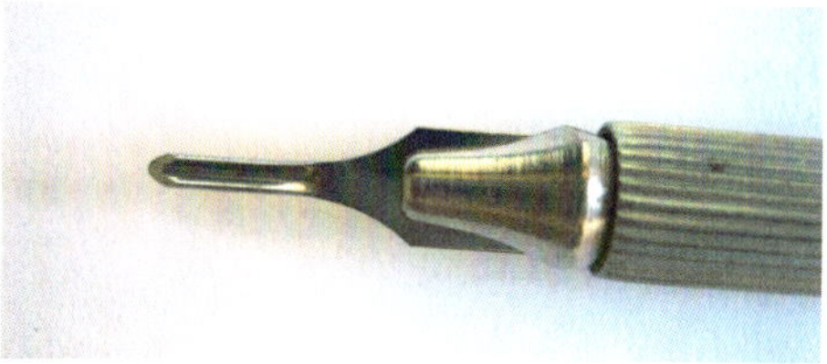

Image 8.32

For the safe removal of grypotic nails and the shaping and smoothing of fungal infected nails, using rotating cutters is often inevitable. Caution must be taken not to damage the lunula during the cutting process. I recommend the carbide cutters manufactured by Acurata. The patented combination toothing (coarse and fine segments on one cutter) offers an unmatched cutting performance while creating smooth, even surfaces (images 8.33 to 8.35).

Corundum burs and diamond burs (image 8.36)
Corundum is a white abrasive stone and is used for smoothing nail margins, clavus edges, rhagades and callus. However, for smoothing out edges, diamond burs are more suitable.

Coarse or fine spherical shaped burs, also known as tulip or cylinder burs, are used for nail shaping and smoothing (image 8.37).

Rose-head and fissure burs (Images 8.38 to 8.40)
These types of burs are suitable for work in the nail fold area and for working on unguis convolutus, unguis incarnatus, onychomycosis and clavus under the nail or in the sulcus area. A carbide disc cutter works well on severely grypotic nails. I carefully cut the nail above the hyponychium and then use a carbide bur with a coarse and fine combination toothing to reduce the nail's thickness (image 8.41).

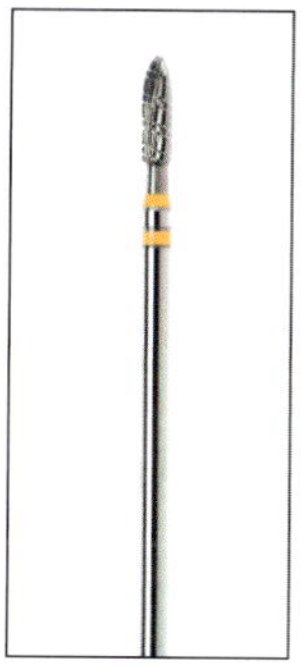

Image 8.33

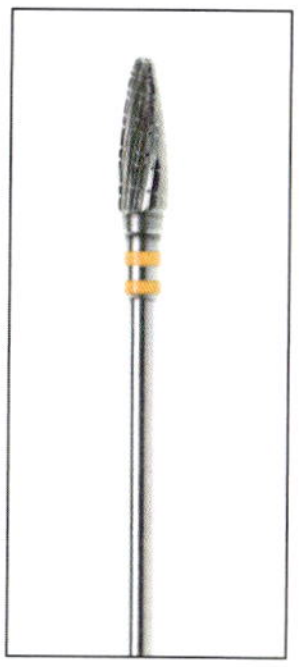

Image 8.34

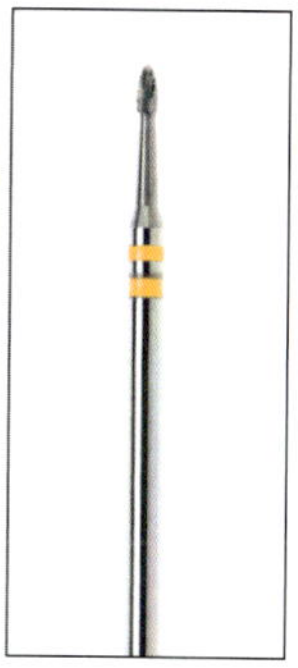

Image 8.35

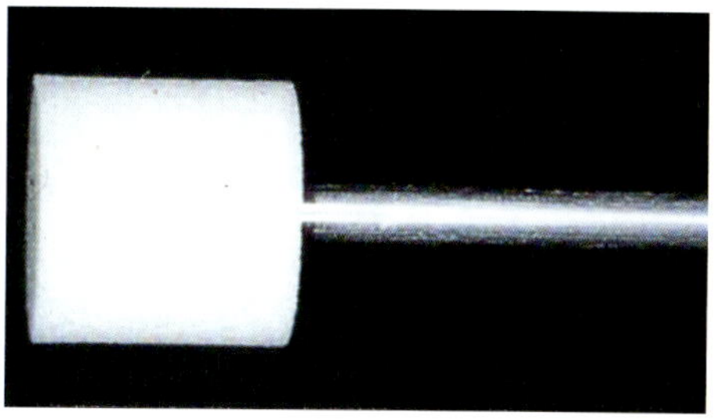

Image 8.36

Source Image 8.31 and 8.36: Podo-Wörterbuch, Verlag Neuer Merkur GmbH

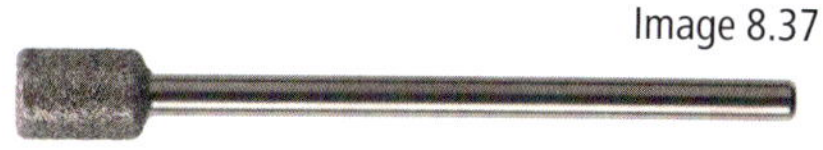

Image 8.37

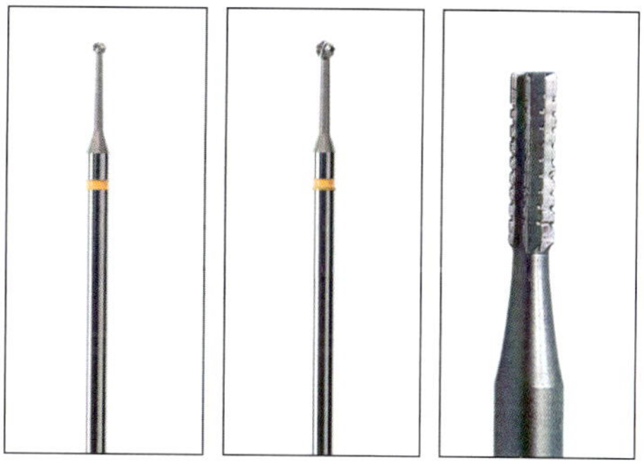

Images 8.38 to 8.40 (left to right)

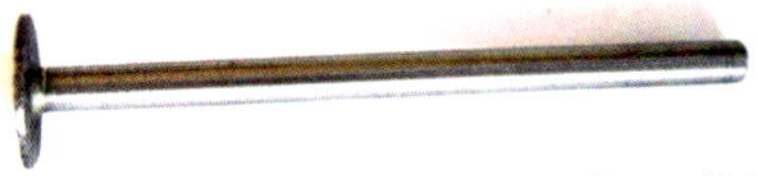

Image 8.41

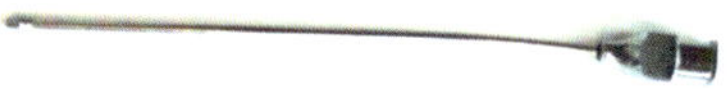

Image 8.42

The irrigation cannula (image 8.42)
Ideal for wound rinsing and liquid aspiration. It ensures proper cleaning and rinsing of onycholysis sites.

8.3 Using rotating instruments

The correct rotation speed
The maximum rotation speed of grinding/cutting instruments must be respected to prevent patient injuries and motor, handpiece and bur damage. Therefore, the following rule applies: The larger the grinding body, the lower the rotational speed. Individual grit particles on a large grinding body create tremendous friction heat at a high rotational speed.

For example: If a grinding body with a 5 mm diameter reaches a rotational speed of 40,000 rpm, then each grit particle moves at a speed of 38 km/h while the grit particles of a grinding body with a 20 mm diameter would reach a speed of 150 km/h at 40,000 rpm! This produces dangerous friction heat and can cause painful burn injuries to the patient. Patients who suffer from polyneuropathy are especially vulnerable, since they have a low or no sensation of pain. It is, therefore, recommended to use rotating instruments at half their rotational speed which ensures patient safety, prolongs the service life of the instruments and creates overall satisfying results.

Regular inspection of the instruments
It is also important to check the rotating instruments regularly. An instrument gauge is a helpful tool for verifying the concentricity of instruments. The instrument shaft should glide smoothly and without added pressure into the stainless steel gauge. Any resistance felt while inserting the instrument shaft means that the instrument has lost its concentricity; it vibrates or jumps during the grinding process and should be disposed off since it no longer functions properly. The patient feels an increased vibration sensation, precise accurate work can no longer be performed, and the bearings of the handpiece are gradually damaged.

Do not apply pressure during grinding
It is important not to apply pressure during grinding because the coarse and sharp-edged grit particles on the grinding body are extremely abrasive and produce additional friction heat which damages the bearings of the handpiece and causes the grinding body to wear down faster.

Instrument sterilization
Proper hygiene measures are of uttermost importance. All instruments must be cleaned, disinfected and sterilized before first use and immediately after each use. Start by placing the instruments in a disinfection solution containing a corrosion protection agent suitable for rotating instruments. The instruments must be completely covered with the solution. The concentration, application time and ultrasonic cleaning suitability specified by the manufacturer of the cleaning and disinfection agent must be complied with absolutely. After removing the instruments from the disinfection bath, they are thoroughly rinsed under running water, placed in a heat seal envelope and sterilized. All instruments must be stored in a dust- and moisture-free and contamination-protected environment.

Overview of various rotating instruments and their applications

Instrument	Images	Maximum rpm	Application	Working process
ball cutter	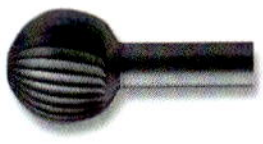	depending on the size max. 50,000 rpm	nail plate	for drilling the nail plate and the treatment of subungual clavus or hematoma
cross cut ball cutter	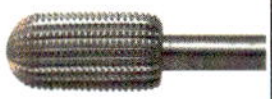	depending on the size max. 42,000 rpm	nail plate, skin	for the treatment of mycosis and clavus under the nail and in the nail fold
cross cut callus remover	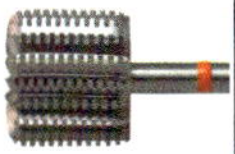	depending on the size max. 21,000 rpm	skin	for the removal and smoothing of callus and clavus in the nail fold
Ony-Clean		15,000 rpm	skin	for the gentle and effective cleaning of the nail fold
trephine	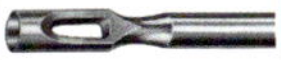	6,500 rpm	skin	for the careful removal of painful clavus, callus and rhagades
diamond burs	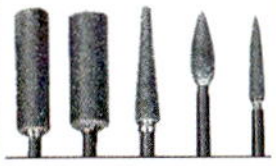	depending on the size between 10,000 and 85,000 rpm	skin, nails	• super coarse grit: removes thick callus skin • coarse grit: removes callus skin and thick nails • medium grit: smoothes callus and nails • fine grit: for delicate finishing work on nails • extra fine grit: for prepolishing natural and artificial nails
DiaTwister	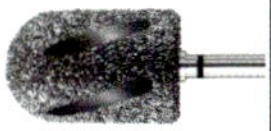	20,000 rpm	skin	for effective callus removal
white sanding stones (corundum)	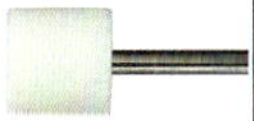	50,000 rpm	nails	for gently shaping nail plate and nail margins
pink sanding stones	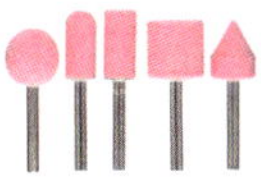	depending on the size max. 85,000 rpm	skin, nails	for the delicate refining work on skin and nails
blue callus sander	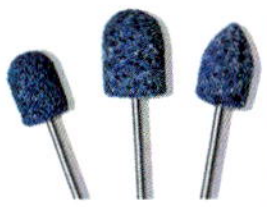	10,000 rpm	skin	callus sander which can be re-roughened

Instrument	Images	Maximum rpm	Application	Working process
carbide cutters	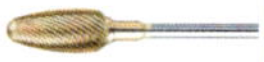	depending on the size between 10,000 and 70,000 rpm	skin, natural nails, orthosis material, acrylic nails, gel nails	• fine cross cut: for the delicate treatment of the nail surface prior to polishing • medium cross cut: for the removal and shaping of fungal infected nails • coarse cross cut: for the coarse shaping of nails • super coarse cross cut: for the effective removal of thick nails • ball cutter: for callus removal and clavus treatment • Rocket SNC cutter: for the shaping and refining of acrylic nails • GQSR cutter: for the treatment of extremely thick nails and for orthosis material • X-toothing: for delicate work on the nail fold and for the treatment of fungal infected nails
rubber burs with sanding caps	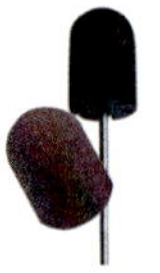	8,000 rpm	skin, nails	For the removal and smoothing of cracked, dry callus after preparatory work with the scalpel, removal and reduction of thick nails. The sanding caps are disposable, the rubber burs are considered a certified medical product and can be autoclaved.
prepolishers	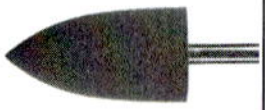		acrylic nails	creates a matt shine on the nail surface
high-gloss polishers	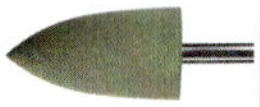		natural nails, acrylic nails	creates a high gloss shine at the end of a manicure
polishing brushes and buffing wheels	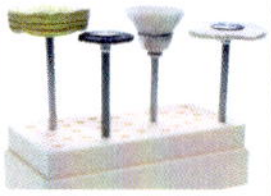		nails, nail fold	for the effective cleaning and polishing of the nail

Brief Summary

9

9 Brief summary of various nail diseases

9.1 Diabetic neuropathic onychopathy (dno)

Cause

Neuropathic component of the pathogenetic neural disorder of the nail

Treatment

- Always test the patient's sense of touch with a tuning fork, monofilament and Tip Therm® at the beginning of the treatment.
- Use a very gentle approach.
- Do not leave the tamponade longer than 24 hours in the sulcus.
- Only apply adhesive braces, not wire braces.

9.2 Unguis incarnatus (ingrown toenail)

Causes

- incorrect cutting of the nail
- nail splintering
- Treatment
- wound care
- cut correction
- remove sharp tips
- apply tamponade
- apply brace
- consult a physician

9.3 Paronychia/panaritium (nail wall)

Causes

- shoes are too tight
- trauma or injury
- medication intolerance
- moist environment
- diabetes
- can penetrate deeper skin layers

Treatment

- wound care
- for tamponade application, consult a physician

9.4 Unguis convolutus (pincer nails, rolled nails)

Causes

- incorrect cutting
- pressure (shoes, toe deformity)
- heredity

Treatment

- apply tamponade
- orthonyxie treatment

9.5 Onychomycosis (nail mycosis)

Causes

- weakened immune system.
- microlesions.
- systemic diseases.
- moist environment in footwear or poor hygiene
- pathogenic fungi colonization on or in the human organism
- An infection is always preceded by cellular damage caused by trauma, diabetes or metabolic disorders (e.g., angiopathy).

Treatment

- assessment by a physician to determine the type of mycosis
- removal of the affected parts of the nail
- reliable cooperation of the patient to apply antimycotic medication consistently at home

9.6 Psoriasis nails (psoriasis vulgaris)

Causes

- autoimmune disease
- pitted nails
- subungual hematoma
- "beading"
- onycholysis

Treatment

- smoothing
- removal of loose particles

9.7 Koilonychia (spoon nail)

Causes
- hereditary
- eating disorders
- deficiency of Fe, vitamins B2 and C
- anemia
- in rare cases, caused by trauma (e.g., incorrectly applied brace)

Treatment
- smoothing

9.8 Leukonychia (white discolouration of the nail)

Causes
- minor trauma
- altered light reflection caused by impaired hornification
- small blisters in the nail substance
- hereditary
- loosening of the nail plate
- contact with concentrated table salt
- symptom of poisoning
- incorrect cutting
- braces

Treatment
- permanent – no effective treatment

9.9 Onychauxis (thickening of the nail without deformity)

Causes
- slowed growth, circulation disorder, ageing

Treatment
- circulation stimulation

9.10 Onychogryposis (thickening and deformity of the nail, ram's horn nail)

Causes
- claw-like thickening
- bending and twisting of the nail (often caused by trauma)

Treatment
- reduce the thickness by grinding
- mycosis prophylaxis

9.11 Pachyonychia (growth disorder of the nail bed)

Causes
- prolonged trauma
- toe deformities, e.g., hammer toe
- frostbite

Treatment
- no grinding
- carefully remove the callus skin, apply etching agent to the papillae rims and gently push them back to the level of the free nail margin

9.12 Onychodystrophy (changes in the nail's colour, shape and texture)

Causes
- various causes, depending on the type of damage

Treatment
- according to the existing damage

9.13 Unguis inflexus (overcurvature of the free nail margin)

Causes
- impaired nail growth, e.g., onychogryposis
- tight footwear
- abnormally shortened terminal phalanx

Treatment
- keep nail short
- remove hyperkeratosis
- nail prosthetics

9.14 Unguis retroflexus (dorsal curvature of the nail)

Causes
- tight footwear
- the nail plate substance is not affected

Treatment
- keep nail short
- remove loose hyperkeratosis particles under the nail

9.15 Onychorrhexis/onychoclasis (longitudinal grooves and splitting)

Causes
- abnormal groove formation caused by lichen ruber
- hepatopathy
- inner secretory disorders
- deposit dermatoses
- anemia
- trauma to the nail plate or matrix
- vitamin B deficiency
- gout
- using alkaline and anti-grease cleansing lotions on the feet
- noxious chemical agents
- radiation and heat damage
- nutritional and hormonal disorders with associated skin diseases

Treatment
- smoothing and/or applying filler material
- consultation
- mycosis prophylaxis

9.16 Onychoschizia (brittle splitting of the free nail margin)

Causes
- chemicals, e.g., alkaline solutions and cleaning detergents
- mineral deficiency and metabolic disorders

Treatment
- consultation
- smoothing
- nail prosthetics
- mycosis prophylaxis

9.17 Onychoatrophy (underdevelopment of the nail plate)

Causes
- unknown

Treatment
- consultation
- smoothing
- nail prosthetics
- mycosis prophylaxis

9.18 Onychomadesis (nail loss)

Causes
- epithelium inflammation
- trauma
- arterial disorders
- febrile infections
- scarlet fever
- sepsis
- influenza
- pneumonia
- blistering diseases
- chemotherapy
- alopecia areata
- psoriasis
- drug-induced toxic epidermal lysis of severely generalized diseases
- bullous dermatoses
- medication exanthema
- intense X-ray radiation
- acute paronychia or severe psychological stress
- idiopathy
- dominant genetic disorder (e.g., associated with the abnormal enamel formation of teeth)

Treatment
- artificial nail
- nail prosthetics

9.19 Onycholysis (nail plate separates from the nail bed)

Causes
- trauma
- mycosis
- pressure
- frostbite
- hematoma

Treatment
- pressure relief
- mycosis prophylaxis
- circulation stimulation

9.20 Onychophosis (wax-like callus build-up on the nail fold)

Causes
- improperly fitting footwear
- overlapping of neighbouring toes (subcause)

Treatment
- removal of the callus build-up

9.21 Beau's lines (deep horizontal ridges)

Causes
- serious sudden illness
- surgery
- psychological stress
- arterial circulation disorder
- zinc deficiency

Treatment
- smoothing and/or applying filler material

9.22 Subungual hematoma

Causes
- pressure caused by trauma

Treatment
- nail trepanation to relieve hematoma pressure (small hole is drilled into the nail)
- antiseptic treatment

9.23 Onychia (inflammation of the nail bed)

Causes
- consistent application of strong pressure

Treatment
- wound care
- tamponade application only in cooperation with a physician

9.24 Subungual granulation tissue/ulcers

Causes
- pressure and friction under the nail plate or on the nail fold
- injury

Treatment
- wound care
- tamponade application only in cooperation with a physician

9.25 Subungual exostoses (bony overgrowth underneath the nail)

Causes
- repeated traumas

Treatment
- wound care only in cooperation with a physician

9.26 Subungual clavus

Causes
- pressure and friction underneath the nail plate

Treatment
- exposure of the subungual clavus by cutting or grinding the affected nail area
- pressure relief

9.27 Subungual hyperkeratosis

Causes
- pressure and friction underneath the nail plate

Treatment
- removal of the hyperkeratosis
- pressure relief

9.28 Trachyonychia (sandpaper nails)

Causes
- suspected damage to the nail matrix

Treatment
- consultation
- smoothing
- nail prosthetics
- mycosis prophylaxis

9.29 Pterygium (abnormal overgrowth of the cuticle)

Causes (dorsal)
- congenital
- bullous dermatoses (e.g., scarred pemphigoid)
- burn injuries
- Dyskeratosis congenital (DKC)
- Graft-versus-host disease (GvHD)
- lichen ruber planus (most commonly)
- onychotillomania
- radiodermatitis
- Raynaud's disease and pad

Causes (ventral)
- congenital
- familial
- idiopathic
- peripheral neuropathy
- Raynaud's disease and systemic scleroderma
- trauma
- mostly found on the small toe

Treatment
- removal of the excess cuticle

9.30 Brachyonychia (abnormally short nail)

Causes
- abnormally short distal phalanx

Treatment
- avoid cutting the nail too short
- nail prosthetics to prevent bulging of the nail

9.31 Scleroderma (permanently slowed nail growth)

Causes
- unknown

Treatment
- consultation
- smoothing
- prosthetic nail
- mycosis prophylaxis

9.32 Tumors in the nail area

Causes
- various

Treatment
- can only be treated by a physician

9.33 Scleronychia

Causes
- often unknown, usually accompanied by respiratory diseases

Treatment
- carefully grinding the nails' edges

9.34 Dyschromia

Causes exogenous
- colouring agents
- medication
- toxins
- callous skin
- foreign particles
- hematomas

Causes endogenous
- heart disease
- kidney insufficiency
- hepatopathy
- liver disease

Treatment
- podiatric treatment, depending on the cause
- no therapeutic treatment options

10

Differential diagnoses of nail abnormalities

Possible causes for nail abnormalities – differential diagnoses

Nail separating from the nail bed
- onycholysis
- iron deficiency anemia
- hemochromatosis
- Raynaud's disease
- systemic lupus erythematosus (SLE)
- psoriasis
- toe deformities
- scleroderma
- erythroderma
- traumatic injuries
- eczema

Blue nails
- normal condition in dark-skinned people (can be found in 70% of dark-skinned people older than 20 years of age)
- malignant melanoma or benign nevus
- subungual hematoma

Brown-black nails
- melanonychia, can be caused by various conditions – malignant melanoma or more harmless causes
- black melanonychia
- nevus
- adriamycin
- cyclophosphamide
- bleeding
- malignant melanoma
- black onychomycosis
- medication and colourants
- adrenocortical insufficiency
- fetal hydantoin syndrome
- hemochromatosis
- Laugier-Hunziker-Baran syndrome
- malnutrition
- lymphoedema
- pleural effusion
- immune deficiency
- bronchiectasis
- sinusitis
- rheumatoid arthritis
- nephrotic syndrome
- thyroiditis
- tuberculosis
- Raynaud's disease
- nail polish and hardeners
- Peutz-Jeghers-Touraine syndrome
- pregnancy
- thyroid disorders
- onychomycoses

Brittle and dry nails
- Arsenic poisoning
- Cachexia
- Chronic arthropathy of the fingers or toes
- Iron deficiency
- Neurological causes:
- Hemiplegia
- Neuropathy
- Oral retinoids
- Osteoporosis
- Osteomalacia
- Peripheral Arterial Occlusive Disease (PAOD) syndrome
- Sulphur deficiency
- Systemic amyloidosis
- Vitamin A, C and B6 deficiency

Dark longitudinal streaks
- specific for hypoalbuminemia (low levels of albumin in the blood)

Yellow nails
- nail mycosis
- aging process
- alopecia areata
- vitiligo
- neurodermatitis or psoriasis
- yellow nail syndrome or "smoker's nails"

Pitted nails
- psoriasis
- parakeratosis
- alopecia areata
- tachyonychia
- rheumatoid arthritis
- spoon nails
- tuberculosis
- chronic inflammatory bowel diseases, such as Crohn's disease and colitis

Partly brownish-red and white discolouration
- half-and-half-nails
- minor injuries during cosmetic treatments
- arsenic, thallium and carbon monoxide poisoning
- heart failure
- Hodgkin's disease
- malaria
- leprosy
- chemotherapy

Light-blue Lunula
- normally skin-free, whitish translucent base of the nail bed
- common side effect of chloroquine (anti-malaria medication)

Curved nails
- socks and shoes that are too small
- hourglass nails
- heart-lung disease
- liver disease
- thyroid disorders

Longitudinal cracks
- traumatic injuries to the matrix
- vitamin B deficiency
- lichen planus (LP)
- hepatopathies
- endocrine disorder
- anemia
- plaque dermatoses
- genetic factors

Longitudinal streaks or depressions
- any severe disease affecting nail growth
- Raynaud's disease
- pemphigus
- traumatic injuries

Koilonychia (spoon nails)
- chronic inflammatory bowel diseases: Crohn's disease and ulcerative colitis
- bronchial carcinoma
- asbestosis
- chronical bronchitis
- chronic obstructive pulmonary disease (COPD)
- cystic fibrosis
- cirrhosis
- congenital heart defects
- endocarditis
- heart valve defects

Small blood spots under the nails
- Wilson's disease (copper-storage disease)
- silver poisoning
- subacute bacterial endocarditis
- systemic lupus erythematosus (SLE)
- rheumatoid arthritis
- stomach ulcers
- cancer
- psoriasis
- traumatic injuries
- pregnancy

Pitting
- traumatic injuries
- psoriasis
- chronic infections
- sarcoidosis
- hyperthyreosis
- amyloidosis
- connective tissue disease

Beau's lines (horizontal ridges)
- psoriasis
- Reiter's disease
- alopecia areata
- eczema
- serious illness (chemotherapy)

Thickening of the nail
- onychauxis
- natural part of aging
- poor circulation
- decreased nail growth

Scarring of the nail bed
- traumatic injuries
- psoriasis
- lichen ruber
- medication exanthema
- epidermolysis bullosa

Soft nails (egg-shell nails)

= Hapalonychia, no causative primary specific nail disease; congenital

- also caused by the following diseases, deficiencies and disorders:
  sulphur deficiency syndrome, a thin nail plate, occupational diseases, chronic arthritis, leprosy, hypothyroidism, PAOD, peripheral neuropathies, hemiplegia, cachexia
- eczema
- lichen ruber planus
- rarely with psoriasis, PAOD, alopecia areata

White spots

- leukonychia
- onychomycosis
- microtraumas
- iron deficiency
- mineral deficiency

White lines

These extend across the nail and disappear when pressure is placed on the nail.

- Muehrcke's lines, specific for kidney insufficiency

White nails

- traumatic hematoma
- bruising
- Peutz-Jeghers-Tourain syndrome
- vitamin B12 deficiency
- post radiation treatment

White horizontal lines

- Mees' lines
- liver failure
- liver cirrhosis
- diabetes mellitus
- hyperthyroidism
- heart failure
- vitamin deficiency